ADOLESCENT STRESS

Causes and Consequences

SOCIAL INSTITUTIONS AND SOCIAL CHANGE

An Aldine de Gruyter Series of Texts and Monographs

EDITED BY

Michael Useem • James D. Wright

Mary Ellen Colten and Susan Gore (eds.), **Adolescent Stress: Causes and Consequences**

Paul Diesing, **Science and Ideology in the Policy Sciences**

G. William Domhoff, **The Power Elite and the State: How Policy is Made in America**

Glen H. Elder, Jr. and Rand D. Conger, **Families in a Changing Society: Hard Times in Rural America**

Paula S. England, **Comparable Worth**

Paula S. England, **Theory on Gender/Feminism on Theory**

Paula S. England and George Farkas, **Households, Employment, and Gender: A Social, Economic, and Demographic View**

George Farkas, Robert P. Grobe, and Daniel Sheehan, **Human Capital or Cultural Capital?**

F. G. Gosling (ed.), **Risk and Responsibility**

Richard F. Hamilton and James D. Wright, **The State of the Masses**

Gary Kleck, **Point Blank: Guns and Violence in America**

James R. Kluegel and Eliot R. Smith, **Beliefs About Inequality: Americans' Views of What Is and What Ought to Be**

David Knoke, Organizing for Collective Action: **The Political Economies of Associations**

Dean Knudsen and J. L. Miller (eds.), **Abused and Battered: Social and Legal Responses to Family Violence**

Robert C. Liebman and Robert Wuthnow (eds.), **The New Christian Right: Mobilization and Legitimation**

Clark McPhail, **The Myth of the Madding Crowd**

Clark McPhail, **Acting Together: The Organization of Crowds**

John Mirowsky and Catherine E. Ross, **Social Causes of Psychological Distress**

Carolyn C. and Robert Perrucci, Dena B. and Harry R. Targ, **Plant Closings: International Context and Social Costs**

Robert Perrucci and Harry R. Potter (eds.), **Networks of Power: Organizational Actors at the National, Corporate, and Community Levels**

David Popenoe, **Disturbing the Nest: Family Change and Decline in Modern Societies**

James T. Richardson, Joel Best, and David Bromley (eds.), **The Satanism Scare**

Bernard C. Rosen, **The Industrial Connection: Achievement and the Family in Developing Societies**

Alice S. Rossi and Peter H. Rossi, **Of Human Bonding: Parent-Child Relations Across the Life Course**

Roberta G. Simmons and Dale A. Blyth, **Moving into Adolescence: The Impact of Pubertal Change and School Context**

David G. Smith, **Paying for Medicare: The Politics of Reform**

Walter L. Wallace, **Principles of Scientific Sociology**

Martin King Whyte, **Dating, Mating, and Marriage**

James D. Wright, **Address Unknown: The Homeless in America**

James D. Wright and Peter H. Rossi, **Armed and Considered Dangerous: A Survey of Felons and Their Firearms**

James D. Wright, Peter H. Rossi, and Kathleen Daly, **Under the Gun: Weapons, Crime, and Violence in America**

ADOLESCENT STRESS

Causes and Consequences

Mary Ellen Colten

Susan Gore

Editors

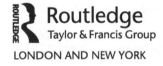

Routledge
Taylor & Francis Group

LONDON AND NEW YORK

ABOUT THE EDITORS

Mary Ellen Colten is Director of The Center for Survey Research, University of Massachusetts at Boston. She received her M.A. from Yale University and her Ph.D. from The University of Michigan.

Susan Gore received her M.A. and Ph.D. from the University of Pennsylvania. She is presently in the Department of Sociology, University of Massachusetts, Boston, and is Senior Research Associate, The Center for Survey Research, University of Massachusetts, Boston.

First published 1991 by Transaction Publishers

Published 2017 by Routledge
2 Park Square, Milton Park, Abingdon, Oxon OX14 4RN
711 Third Avenue, New York, NY 10017, USA

Routledge is an imprint of the Taylor & Francis Group, an informa business

Library of Congress Cataloging-in-Publication Data

Adolescent stress: causes and consequences / Mary Ellen Colten and
  Susan Gore, editors.
      p.   cm.—(Social institutions and social change)
    Some of the papers originally presented at a conference, held in
  Nov. 1988, organized by the editors.
    Includes bibliographical references and index.
    ISBN 0-202-30420-5 (alk. paper). — ISBM 0-202-30421-3 (pbk. :
  alk. paper)
    1. Stress in adolescence—Congresses.   2. Interpersonal relations
  in adolescence—Congresses.   3. Teenagers—Mental health—
  Congresses.   I. Colten, Mary Ellen.   II. Colten, Mary Ellen.
  III. Gore, Susan.   IV. Series.
  BF724.3 S86A36   1991
  155.5′ 18—dc20   90-47963
                                                                              CIP

ISBN 13: 978-0-202-30421-2 (pbk)

To Our Parents

CONTENTS

Foreword
Robert J. Haggerty   ix

Preface   xi

1. Introduction: Adolescent Stress, Social Relationships,
   and Mental Health
   Susan Gore and Mary Ellen Colten   1

Part I. Editors' Overview
Development, Stress and Relationships   **15**

2. Anger, Worry, and Hurt in Early Adolescence:
   An Enlarging World of Negative Emotions
   Reed Larson and Linda Asmussen   21

3. Conflict and Adaptation in Adolescence:
   Adolescent-Parent Conflict
   Judith G. Smetana, Jenny Yau, Angela Restrepo, and
   Judith L. Braeges   43

4. Psychosocial Stress during Adolescence: Intrapersonal
   and Interpersonal Processes
   Bruce E. Compas and Barry M. Wagner   67

Part II. Editors' Overview
Sources of Variation in Stress and Stress Responses   **87**

5. Coping with Adolescence
   Anne C. Petersen, Robert E. Kennedy, and
   Patricia Sullivan   93

6.   Stressful Events and Their Correlates among
     Adolescents of Diverse Backgrounds
         Sanford M. Dornbusch, Randy Mont-Reynaud,
         Philip L. Ritter, Zeng-yin Chen, and Laurence Steinberg   111

7.   How Stressful Is the Transition to Adolescence for Girls?
         Jeanne Brooks-Gunn   131

Part III. Editors' Overview
Youth at Risk: The Social Situation and Mental Health
of Adolescents Under Adversity   **151**

8.   The Patterning of Distress and Disorder in a
     Community Sample of High School Aged Youth
         Mary Ellen Colten, Susan Gore, and Robert H. Aseltine, Jr.   157

9.   Minority Youths at High Risk: Gay Males and Runaways
         Mary Jane Rotheram-Borus, Margaret Rosario, and
         Cheryl Koopman   181

10. Childhood Victimization: Risk Factor for Delinquency
         Cathy Spatz Widom   201

11. Psychoactive Substance Use and Adolescent Pregnancy:
     Compounded Risk among Inner City Adolescent Mothers
         Hortensia Amaro and Barry Zuckerman   223

12. Stress in Mentally Retarded Children and Adolescents
         Gary N. Siperstein and Melodie Wentz-Gross   237

Part IV. Editors' Overview
Strategies for Intervention   **257**

13. A Multilevel Action Research Perspective on
     Stress-Related Interventions
         Maurice J. Elias   261

14. Social Support in Adolescence
         Benjamin H. Gottlieb   281

     Biographical Sketches of the Contributors   307

     Author Index   312

     Subject Index   322

FOREWORD

If you ask the average person what stress is, he seems to know; and almost everyone believes that his life is in some way stressful. However, it has been very hard for the research worker to define stress precisely. As the rays of the sun are bent by a lens, so too is the stressful event (the stressor) bent by the personality and life experiences of the individual, and experienced differently from one person to another.

On a trip to the People's Republic of China a few years ago, I was giving a lecture on stress and coping to a group of Chinese pediatricians. At the end of my speech, several of them looked very puzzled, and commented that they did not feel that it was stressful for one to lose one's job, or have a death in the family. I then asked them, "What about the failure of one of their children in an examination?" They all jumped up and excitedly exclaimed, "Yes! That is stress!" Stress is in the eye of the beholder.

It is a courageous researcher and editor, therefore, who attempts a book on stress. The editors of *Adolescent Stress: Causes and Consequences* have made a major contribution to the field of stress research by emphasizing two previously ignored factors. The first is the developmental aspect of the human response to stress. Adolescence as a time of change has rarely been studied from the point of view of the changes in perception of stress related to the developmental changes occurring during this period. The second is the book's emphasis on the environment, both social and physical, as independent and intervening variables, which are so important in assessing the impact of stressful events.

The emphasis on the developmental aspect of stress is elegantly illustrated in this collection of papers by the data showing that what is stressful at one stage of life may not be at another. For instance, during adolescence, it is no longer the family that is the major source of stress, but friends and heterosexual relationships. The complexity of this relation is illustrated by the fact that friends not only cause stress, but are also the source of social supports that moderate stress, in contrast to the pre-adolescent period.

The second major theme is that the environment, or the social context, is a crucial variable in the perception of whether events are stressful or not, and their relation to mental health and illness.

This compilation of the papers given at the Conference on Adolescent Stress therefore extends the theoretical base for understanding stressful events and their impact on adolescents. In addition, the importance of interventions, particularly the provision of social support and social competence training, is emphasized. Although it is fair to say that our knowledge of how most effectively to help young people avoid the harmful effects of stressful events, and at the same time gain from the potentially uplifting and creative aspects of novel and stressful events, has not yet been fully elucidated, the results of this conference have made progress in this field. The challenge is now to apply this knowledge to assist young people to achieve their full potential rather than to be ground down by their destructive responses to stressful events.

Robert J. Haggerty
President, William T. Grant Foundation

PREFACE

Research on adolescent stress and its consequences for mental health is undertaken from diverse perspectives, often tackling very different questions, despite the common subject matter. This volume focuses on the interface of research on adolescent development and social stress and it underscores the richness of conceptual and methodological approaches to understanding how both positive and negative trajectories of mental health are set in motion at this time in life.

Our scope is defined still further by a special emphasis on the importance of social relationships as independent, intervening and dependent variables in these various models of stress and mental health. It is widely known that relationships are the driving force of growth and risk in adolescence, and that adaptation results from the complex interplay of their supportive and injurious features. The chapters that follow explore the complexity of these influences and cover recent research developments on a range of significant issues: the nature of stress, important sources of variation, subgroups of youth at severe risk, and intervention strategies.

To encourage better communication among researchers in this area, the editors held a Conference on Adolescent Stress, Social Relationships and Mental Health in 1987, and several of the volume's contributors spoke at this meeting. The chapters produced after this gathering benefited from this exchange, and several other individuals were invited to submit papers, making a rich and coherent volume.

Here, we want to express our appreciation to these colleagues, and to others who have supported and worked with us on the conference and this book. First, we find this an impressive set of papers and we are grateful for the authors' hard work and positive responses to our editorial feedback, including our nudges on deadlines. We wish to thank Dottie Cerankowski, Nancy Farinella, Ansti Benfield, Virginia MacKay and

Pearl Porter for their assistance with the Conference and with manuscript preparation. Appreciation to Robert Aseltine Jr. and Wendy Miller Sullivan for research assistance.

Special acknowledgment should be made to the William T. Grant Foundation and the University of Massachusetts-Boston for sharing the costs of the Conference. In particular, we wish to thank Dr. Robert Haggerty and Mrs. Linda Pickett of the Grant Foundation and Chancellor Sherry Penney of the University of Massachusetts. The William T. Grant Foundation has also supported Dr. Gore's membership in its Consortium for Study of Stress Processes, and this group as well as members of other Grant Foundation Consortia played an important role in formulating the volume. Our own study of adolescent stress and mental health reported on in Chapter 8 is supported by a grant from the National Institute of Mental Health (R01 MH42909); and work on this volume was supported under this grant as well.

1

Introduction: Adolescent Stress, Social Relationships, and Mental Health

Susan Gore and Mary Ellen Colten

In this volume we bring together a series of papers that focus on the multifaceted nature of adolescent stress and its consequences for mental health and well-being. The topic, of course, is timely, in light of documented increases in rates of both suicide (Murphy & Wetzel, 1980; USDHHS, 1986) and depression (Klerman & Weissman, 1989) among adolescents and young adults. The high rates of substance use and abuse in junior high and high school aged youth (Wetzel, 1987; Johnston, O'Malley & Bachman, 1987) as well as other risk-taking behaviors are negative health outcomes in and of themselves, and reflect the dysfunctional strategies many youth use (Huba, Winegard, & Bentler, 1980) to cope with stressful life conditions and emotional distress.

The concept of stress is an important tool for organizing research seeking to understand development during the adolescent years, how development is shaped within the wider contexts of individual experience and societal forces, and the processes that lead to well being on the one hand or to distress and life problems on the other. The thirteen papers in this volume consider stress and adaptation during the adolescent years in the broadest possible way, drawing on key concepts and the wealth of existing research across a number of disciplines. In combination, they characterize the origins, nature and means for addressing some of today's most vexing problems.

1

There is already such a rich body of research on child and adolescent mental health (see the special issue of the *American Psychologist*, 1989) that we should first consider the place of this volume in the larger field and characterize its special niche. In many ways the volume reflects continuity within established lines of investigation. Several of the authors are senior researchers in the field of adolescent mental health and have developed some of the major frameworks and data sets (Dornbusch et al., 1985; Petersen & Spiga, 1982; Brooks-Gunn, 1987; Csikszentmihalyi & Larson, 1984) for conceptualizing and studying the interrelationships among development, stress, and mental health. In addition, many of the papers reflect an underlying concern with the twin concepts of risk (exposure to stress) and resilience (resistance to stress), which have been a critically significant organizing tool for theory and research on child mental health (Werner & Smith, 1982; Rutter, 1979; Anthony, 1974; Garmezy, 1981; Felner, 1984). Finally, in keeping with much of the research on the developmental "tasks" of adolescence (Hamburg, 1974; see Petersen, 1988, for a review) and on the transformation of parent and peer relationships during these years (Youniss, 1980), the papers highlight both positive and negative processes in relationships with family and peers, yielding clues to the complex dynamics between stress and social support processes that are the subject of much current research attention. In these and other ways, this volume is clearly informed by significant existing traditions.

At the same time, these papers speak from new data, methodologies, and ideas, departing from these established traditions in several ways. First, they envision both stress and adaptation as occurring along a continuum ranging from "low-risk" normal developmental processes to potentially more maladaptive "high-risk" situations that constrain coping resources and place youth at even greater risk for other difficulties and a problematic life course. Although the papers implicitly and explicitly concern adolescent mental health, the diverse perspectives taken do not seek to provide a profile of optimal behavior or of psychopathology. Rather, as Powers, Hauser, and Kilner note (1989, p. 201), there is much need for dialogue that can help to "define the limits of the range of functioning that is adaptive in adolescence." The papers address this need and also elucidate individual and subgroup differences, which, as Powers and associates also note, should facilitate discovery of various patterns of positive mental health. In this way, the papers also draw our attention to the many conceptual and operational definitions of both the independent variable, stress, and the dependent variable, adaptation, thus broadening our definitions of each.

The papers also report on a wide range of populations, including representative cross-sections of community populations and convenience samples of both well and troubled youth, underscoring the importance of considering the gamut of stress responses that define mental health and well being in the adolescent years. According to Aneshensel (1988), this attentiveness to a number of theoretically relevant stress responses contrasts with the disease–specific orientation of etiological research that is often superimposed on stress research. Unfortunately, many of the major studies of life stress have focussed on a single dependent variable, making it impossible to chart alternative expressions of distress and the clustering of multiple risks and problems in the same individuals. This volume accords an important corrective by considering a range of stressors and outcomes and providing frameworks for understanding processes both specific to and across diverse populations of youth.

Another special feature of this volume is the attention given in several chapters to understudied populations of at-risk adolescents such as runaways, victims of child abuse, gay, educationally handicapped youth, and teenage mothers in a drug-centered social milieu. Understanding the social situation and mental health of youth in these groups is important in its own right, and draws our attention to the importance of interventions for youth who are not only at-risk, but also for those who have already experienced significant mental health and behavioral problems and other trauma that jeopardize their futures. Too often these groups are studied only from a problem-oriented perspective that ignores the larger context, uninformed by either of the traditions of stress or developmental research. At the same time, the extreme adversity faced by these youth forces us to reconsider some of our existing models of developmental stress, an issue we will address later in this chapter.

Finally, the range of topics and formulations advanced in these chapters is the direct result of our effort to select authors who represent a number of disciplines with unique concepts and concerns regarding stress and development and, in each case and as a whole, the papers reveal the potential for cross-fertilization of several rather distinct lines of investigation. In the Editors' summary that precedes each section of readings we will emphasize the specific perspectives and contributions of each reading, and suggest linkages and further ideas generated by the group of papers as a whole. Also, in the final section of this introduction we will present an overview of the volume's organization, but here we would first like to return to the issue of the many understandings of adolescent stress processes, considering several of the ways in which a more coherent field of adolescent stress research follows from the integration of child and adolescent development studies with life stress and coping perspectives on mental health.

Development, Stress and Mental Health

As noted above, there are many different conceptual and operational definitions of stress in the volume chapters. An important distinction lies in whether stressful life transitions and experiences are seen as stemming directly from adolescent development or whether the life stresses of *adolescents*, rather than of *adolescence*, are being studied. These italicized terms convey the distinctive emphases of the life stress and child development fields, which have differed significantly in their orientation, while sharing a focus on the problems of adaptation during the adolescent years. Life stress researchers have most often emphasized study of non-normative stressful life events, that is, stressful experiences that can happen to different people at different times. In seeming contrast, developmentalists have taken life stage as the point of departure, seeking to understand—in the case of adolescence—the normative developmental changes that all youth experience. Some of these life transitions are experienced with a cohort, such as the change from elementary to junior high school, while others, like pubertal change, have a variable timing within the age cohort. Interestingly, this feature of variable timing can turn "normative" events into "non-normative" events for individuals, providing a basis for studying the non-normative nature of some transitions for subgroups of individuals, and thus suggesting greater similarities between stress and child development research than are often recognized.

These two traditions have always shared a common concern with the two fundamental problems in the study of risk and resilience: (1) establishing the influence of stress on mental health—the study of stress exposure and its effects, and (2) uncovering processes that mediate these stress responses, as well as those that determine resilience or vulnerability by moderating or "buffering" the effects of stress. Despite this mutuality of concerns, early research in both the life stress and adolescent development fields was narrowly focussed. In the life stress field, an initial understanding of stressors as "fortuitous" or "eventful," and as influencing health status only in the aggregate, discouraged sensitivity to the distinctiveness of life experience and stress for different population subgroups and at each stage in the life course. As noncontextual as this "pure stress" research model was, the early "pure development" research orientation was its match. Petersen and associates remind us in their chapter that early research on adolescent stress was guided by the hypothesis that the hormonal changes of puberty were solely responsible for psychological status during early adolescence, a view that exemplifies this disregard for social context as well as other individual variables.

The papers in this volume demonstrate the considerable movement toward convergence of interests and a mutual strengthening of developmental and stress research traditions. Progress is evident in modeling the interrelationships between the myriad of developmental and nondevelopmental stresses experienced by adolescents. For example, from developmental perspectives, Rutter (1979) and Simmons and colleagues (Simmons, 1987; Simmons, Burgeson, Carleton-Ford, & Blyth, 1987) have been concerned with the effects of *simultaneous developmental changes*, in contrast to *singular developmental events*, as their evidence shows that particular transitions by themselves do not pose a major threat for most youth, but that transitions in the context of other developmental events can increase the risks for some. This shift in research orientation has great theoretical and practical potential, as this may be an important basis for differentiating high and low risk populations, and between situations that are likely to be challenging to youth and promote mastery experiences, versus those that are overwhelming and cannot, objectively, be mastered.

The problem of coming to grips with the linkages between development, stress and context is not limited to the tradition of child and adolescent development studies. The paper by Compas and Wagner in this volume, takes the framework of stress research as its point of departure and seeks to enrich this perspective through attention both to age differences and the developmental relevance of different clusters of stressors. Specifically, their data establish that the pattern of correlations between the kinds of stressors and symptoms of distress for different age groups follows a developmentally meaningful pattern: only negative *family events* predicted to distress in the junior high sample, only negative *peer events* in the high school sample, and only negative *academic events* were predictive of distress in the college sample.

In each research tradition, whether developmental or other stressers are the point of departure, questions about the overall stress context are highlighted. What are the other stressful events and conditions in the lives of adolescents that add to or interact with a particular developmental or nondevelopmental stressor? This problem of the multiple stress arenas of adolescent functioning must be distinguished from a different contextual issue, namely the importance of protective factors, such as social support or individual characteristics, that promote resilience in the face of stress. These are usually understood as moderator variables, and they are another piece of a complex picture that is illustrated in Figures 1 and 2.

These two figures are identical in depicting key aspects of the stress process, but they differ in one important regard, which is whether developmental stressors or other non-normative stressful life events and conditions should be modeled as the independent variable or the moderator variable. Figure 1 depicts a concern with the effects on adolescent health of a particular normative developmental change, such as a school transition, which occurs in the context of other life stresses, such as parental divorce, or other developmental changes (e.g., puberty). Here we are investigating the conditions under which a transition such as school change has a negative versus a benign or even positive influence. In Figure 2, our perspective is somewhat modified, in that we now ask whether the effects of non-normative life stresses are conditional upon other contextual and individual factors, including developmental stages

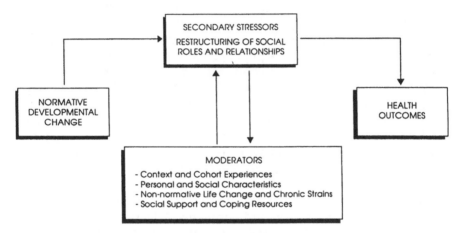

Figure 1. Health effects of developmental transitions: mediating and moderating processes.

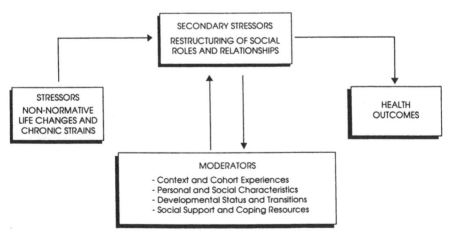

Figure 2. Health effects of life stress: mediating and moderating processes.

or transitions. For example, this has been an important question in research on the effects of parental conflict and divorce on children's mental health (Emery, 1982). Much research documents that the nature, severity and persistence of children's negative responses to life stresses within the family domain are dependent on the developmental status of the child.

Moreover, it is important to keep in mind that many subgroups of youth face extremely adverse life conditions, such as poverty, a climate of violence or familial homelessness. For these youth it is not entirely appropriate to focus on the processes in Figure 1, that is, the relationship between developmental changes and health and behavioral outcomes, since the effects of major nondevelopment related risk factors are clearly more influential in shaping their mental health than are developmental transitions. In addition, models of developmental transitions, such as that depicted in Figure 1, assume some level of prior growth in a normative fashion, and an existing set of social roles that gave order to the previous period of development. However, for many youth the conditions of living are so adverse that we are likely to find extreme lack of parental support or detachment from parents, an overwhelming negative peer influence when peers are present, and a life course that is "off-track" in many respects. Thus, we must keep in mind that Figure 2 may be a more appropriate representation of the stress process for youth whose course of development has already been jeopardized, and who continue to face an atypically high number of life changes and adversities. For example, the papers by Amaro and Rotheram-Borus and their colleagues in this volume focus on two groups—runaways and teenage single parents—for whom adaptation cannot be understood through a primary focus on normative developmental experiences. Thus, in light of the great diversity of experience in the adolescent population, and the increasing numbers of youth who do not face the usual transitions of development with their cohort, we see the need for several visions of both risk and protective mental health processes, and the importance of secondary as well as primary prevention efforts.

Clearly, we are suggesting here that the precise nature of the research question will shape the specific model and analytic strategy chosen, that is, which factor should be modeled as the independent variable and which as the moderator variable, and that there are no a priori rules for making this decision. In addition, it is most important to recognize that no event or transition can be studied in isolation from related events and transitions, both social and developmental. This more contextual orientation in research on adaptation to life stress is now strongly evidenced in the study of children's adjustment to marital separation and divorce. Wertlieb nicely chronicles the shift in the field that has moved from a sole concern with the effects of the divorce event per se to a recognition that there are "multiple and cumulative 'events' underlying the divorce adjustment process" (Wertlieb, 1991).

The Social Arenas of Developmental Stress

Issues regarding this multiplicity of relevant stressors and their various sources are but one facet of the problem of integrating stress theory with the concepts and methods of child and adolescent development studies. Perhaps also, we too strongly emphasize the distinction between developmental and nondevelopmental stressors, lines that become blurred considerably when more transactional approaches are taken to understanding why these events and transitions are so stressful. In the field of stress research we refer to this unfolding series of responses and further life change as *mediating processes* in that they provide the link between initial life changes and indicators of health status and functioning. In Figures 1 and 2 we characterize the processes through which developmental transitions as well as other life stresses come to influence mental health and behavior. Our figures also differentiate these intervening responses from so-called protective or stress-buffering factors. These are depicted as *moderator variables* because they are understood to attenuate the negative health effects in groups exposed to high degrees of stress.

Looking first to the issue of stress mediation, the papers by Larson and Asmussen and by Smetana impress on the reader that it is not cognitive development and the social transitions of adolescence per se that are stressful, rather it is the nature in which they transform the bases for existing relationships, expand significantly the world of relationships by introducing intimacy, and enlarge the possibilities for thinking about these relationships. Therefore, in Figures 1 and 2 we emphasize that the implications of these developmental transitions are played out in social domains and that these represent role transitions in the broadest sense as they disrupt the rules governing prior relationships. In addition, as Larson and Asmussen note, these changes also create new relationships and in doing so "expand the world of what matters," thus changing the view of the self and others in that world.

Research within the stress and coping research tradition focuses in a parallel manner on the developmental context of stress processes. In their paper, Compas and Wagner establish that there is a strong relationship between interpersonal stressors and symptoms of psychological distress. They indicate that many of the kinds of stressors we find in inventories of life events (such as having more arguments with parents, loss of a friend, bad grades in school) are in fact developmentally mediated stresses. That is, these experiences are generated by developmental changes and/or their meaning to youth is established within these changing social contexts. Thus, many so-called life events that have been studied in stress and coping research are in fact the "secondary stressors" of developmental transitions. Of course, many other stressors, including illness, parental and sibling problems, are not, and this is why it is important to assess these situations as well.

Social Support, Coping and Relationships

These papers are suggestive of yet other ways in which the themes in child development studies and in stress and coping studies are not only compatible but mutually informative. Specifically, this discussion of developmentally mediated social stress raises questions about the nature and functions of protective mechanisms, especially since social support, a key protective factor, seems to be so jeopardized by the stresses of these new and changed roles. Indeed, this appears to be well documented in other major research studies as well (see the review by Gore & Colten, 1991), and much of the data (Simmons & Blyth, 1987; Bush & Simmons, 1987), including this volume's findings, indicates that relationships present the greatest hardships for adolescent girls. Because stressors have the capacity to undermine coping resources, especially self esteem and social support, we include a bidirectional arrow in Figures 1 and 2 linking the stress process to these moderators.

This type of data about the social relational basis for both the stresses and protective resources of adolescence provides an important counterpoint to the dominant concern in life stress research with social support, the protective side of social networks. While the field of stress research has been critiqued for not attending to a set of social relational processes broader than the concept of social support denotes (Rook, 1984), research on the developmental significance of friendships has not traditionally spoken to the importance of social support, that is, the role of relationships in protecting youth against the health damaging effects of stress, though new studies of the social networks of youth (see the volume edited by Belle, 1989) show this orientation to be changing. Thus, it appears that while each field has picked up on one or two foci concerning relationships, in neither field has there been thoroughgoing attention to the embeddedness of many key stress and coping processes in personal relationships. This issue is covered in more detail by Gottlieb in his chapter on social support, but here we might note some of the issues regarding relationships, social support and coping resources that might inform and be informed by the study of adolescent stress.

Foremost on this agenda, we think, is the need to focus on theoretically guided questions about stress, relationships and other protective individual and social resources, as is reflected, for example, in an accumulating body of research on gender, stress and coping. In their chapter, Petersen and colleagues report patterns suggesting a correlation between increases in the depressive symptoms of the girls over the high school years and instability in their sense of mastery. These findings are consistent with the view (Bush & Simmons, 1987) that the stresses of adolescence are different and more difficult for girls than boys. The early developing girl is unhappy with her appearance and faces unwanted sexual pressures. For boys, early pubertal change is perceived as a physical and social asset. In addition, the research literature on the differing socialization of boys and girls documents the greater dependency of adolescent girls on their friends for self image and self esteem (Douvan & Adelson, 1966), and strongly suggests that the tensions, conflicts and rejections that characterize girls' friendships during these years are stressful in and of themselves and delay or undermine the development of positive coping related beliefs about one's self, such as a sense of mastery and a stable self image. Although this summary of current thinking on gender and stress in adolescence is necessarily brief, it is suggestive of reasons for the higher rates of depression among adolescent girls than boys, and why girls' close friendships at this time may function to exacerbate rather than alleviate these feelings.

The question of how social relationships can shape coping characteristics like a sense of mastery—in either a positive or negative direction—provides a new and needed direction for social support research in that it recognizes the significance of both "external" (social support) and "internal" (personal characteristics) coping resources and the processes that may link them. It is only during the last decade that we see an accumulation of social support reseach in adolescent populations (see as examples: Felner, Ginter, & Primavera, 1982; Hirsch, 1985; Barrera, 1981; Compas et al., 1986). There is already evidence of the health-relevance of negative peer processes (Cauce, 1982) and of social isolation (Wells, Deykin, & Klerman, 1985). The sum total of this research on both the positive and negative sides of social ties shows how much there is to be learned about the role of social relationships in health and well being, and this is exceptionally important for consideration of interventions to reduce risk and promote resilience, themes that Gottlieb and Elias discuss in their chapters.

Volume Outline

We have already provided an introduction to some of the articles in this volume and will provide additional overviews before each of the following three sections of readings. Here, we will briefly describe the volume's organization.

The volume begins with a set of readings by Larson and Asmussen, by Compas and Wagner, and by Smetana, Yau, Restrepo and Braeges, which emphasize the ways in which the stresses of developmental change play themselves out in significant social arenas. Specifically, the papers emphasize the transformations of social roles and the relationships of these processes to mental health. Here we see an interesting range of perspectives and methodologies, yet they generate compatible understandings of the stress-mediation processes we characterized earlier in this chapter.

These themes are further elaborated in the next set of papers in Part II that emphasize the longitudinal trajectories that are set in motion by particular developmental transitions, as well as subgroup differences in patterns of stress and in the relationship between stressors and indicators of mental health. We see in the papers by Petersen, Kennedy and Sullivan, and by Brooks-Gunn, models that depict the interacting ingredients of the stress process and a focus on gender differences. In partial contrast, Dornbusch, Mont-Reynaud, Ritter, Chen, and Steinberg consider these stress processes within the significant sociodemographic contexts that have been identified in major epidemiological studies of mental health and illness. Much of the research on child and adolescent development is based on small convenience samples and, although gender has been a popular focus, attention to other social structural forces has been relatively neglected. The approach taken by Dornbusch and associates provides an important corrective in this regard.

The papers in Part III zero-in on specific subgroups of youth, some evidencing a singular problem of significant magnitude and others experiencing a cluster of mental health-related problems. In a first chapter by the editors we describe various configurations of stress-related disorders in a representative sample of high school aged youth. In the chapters that follow, by Rotheram-Borus, Rosario and Koopman, by Widom, by Amaro and Zuckerman, and by Siperstein and Wenz-Gross, the authors take a closer look at a variety of populations under stress.

In the final section, the papers by Elias and Gottlieb focus on two concepts that have been important bases for thinking about prevention and intervention: social support and decision-making/problem solving skills. As the final papers in the volume, they provide a sense of the tools needed for reducing exposure and vulnerability to the stresses described in earlier chapters.

References

Aneshensel, C. (1988). *Disjunctures between public health and medical models.* Paper presented at the annual meeting of the American Public Health Association.

Anthony, E. J. (1974). The syndrome of the psychologically invulnerable child. In E. Anthony & C. Koupernick (Eds.), *The child in his family. Vol. 3: Children at psychiatric risk.* New York: John Wiley.

Barrera, M. (1981). Social support in the adjustment of pregnant adolescents: Assessment issues. In B. H. Gottlieb (Ed.), *Social networks and social support* (pp. 69–96). Beverly Hills, CA: Sage.

Belle, D. (1989). *Children's social networks and social supports.* New York: Wiley.

Brooks-Gunn, J. (1987). Pubertal processes and girls' psychological adaptation. In R. M. Lerner & T. T. Foch (Eds.), *Biological-psychosocial interactions in early adolescence* (pp. 123–153). Hillsdale, NJ: Erlbaum Associates.

Bush, D. M. and Simmons, R. (1987). Gender and coping with the entry into early adolescence. In R. C. Barnett, L. Beiner, & G. Baruch (Eds.), *Gender and stress* (pp. 185–217). New York: The Free Press.

Cauce, A. M. (1982). Social support in high risk adolescents: Structural components and adaptive impact. *American Journal of Community Psychology, 10,* 417–428.

Csikszentmihalyi, M., & Larson, R. (1984). *Being adolescent.* New York: Basic Books.

Compas, B. E., Slavin, L. A., Wagner, B. M., & Vannatta, K. (1986). Relationship of life events and social support with psychological dysfunction among adolescents. *Journal of Youth and Adolescence, 15,* 203–219.

Dornbusch, S. M., Carlsmith, J. M., Bushwall, S. J., Ritter, P. L., Leiderman, H., Hastorf, A. H., & Gross, R. T. (1985). Single parents, extended households, and the control of adolescents. *Child Development, 56,* 326–341.

Douvan, E., & Adelson, J. (1966). *The adolescent experience.* New York: Wiley.

Emery, R. (1982). Interparental conflict and the children of discord and divorce. *Psychological Bulletin, 92(2),* 310–330.

Felner, R. D. (1984). Vulnerability in childhood. A preventive framework for understanding children's efforts to cope with life stress and transitions. In M. C. Roberts & L. Peterson (Eds.), *Prevention of problems in childhood: Psychological research and applications.* New York: Wiley-Interscience.

Felner, R. D., Ginter, M., & Primavera, J. (1982). Primary prevention during school transitions: Social support and environmental structure. *American Journal of Community Psychology, 10,* 277–290.

Garmezy, N. (1981). Children under stress: Perspectives on antecedents and correlates of vulnerability and resistance to psychopathology. In I. A. Rabin, J. Aronoff, A. M. Barclay, & R. A. Zucker (Eds.), *Further explorations in personality.* New York: Wiley.

Gore, S., & Colten, M. E. (1991). Gender, stress, and distress: Social relational influences. In J. Eckenrode (Ed.), *The social context of stress and coping.* New York: Plenum Press.

Hamburg, B. (1974). Early adolescence: A specific and stressful stage of the life cycle. In G. V. Coehlo & J. E. Adams (Eds.), *Coping and adaptation* (pp. 101–124). New York: Basic Books.

Hirsch, B. J. (1985). Adolescent coping and support across multiple social environments. *American Journal of Community Psychology, 13,* 381–392.

Huba, G. J., Winegard, J. A., & Bentler, P. M. (1980). Applications of a theory of drug use to prevention programs. *Journal of Drug Education, 10,* 25–38.

Johnston, L. D., O'Malley, P. J., & Bachman, J. G. (1987). *National trends in drug use and related factors among American high school students and young adults, 1975–1986.* Washington, D.C.: U.S. Government Printing Office.

Klerman, G. L., & Weissman, M. M. (1989). Increasing rates of depression. *JAMA, 261* (15), 2229–2235.

Murphy, G. E., & Wetzel, R. D. (1980). Suicide risk by birth cohort in the U.S., *Archives of General Psychiatry, 37,* 519–523.

Petersen, A. C. (1988). Adolescent development, *Annual Review of Psychology, 39,* 583–607.

Petersen, A. C., & Spiga, R. (1982). Adolescence and stress. In L. Goldberger & S. Bresnitz (Eds.), *Handbook of stress: Theoretical and clinical aspects.* NY: The Free Press.

Powers, S. I., Hauser, S. T., & Kilner, L. A. (1989). Adolescent mental health. *American Psychologist, 44* (2), 200–208.

Rook, K. S. (1984). The negative side of social interaction: Impact on psychological well-being. *Journal of Personality and Social Psychology, 46,* 1097–1108.

Rutter, M. (1979). Protective factors in children's responses to stress and disadvantage. In M. W. Kent & J. E. Rolf (Eds.), *Primary prevention of psychopathology: Social competence in children (Vol. 3).* Hanover, New Hampshire: University Press of New England.

Simmons, R. (1987). Social transition and adolescent development. In C. E. Irwin (Ed.), *Adolescent social behavior and health* (pp. 33–62). San Francisco: Jossey-Bass, Inc.

Simmons, R., Burgeson, R., Carleton-Ford, S., & Blyth, D. (1987). The impact of cumulative change in early adolescence. *Child Development, 58,* 1220–1234.

Simmons, R. S., & Blyth, D. (1987). *Moving into adolescence: The impact of pubertal change and school context.* Hawthorne, NY: Aldine.

The American Psychological Association. (1989). Special issue: Children and their development: Knowledge base, research agenda, and social policy application. *American Psychologist, 44* (2).

United States Department of Health and Human Services, Centers for Disease Control. (1986). *Youth Suicide in the United States, 1970–1980.* Washington, DC: U.S. Government Printing Office.

Wells, V. E., Deykin, E. Y., & Klerman, G. (1985). Risk factors for depression in adolescence. *Psychiatric Developments, 3,* 83–108.

Werner, E. E., & Smith, R. S. (1982). *Vulnerable but invincible: A study of resilient children.* New York: McGraw Hill.

Wertlieb, D. (1991). Children and divorce: Stress and coping in developmental perspective. In J. Eckenrode (Ed.), *The social context of stress and coping*. New York: Plenum.

Wetzel, J. R. (1987). *American youth: A statistical snapshot*. Washington, D.C.: William T. Grant Foundation Commission on Youth and America's Future.

Youniss, J. (1980). *Parents and peers in social development*. Chicago: University of Chicago Press.

I

Editors' Overview

Development, Stress and Relationships

Part I consists of three papers that characterize the social world of adolescents and its inherently stressful nature. In these papers we see distinct yet compatible conceptual and analytic frameworks which, taken together, speak to several unifying themes of this volume which we shall briefly describe.

First, the papers focus on the nature of family and peer relationships, establishing their central place in daily life, and their formative role in mental health. As we noted in Chapter 1, this emphasis contrasts with much of the research on adolescence as a stressful life stage, which has emphasized the biological, cognitive and school changes of early adolescence. In our view, these kinds of developmental changes are all important markers of transition and stress, but variables whose effects on mental health are likely to be both mediated and moderated by complex interpersonal processes. Thus, in Figures 1 and 2 in Chapter 1 we suggested that much of the mental health impact of both developmental and nondevelopmental transitions and stresses can be traced back to the interactions occurring in critical social arenas, and it is the new social roles that give meaning to changes in biology, cognition and environment, and provide resources for managing stress. The chapters in Part I elaborate this theme, describing the pivotal role of change and adaptation to change in parental and peer relationships, and the mental health significance of these processes.

A second theme of the volume is diversity in perspective and methodology. Research on adolescent mental health is increasingly a multidisciplinary undertaking, and this is particularly evident in discussions of stress. As we noted in Chapter 1, much of the research is identified with either the tradition of stress and coping research or the tradition of child development studies. In the following chapters and throughout the volume we see how each tradition has expanded its perspectives, drawing somewhat from the other through attention to relevant contextual data, thus blending the earlier "pure stress" and "pure development" models.

The life events tradition of stress research has made significant contributions to research on the etiology of particular disorders, such as depression, and has contributed to a large body of research on a broad spectrum of mental and physical health responses to stress. It has been critiqued, however, for its relative lack of descriptive detail on the nature of stress and its inattention to the sources of stress, that is, the life contexts that give rise to problems. The increasing use of the life stress framework for the study of adolescent populations makes the problem of context even more pressing because the challenge is not limited to finding appropriate lists of stressors or developing indicators of social support; rather the major variables of the traditional research model—stressors, coping resources and health outcomes—all must be seen as developmentally mediated (Aneshensel & Gore, 1991).

* * * * *

The paper by Compas and Wagner nicely exemplifies the life events tradition of study, focussing on the relationship between life events and mental health. It is also attentive to the developmental context of these processes and outlines several themes that cut across both developmental and stress studies. Of particular interest is the dual emphasis on the *interpersonal dimensions* of life event stressors and the *interpersonal effects* of life event stressors. Whereas the former refers to the social nature of experienced stress, the latter addresses the association between the stresses or symptoms reported by one individual and the symptoms reported by a significant other. In stress research, this problem of the cross-person (and cross role) effect of stress and distress has been an important innovation for exploring issues pertaining to the multiple sources of stress, stress contagion and stress-buffering processes (Eckenrode & Gore, 1990). Compas and Wagner consider these cross-person stress effects in the family context, exploring the effects of fathers' and mothers' stresses and distress symptoms on adolescents' distress symptoms. Their findings, that fathers' (but not mothers') symptoms were significantly related to their *children's reports* of emotional and behavioral problems, while mothers' symptoms were predictive of *mothers' reports* of their children's problems, contributes greatly to our understanding of parental variables affecting adolescent mental health, and underscores the importance of the reporting source in the research design. How family structure and functioning affects the adolescent and how the adolescent affects his or her family is also a well established area of investigation in child and adolescent development studies. Compas' and Wagner's analyses exemplify one model for integrating the concepts and methodologies of stress and coping research with those of developmental studies.

The paper by Smetana, Yau, Restrepo and Braeges seeks to uncover the bases for parent-adolescent conflict and disagreement, a widely discussed feature of the adolescent period. Using the framework of social cognitive development, Smetana and associates discuss the basis for the parent-child conflict so prevalent during adolescence: their different reasoning about the issues that are the source of family conflict. Specifically, their data, based on both observation and interviews with adolescents and their parents, support the following description of parent-child disagreement:

> Preadolescents and adolescents understood but rejected or subordinated their parents' conventional interpretations of conflictual issues and reinterpreted them as issues of personal jurisdiction. Parents similarly understood but rejected or subordinated their adolescents' claim to personal jurisdiction, restating the issues in conventional terms.

Here we see that arguments with parents, one of the most frequently reported stressors in checklists of life events developed for adolescent populations, are not just a social stress happening to adolescents, rather they are developmentally mediated stressors. In other words, developmental changes, in this case in cognitive capacity, give rise to and shape the meaning and intensity of the stressors experienced by virtue of these life changes. Interestingly, these data show that girls manifest a significant decline in understanding their parent's "social conventional" viewpoints from preadolescence to adolescence, data that might explain why many studies report more conflict between mothers and daughters at this time.

The paper by Larson and Asmussen draws from both developmental and stress research traditions and further exemplifies the importance of cross-fertilization between these two lines of investigation. Critically, they impress on the reader the linkage between cognitive development and an expanding and changed peer arena. Like Smetana and associates, they show it is not cognitive development and social transitions per se that are stressful, rather it is the nature in which they transform the bases for existing relationships. Thus, developmental transitions are role transitions in the broadest sense as they disrupt the rules governing prior relationships. Moreover, these psychological changes bring about even more profound social change: they expand significantly "the world of what matters" by introducing intimacy, they magnify the possibilities for thinking about these relationships, and they change the view of the self and others in that world. While Smetana and colleagues focus on the family arena, which also has expanded possibilities for understanding and conflict, Larson and Asmussen's data establish that peer relationships are most central to the preoccupying thoughts of older adolescents. These preoccupations contrast with the less abstract "activity orientation" of younger children. Their data show that thoughts regarding this social world become more negative over the adolescent years, and this negative emotion is related to symptoms of depression. Here again we see that it is not cognitive growth itself that is the stressor, rather it is having this psychological capability in the context of the new possibilities for intimate relationships. Thus, Larson and Asmussen speak of the increased empathic ability of youth as evidenced in worry about their friends, as well as the expanded possibilities for jealously in those same relationships. In contrast, they also document some benefits of this cognitive growth. The data show that older adolescents are more often alone than younger adolescents, but that they experience less negative emotion associated with it. The aloneness of these youth is not directly related to the experience of loneliness—a risk factor for suicide (Wells, Deykin, & Klerman, 1985)—because their additional years also gives them the capacity to manage and benefit from time spent alone.

A final feature of these papers that should be highlighted is the diversity of methodological approaches that are utilized. Note that Compas and Wagner rely on survey research to obtain the reports of the adolescents themselves, and of their mothers and fathers. In addition to interviews, Smetana and associates use observational techniques for obtaining additional data on parent and child perspectives, and for studying the dyadic behavior as it unfolds. Most research on adolescents focuses on the adolescents themselves and not significant others, but we see in both of these papers that the combination of parent's and child's perspectives is the important ingredient in the growing body of literature on family stress. Finally, Larson and Asmussen use what is called the Experience Sampling Method to sample the thoughts, activities, and emotional states of youth during each two hour interval between 7:30 AM and 9:30 PM daily for one week. Their research is popularly called the "beeper study" because each adolescent is given a beeper and, upon being signalled, fills out a questionnaire to report these assessments. This methodology yields rich verbatim descriptions of thoughts, and representative samples of activity and mood, thus providing a multiplicity of snapshots of usual as well as unusual experiences. Consequently, analyses can be conducted through aggregating the data both within and across individuals. We see in these three papers an exciting array of methodological strategies.

References

Aneshensel, C., & Gore, S. (1991). Development, stress and role-restructuring: Social transitions of adolescence. In J. Eckenrode (Ed.), *Social contexts of stress and coping*. New York: Plenum Press.

Eckenrode, J., & Gore, S. (1990). *Stress between work and family*. New York: Plenum Press.

Wells, V. E., Deykin, E. Y., & Klerman, G. (1985). Risk factors for depression in adolescence. *Psychiatric Development, 3*, 83–108.

2

Anger, Worry, and Hurt in Early Adolescence: An Enlarging World of Negative Emotions

Reed Larson and Linda Asmussen

Introduction

In an ethnography of the Ifaluk, a Micronesian society, Catherine Lutz (1988) advocates the study of emotions within a cultural group as "a way of orienting us toward things that matter" (p. 5). "Emotions," she writes, "are a way of talking about the intensely meaningful as that is culturally defined, socially enacted, and personally articulated" (p. 5). In the words of Rom Harré (1986), emotions are social constructions, constituted by and reflective of a local cultural and moral order. As "ethnographers" of adolescence, therefore, it behoves us to attend to the emotions that make up the lives of our chosen "cultural group."[1] By identifying what events in their experience elicit emotional reactions we gain access to that which is significant and meaningful to them.

Negative emotions, theorists tell us, reflect breaches in the cultural and moral order—violations of "things that matters." They occur when there is a discrepancy between what is valued and expected and what really happens (Lazarus, Kanner & Folkman, 1980; Mandler, 1980; Rorty, 1980; Roseman, 1984; Scherer, 1984; Soloman, 1976). Quoting Lutz again, they reflect a disjunction between the "ideal or desired world and actual world" (1988, p. 5), a disjunction between life as people expect and want it and life as it actually is.

21

Our research has shown that between preadolescence and early adolescence there is a substantial increase in the experience of negative emotions. Signaled at random times during their daily lives by a pager, junior-high-aged teens reported more occurrences of anger, worry, and hurt than did fifth- and sixth-grade preadolescents; older youth reported many fewer occasions when they felt "very" happy and cheerful (Larson & Lampman-Petraitis, 1989). Furthermore, those adolescents reporting more negative states were more likely to be depressed (Larson, Raffaelli, Richards, Ham, & Jewell, 1990), to do more poorly in school (Leone, 1989), and to have disturbed eating patterns (Richards, Casper & Larson, 1990), findings which indicate that these negative emotions are manifestations of stress. For some these negative states may be a precursor of the severe psychological problems that often begin about this age: affective disorders, delinquency, eating disorders, and suicidal behavior. The question is, what is going on in adolescents' lives that creates more negative emotion than they encountered just a few years earlier?

All of the findings we discuss here are based on an extensive study of 483 randomly selected fifth to ninth graders from a working class and middle class suburb. Following the procedures of the Experience Sampling Method (Csikszentmihalyi & Larson, 1987), these youths were signaled randomly during each 2-hour interval between 7:30 AM and 9:30 PM for 1 week. On receipt of the signal, they filled out a self-report form asking about their thoughts, activities, and emotional states at that point in time. For a more comprehensive description of the study see Larson (1989).

Correlates of Increased Negative Experience

The literature on adolescence offers many explanations for adolescents' more frequent negative states. One of the most common hypotheses is that adolescents' emotional states are attributable to hormonal (or libidinal) changes associated with puberty (Freud, 1946; Petersen & Taylor, 1980). However, in a paper with Maryse Richards we found remarkably little relationship between our adolescents' pubertal statuses and their emotional states (Richards & Larson, 1990). When we controlled for age, there was no substantial relationship between pubertal stage and average mood or the variability of moods. The only exception was a trend toward more positive affect among early maturing boys, which suggests that bigger, more muscular boys enjoy certain social rewards less available to others. Brooks-Gunn and Warren (1989) have also found only a minimal relationship between pubertal status and negative affect.

Another hypothesis is that the more dysphoric moods of adolescents are attributable to stressful events. In support of this hypothesis we found, first, that our adolescents experienced more negative events in their lives than did our preadolescents and, second, that those who reported more negative events experienced a greater frequency of negative states (Larson & Ham, 1989). There is a problem, however, with rushing to the conclusion that these events "cause" the negative states. Recent longitudinal research suggests that dysphoric states may be as likely to cause negative events as the reverse (Cohen, Burt, & Bjorck, 1987; Compas, Wagner, Slavin, & Vannatta, 1986). Thus while stressful events are related to the negative affect of adolescents, there must be more to the story.

Another explanation for adolescents' increased dysphoria is an ecological one. We found that adolescents spent more of their daily lives alone, often in their bedrooms, than did preadolescents, and that being alone was associated with lower mood states (Larson & Richards, 1991). Indeed young adolescents who spent more time alone experienced more negative average mood states (Larson, 1990). Like the life events explanation, however, this explanation leaves the question of causality unanswered: Why do adolescents spend more time alone? Might they be choosing to be alone because their moods are negative?

A limitation of all these explanations is that they attempt to second-guess the reasons for adolescents' negative states. The search for correlates of these states is an experience-distant approach that does not illuminate how these emotions emerge from adolescents' own meaning systems. In this paper, therefore, we attempt a more experience-near approach, examining adolescents own reports on what caused their emotions.

Negative Emotions as Breaches in What Matters

Seymour Epstein (1984) argued that analysis of emotions provides a "royal road" to understanding people's fundamental presuppositions, their preconscious postulates. Employing this "regal" access, adolescents' experiences of anger, worry, and hurt can be understood as responses to breaches of what really matters, as disjunctions between life as they expect and want it and life as it actually is. In Piagetian terms, they reflect disequilibrium between an internal model or representation of the world and the world as it is encountered.

What does it mean, then, that adolescents experience more negative and fewer positive emotions than preadolescents? Clearly it suggests that adolescence is a time of heightened friction between ideal and real, between expected and actual, between an adolescent's internal model of the world and the world as it is encountered. But the important question is why this heightened friction occurs in adolescence.

One explanation is that adolescents, as compared to preadolescents, have expanded the domain of "what matters." The adolescent age period is associated with an expanding horizon, an increased awareness of a wider social, political, and economic world (Inhelder & Piaget, 1958), and also budding interest in romantic relationships. Investments in this wider world of concerns potentially increases their area of vulnerability to worry, disappointment, and hurt.

Another explanation is that adolescents have raised the ante on what they expect from the world, more specifically that cognitive growth has led them to impose a more penetrating set of standards on the events and people around them. Early adolescence is a time when young people develop an ability for abstraction (Inhelder & Piaget, 1958)—for seeing beneath the surface of things, including an ability to perceive the point of view of others and analyze their own and others' emotions (Harris, Olthof, & Terwogt, 1981; Selman, 1980). These abilities may lead to greater sensitivity, to a deeper set of concerns, standards, and expectations—which are more vulnerable to being disappointed.

The relationship of cognitive development to emotional experience is suggested by a set of analyses already done with our data. We found that the adolescents demonstrating more advanced reasoning on the water glass puzzles, a measure of Piagetian stage, reported fewer positive states (Greene & Larson, 1991). This finding supports our counterintuitive hypothesis: that cognitive development during this age period *increases*, rather than diminishes, the stressfulness of daily life.

Here we provide a further test of this relationship, employing a more experience-near approach. By examining the explanations our students gave for their negative emotions, we hope to gain insight into the assumptions and expectations of adolescents that are so frequently dashed.

The Pool of Negative Emotions

Our inquiry deals with responses to a single, open-ended question that occurred on the pager self-report form. Each time participants were signaled, they were asked: "If you were feeling a lot of something, why did you feel that way?" Their instructions were to fill this item out only if they were feeling something strongly. Responses have been coded on three conceptual dimensions.

First we coded the feeling state that the students identified as the object of their explanation. For the purposes of this study, we consider only those occasions when the strong feeling was an *emotional* state, defined broadly to include social emotions (e.g., feeling kindly, hurt, accepted) and arousal states (e.g., feeling calm, excited, tense, bored), as well as more classic emotional states such as anger and happiness. We excluded occasions when they explained physical states, like feeling tired or hungry, and other states that bear little relation to those typically discussed in the emotion literature (e.g., feeling thin, hurried, self-conscious).

In total the students provided explanations for 9405 states of which 6113 were classified as emotional states. Among these we excluded 119 cases in which the beeper or the study were given as the reason for the emotion, leaving a total pool of 5994 cases or 13.2 per person for the 452 people who provided at least one entry. Girls reported significantly more emotional states per person, $F(1,448) = 31.0$, $p < .001$, a pattern that is consistent with our earlier finding that the girls identified a greater frequency of extreme states on the fixed response rating scales (Greene & Larson, 1991; Larson & Lampman-Petraitis, 1989). There was not a significant difference in the average number of states reported between preadolescents (fifth and sixth graders) and young adolescents (seventh to ninth graders).

The total pool of negative emotions included 2012 cases. Congruent with prior findings, we found that the rate of negative emotions was significantly higher among the adolescents (37%) than the preadolescents (33%), $F(1,448) = 11.4$, $p < .001$. Anger, worry, and hurt seemed to be a larger part of their lives. For the girls this age difference was somewhat larger, although the interaction between age and sex was not significant.

The types of negative emotions that the students reported were generally quite similar across age and sex groups. The frequency of feeling bored was somewhat less among the young adolescents (14.7% of all negative emotions vs. 24.8% for preadolescents), while the frequency of feeling lonely was somewhat greater (8.7 vs. 6.2%). Boys reported more activation states, such as anger and boredom, while girls reported more social emotions, such as irritability, awkwardness, and worry, a sex difference consistent with findings of Lewis and Michaelson (1983).

The Life Domains That Elicited Negative Emotions

An important question for us was whether there were age differences in what segments of daily experience generated negative emotion. Hence, we coded the domain of life that the student identified as the context creating these negative states. The domain categories were developed inductively; we describe each to give the reader an understanding of the types of explanations students gave.

1. The first domain, "Self," which was surprisingly small, encompasses intrapersonal explanations, such as those that relate the emotion

to appearance, looks, physical states, abilities, and desires. Typical examples include "because I'm tired" and "because I stink at drawing."

2. "School," the next domain, was the most common context of negative emotions for both boys and girls, accounting for over one quarter of negative states. This domain includes responses such as "because I got a bad grade on my spelling test," "because my math teacher is a jerk," and references to extracurricular activities and getting in trouble with school authorities.

3. Leisure pursuits, competitive games, special outings and non-leisure tasks, as well as "nothing to do," comprise the "Activity" domain. Examples of responses classified under the activity domain would be "because I have to set the table" and "because I hate cleaning my rabbit's cage." Explanations in this category were quite frequent and were given more often by boys than by girls, $z_{proportion} = 7.07$, $p < .001$.

4. The "Media" domain, including subcategories such as television, books and magazines, and music, accounts for relatively few negative emotions for either boys or girls.

5. Likewise, few negative emotions are attributed to food, machines, and other material objects, coded in the next category, "Material Objects." Responses such as "I felt angry because I lost my favorite pen" were coded here.

6. "Family" includes references to the family as a whole and reference to particular family members (including extended relatives and pets). Examples include "because my sister is ignoring me" and "because my dad grounded me for a week." Family was given as a significantly more common domain of negative emotion for girls than boys, $z_{prop.} = 2.15$, $p < .05$.

7. The "Friends" domain includes emotions attributed to the peer group and to friends of the same and opposite sex. Friends were cited significantly more often by girls than by boys as the domain of negative emotion, $z_{prop.} = -8.09$, $p < .001$.

8. The domain "Others" includes emotions attributed to the mail carrier, a neighbor, people who are unknown to the adolescent (e.g., strangers on a bus, kids on a playground), and people whom the adolescent knows but does not identify (e.g., when the child referred to others only as "they" or "he/she").

9. A catch all, "Other" domain included weather, environmental conditions, time, jobs, and origins that were uncodable under any other domain.

10. Finally, for 4% of the negative emotions the students gave us what we coded as a "nonexplanation," such as: "I just felt that way." "I just am." "Why shouldn't I?" These have been excluded from this and subsequent analyses.

Table 1 shows age differences in the rates of these different types of explanations. For both boys and girls, the frequency with which activities were identified as the context of negative states was dramatically less among the older students.[2] Compared to their preadolescent counterparts, activities accounted for one-third fewer negative emotions among adolescent boys and almost one-half fewer among adolescent girls. With age a child's immediate activity appears to diminish as an area of vulnerability to emotional hurt. Interview studies have established the tendency of younger children to see emotions as inseparable from the situations that create them; younger children appear less able to abstract the internal emotion from its external precipitants (Harris et al., 1981; Nannis & Cowan, 1987). Our findings confirm that in real life preadolescent's emotions are more yoked to the immediate situation.

Contrary to popular stereotypes, the family was *not* a greater source of negative experience for the adolescents as compared to the preadolescents (Table 1). Although some studies have found an increase in family conflict associated with adolescence (Steinberg, 1987), our data suggest that if such an increase occurs, it does not have a very marked impact on the daily emotional life of the average boy or girl.

It is friends, not the family, that expand as the domain of more frequent negative emotion. For preadolescent boys, friends were rarely a source of negative stress; among the older boys this rate is more than double.

Table 1. Domains of Negative Emotions

	Boys		Girls	
	Preadolescent (N = 352) (%)	Adolescent (N = 386) (%)	Preadolescent (N = 466) (%)	Adolescent (N = 808) (%)
Self	8.0	9.8	11.2	10.5
School	29.0	25.9	26.4	23.5
Activities (nonschool)	30.7	19.4***	17.2	9.4***
Media	2.6	2.8	1.5	2.2
Material objects	3.1	3.1	2.8	2.4
Family	9.7	9.1	13.9	13.9
Friends	4.3	11.1***	14.4	25.4***
Others, including unidentified others	10.8	13.7	10.3	10.3
Other	2.0	4.9*	2.4	2.5
	100.0	100.0	100.0	100.0

Significantly different from preadolescents using the test of proportions:
*<.05.
**<.01.
***<.001.

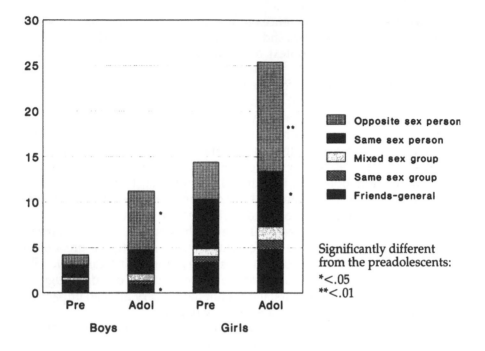

Figure 1. Negative emotions in the domain of friends.

Among girls we see a comparable age difference (Table 1). It is well known that friends increase in importance from childhood to adolescence (Bowerman & Kinch, 1959; Steinberg & Silverberg, 1986; Larson & Richrds, 1990). These findings indicate that more frequent experiences of anger, anxiety, and distress are a part of this change.

In sum, the data show that for boys and girls there is a substantial shift between preadolescence and early adolescence in the locus of emotional trauma from concrete immediate activities to the more abstract social realm. It is tempting to offer a cognitive explanation for this change; indeed we will come back to this theme. A finer breakdown, however, indicates that the more frequent negative emotions related to friends were almost entirely due to one category of friends: single individuals of the opposite sex. Figure 1 presents frequencies for the subcategories of "friends." The total height of the bars here shows the age increase we have already discussed, with girls at both ages showing a much higher norm. One can see, however, that for both boys and girls nearly all of the age difference is due to the top dotted part of the bar, which is explanations relating the negative emotion to the opposite sex.

As children move into the adolescent years, a larger portion of their anger, frustration, and worry emanates from the area of heterosexual concerns, including real relationships and fantasized ones. They have acquired a new area of concern, a new area of "what matters," and along with this they have a new source of vulnerability to hurt.

Perceived Causes of Negative Emotions

Lastly we looked at the causes the students gave for their negative states. We coded where the child pinned the blame for his or her negative emotion. Where did he or she perceive a breach in the normal fabric of life? Our distinction between domain and cause is approximately the distinction Rorty (1980) makes between the "object" of an emotion and its "cause," although the reader will notice overlap between the findings we present for each.

At the broadest level, we were interested in the frequency with which negative states were attributed to the self, to the situation, or to a social dynamic (a triad that approximates one defined by Roseman, 1984). Adolescence is often pictured as a time of inward-turning, in fact, Simmons et al. (1973) documented a major increase in self-consciousness with adolescents. We might, therefore, have expected that the older students would attribute more negative emotions to our first broad category: to traits, states, actions, and performances of the self. The rate of attributions to the self, however, did not differ between preadolescents and adolescents (Table 2). We do not see an increase in scenarios of self-blame and self-recrimination across this age span.

The second global category of causes, "Situation," includes attributions of the emotion to activities, circumstances, and events. Consistent with our findings for the domain codings, these decline between preadoles-

Table 2. Perceived Causes of Negative Emotions

	Boys		Girls	
	Preadolescent (N = 346) (%)	*Adolescent* (N = 378) (%)	*Preadolescent* (N = 455) (%)	*Adolescent* (N = 791) (%)
Self	24.9	24.9	25.3	22.8
Situation	56.4	49.5	49.5	36.0***
Social	18.8	25.7**	25.3	41.2***
	100.0	100.0	100.0	100.0

*<.05.
**<.01.
***<.001.

cence and early adolescence, though the difference is significant only for girls. The concrete, immediate situation appears to diminish as a source of pain.

It is the final category, "Social," that shows a substantial increase with age. This category includes attributions of negative emotion to affiliations, the feelings of others, social give and take, and general social circumstances. A majority of these occur in the domain of friends. Adolescents report significantly more negative states that are due to these social causes than do preadolescents, with girls reporting more than boys in both age groups. These social causes, then, would appear to account for the increase in negative experience associated with entry into adolescence.

It is useful, therefore, to consider more closely the subcategories of social explanations to examine where this increase in worry, anger, and depression comes from. Although social explanations as a whole increase with age, several subcategories decline or show no change between preadolescence and early adolescence. The category "Being alone," as exemplified by "I was lonely because I had nobody to talk to," was a significantly less common explanation for negative emotions among the older group (3.7% vs. 5.7%, $p < .05$). This trend is striking since the adolescents actually spent much more time alone than did the preadolescents (Larson & Richards, 1991). It would appear that they are better able to deal with the experience of solitude than their younger counterparts. Attribution of negative emotions to the subcategories "Fights" and "Social rejection" shows little difference in frequency between age groups. Whereas friction between people may change its form with age, its rate appears to be a developmental constant, at least across this age span.

All of the remaining social causes are more frequent among the older respondents. Examination of examples of each suggest that many involve use of social cognitive abilities developed between preadolescence and adolescence.

Affiliation

"Being with someone" and "Anticipated affiliation" were coded as causes for a much greater number of negative emotions in adolescence than in preadolescence (Being with someone: 4.0 vs. 2.4%, $p < .05$; Anticipated affiliation: 2.2 vs. 1.0%, $p < .001$). Here are some examples for anticipated affiliation, which shows the more dramatic age trend:

> worried—A boy wants me to go to a party with him (he's a sophomore) but my mom probably won't let me go because I'm not old enough and I can't go on dates.

worried and nervous—because Tom is suppose to ask me out. I hope I don't goof.
worried—because I don't want to fight with her. So far nothing has been said about a fight though.

And we can't resist including one example of a positive state in this category:

great—my future boyfriend talked to me.

What is notable to us is that these anticipated affiliations—realistic or fanciful—involve a projection of the self and events into the future in a way that we do not see among the younger students. They reflect the expanded time frame that Inhelder and Piaget (1958) attributed to the cognitive changes of adolescence. While greater extension of time is clearly a developmental achievement, an unfortunate by-product appears to be vulnerability across a longer time span.

It is also notable that these examples, and many below, come from the domain of heterosexual relations. Might it be possible that adolescent love both feeds and is fed by the cognitive advances of this period? It is commonplace to assert that abstract thought makes adolescent love possible; these data suggest that experiences of love, even just anticipation of love, may promote abstract thought.

Feelings Towards Others

Adolescents reported significantly more instances than preadolescents where the cause of their negative state was related to their own feelings toward someone else (4.0 vs. 1.2%, $p < .001$). The following examples illustrate adolescents' feelings directed at others:

nervous—'cuz I like him a lot.
disappointed—because I loved my uncle [just deceased].
irritable—I was sort of mad at Nancy.

In some cases, the adolescent's recognition of feelings for another produced disappointment or sadness; in other cases these feelings ignited more active emotional states like anger and irritation. The acknowledgment that one feeling can cause another reflects these adolescents' deepening psychological sophistication, a developing awareness that abstract internal states—love, worry, anger—have a life of their own.

Undesirable Traits and Behavior of Others

Upsetting behavior or undesirable traits of others account for a significantly greater share of negative emotions in adolescence than in preadolescence (11.1 vs. 7.7%, $p < .05$). Here are several examples of "undesirable traits":

bored—because Mr. Thompson is a jerk and he teaches a boring class.
mad—my sister is sooo . . . dumb it's pathetic. It's sooo . . . nauseating.

Adolescents appear to engage in more frequent labeling of others. One might interpret this increased willingness to label others' undesirable traits as the maturing of the fundamental attribution error. It is possible that cognitive advances give adolescents a greater ability to carry out the inductive process of inferring qualities of others, whether these inductions are accurate or not.

The following are examples of "upsetting behavior of others":

hurt—because they're making up lies about me.
disappointed—Steve is letting our friendship be destroyed.
angry—because someone broke a promise to me that they said they would never do again.

The last two, it should be noted, involve the breach of abstract, principled, expectations. Adolescents appear to be holding others to a more demanding set of behavioral standards. Increased sensitivity to others is also evident in the next category.

Circumstances of Others

The adolescents were more likely than the preadolescents to be moved by a situation that has nothing to do with themselves (2.5 vs. 1.2%, $p < .05$). Examples when the "circumstances of others" were given as the cause for a negative emotion include

mad—because one of my friends got beat up by her brother.
worried—about my dad who is in the hospital.
sorry—for the people in Philadelphia that lost their homes.

Martin Hoffman (1980) has shown that it is somewhere around the beginning of adolescence that cognitive development enables teens to be aware that

others feel pleasure and pain not only in particular situations, but also in their larger pattern of life experiences . . . they can now empathize not only with people's transitory, situation specific distress, but also with what they imagine to be their general condition. (p. 310)

Our data suggest that this greater capacity for empathy results in more daily experiences of distress resulting from identification with the misfortunes of others.

Feelings of Others

This developing awareness that others are centers of thought and feeling also creates more egocentric adolescent misery (4.3% of adolescents vs. 1.4% of preadolescents, $p < .001$). Within this category, we also distinguished a code of "2- and 3-person situations," given the several centers of thought and feeling were named, that provides the most enchanting examples:

> jealous—of Sarah because she gets to sit by a new cute guy.
> worried—because I don't want Stacey to know I like Greg cause she'll beat me up.
> frustrated—that I said sorry to Jason and now he's (I think) trying to make me feel guilty of even other things.

In all of these cases, it is the adolescents' ability to imagine the thoughts and feelings of others that is at the heart of their negative feeling. In the last example, the perceived intention of Jason is central to this girl's negative feeling, yet it is also the perceived reciprocity between her actions, past and probably future, with Jason's intentions that feeds her frustration.

Here's another example with similar complexity:

> disappointed—this guy Paul asked me out but I don't know if he was joking or serious.

If you put yourself in this girl's situation, you will recognize that she faces a two-horned dilemma. If she assumes it was a joke and Paul was serious, she may lose an opportunity; on the other hand, if she assumes it is serious, and it was a joke, she will look like a fool. Acting on either alternative puts her at risk for further pain. Here it is the ambiguity about the other's intentions—and the confusion that creates about how to respond—that is the source of distress. Her capacity to think through the implications of alternate scenarios creates the negative state.

With abstract reasoning, we also find that a fight is no longer just a fight:

> lonely—because when Mike and I fought last night I felt that I was losing a piece of myself because I still love him!

This girl's distress is defined in terms of an internal construction—her beginning imagery of self—a type of construction that did not occur as a source of vulnerability among the preadolescents. No doubt the fight would have caused distress with or without this imagery; this is an example where more abstract cognition is not clearly the cause of injury. Nonetheless we think it likely that this girl's rumination on how her relationship with Mike is connected to her personal identify magnifies her distress.

Finally, among the adolescents, but not the preadolescents, we see many more classical triangular situations in which a person grasps that the feelings and thoughts of three persons are interrelated as a system, a less than perfect system:

> jealous—because a girl I like likes Sean.
> mad—cause my best friend writes her boyfriend his notes back and she doesn't write my notes back.
> worried—because two boys like me very much and I like them and I have to pick one or the other.

These bring to mind Elkind's (1980) discussion of how abstract thought induces adolescents into a new level of "strategic" social interactions. With abstract thought teenagers become capable of deeper analysis of social situations; they become sensitive to the thoughts of others, the discrepancy between appearance and reality, the issues of image management, and the longer term consequences of their actions. Hence, their social lives become a more complex game of chess in which newly discovered levels of social subtlety demand greater calcuation, and, according to Elkind, may require more indirect and devious behavior.

Among the preadolescents, explanations for interpersonal conflict were generally dogmatic and uncomplicated. A terse explanation established the actor's stance toward the situation: he or she had been hurt, disappointed, or wronged. Among the adolescents, however, explanations for negative feelings related to social conflicts were more likely to identify multiple levels, acknowledge ambiguities, and sometimes embody more profound paradoxes that stick in one's mind as allegories on the human condition, such as: "I don't know if he was serious or joking." Rather than establishing the actor's stance toward the situation, they describe his or her dilemma; they are generative and set in motion a round robin of considering alternative points of view and alternative courses of action. As such they create a much more complex playing board, and greater vulnerability to emotional hurt.

Explanations for Positive States

Recent stress research has admonished us to also consider positive events, "uplifts," alongside of stress. Although findings have not always shown that uplifts exert a symmetrical, counteractive effect, it is worth considering them, at least as a kind of control, to see whether domains of increased negative experience are also domains of increased positive experience. If the age shifts we have seen thus far reflect changes in "things that matter," then we might expect parallel shifts in explanations for positive states.

Indeed this is the case. Explanations for positive states exhibit very similar age differences to those seen for negative states. With age, "activities" diminish as a source of positive experience, especially for girls, and "friends," particularly friends of the opposite sex, increase (Table 3). Likewise for both boys and girls, there are significant age increases in the frequency with which the cause of a positive emotion is identified as being social, and increases in the frequency with which the more abstract categories of social explanations—feelings toward others and anticipated affiliation—are given.

This replication of differences for negative and positive states, at first thought, suggests that they may counterbalance each other—and indeed for some individuals they may. Recall, however, that we found an age change in the ratio of negative and positive states, with the adolescents experiencing a higher rate of negative emotions than preadolescents, especially among girls. Thus, with entry into adolescence, the negative side is exerting more impact.

Furthermore, there is no inherent reason why positive and negative experiences will be balanced within a single individual. The girl who is

Table 3. Domains of Positive Emotions

	Boys		Girls	
	Preadolescent (N = 588)	Adolescent (N = 716)	Preadolescent (N = 1016)	Adolescent (N = 1058)
Self	12.6	17.7*	12.2	15.0
School	13.3	13.7	13.2	11.8
Activities (nonschool)	27.4	23.3	22.5	15.7***
Media	12.2	9.8	10.5	7.6*
Material	2.4	3.4	3.1	2.0
Family	6.1	3.6*	7.4	6.8
Friends	10.7	18.0***	19.0	30.2***
Friends-general	1.7	1.8	1.5	2.5
Same sex friend	1.0	1.8	4.5	4.3
Same sex group	1.7	1.0*	2.5	1.3***
Opposite sex friend	4.6	12.6***	8.3	18.3***
Mixed sex group	1.7	.8**	2.3	3.3
Others, including unidentified others	4.9	2.9	5.9	6.0
Other	10.4	7.5	6.1	4.9

*<.05.
**<.01.
***<.001.

jilted by her boyfriend is not necessarily the same one who enjoys the happiness of falling in love. Within the sample we found a complete range, with some people reporting all positive states and others reporting all negative states. Analyses indicate that those at the latter extreme appeared to be at risk. We compared the 10 adolescent boys and 10 adolescent girls from the two opposite ends of this distribution (as a control we included only people reporting at least 10 states in these groups).

As we expected the 20 people with the greatest rate of negative events were experiencing more pain and distress than those 20 people with the lowest rate. Their average self-reported affect scores were dramatically lower [1.35 standard deviation units, $t(39) = 5.23$, $p < .001$] and they rated themselves as much more depressed on the Kovacs Child Depression Inventory [.61 SD units, $t(39) = 2.09$, $p < .05$]. These 20 students reported approximately the same domains and causes for their negative states as we have seen for the entire sample (Tables 1 and 2). We conclude, therefore, that the new sources of negative states we have seen among adolescents—heterosexual strain, more advanced social cognitions—are sources of stress that put some teens at risk.

Conclusion

We began with the position that emotions are social constructions, constituted within an individual's and a group's most strongly held values and beliefs about the world. Negative emotions, we asserted, indicate points of friction between these values and beliefs and the world as it is. In Piagetian terms, they reflect a state of disequilibrium between an internal representation of life and life as it is actually encountered.

Early adolescence, we suggest, is a time when these internal representations are rapidly changing, fueled by cognitive development and an expanding domain of things that matter. The age differences we found indicate increasing mastery of some segments of experience. In adolescence, nonschool activities (household chores, a hobby, a game of baseball) are less likely to cause or deteriorate into negative emotions. Perhaps this reflects an increased ability to accept the concrete rules and structure of such activities; perhaps it reflects diminished investment in them. These old points of friction, however, are replaced by new ones that reflect the emergence of a more penetrating set of values and concerns.

The findings suggest that some of the more frequent negative experiences among adolescents may be a result not of an objectively harder, harsher world, but of subjective changes that make it *seem* harder. The adolescents as compared to the preadolescents more often explained their negative emotions in terms of a more distal world, including the feelings of others and anticipated future events. This shift resembles a Piagetian shift from a concrete, here-and-now world to a more abstract, hypothetical, and constructed reality.

The cognitive advances of adolescence lead to the fundamental insight that other people are centers of thinking and feeling. This insight opens the floodgates to sources of anger and anxiety that were not previously perceived. They experience pain through empathetic identification with others. They suffer the ups and downs associated with new dimensions of strategic social interactions among their peers. Sensitivity to what Suzy told Bob about Jeremy may be beyond the cognitive capability of most fifth graders, yet was a preoccupation of some of our ninth graders.

It is paradoxical that growth leads to expanding possibilities for hurt, yet we are not alone in acknowledging such paradox. Theorists as diverse as Jerome Kagan and Margaret Mahler attributed the emotional turmoil commonly known as "the terrible twos" to cognitive advances of the young child. More pertinent to our study, Weiner and Graham (1984) argue that cognitive development from childhood to adolescence creates the possibility of new emotions, such as guilt, that were not previously possible, and Laursen and Collins (1988) propose that cognitive growth may destabilize family relations. In the long run these cognitive advances may well lead to better adjustment, but in the short run they increase vulnerability. We believe, then, that the increased negative experience in adolescence may be, in part, related to cognitive growth.

At the same time, one cannot fail to recognize that these negative emotions emanate from an expanded set of concerns. The biggest new domain of both positive and negative emotion—and also the domain of their more cognitively advanced emotional explanations—is romantic relationships, both real relationships and fantasized ones. In an analysis of adolescent love, Fischer and Alapack (1987) describe the enormous expectations associated with adolescent love in our culture. These expectations, which form the subtext of movies, TV shows, and music, are founded upon a Western cultural mythosis of romantic love that De-Rougemount (1956) traces back to the age of chivalry. The frequency with which romance is a source of negative emotion indicates, first, that the ideal of romantic love has assumed a place at the very core of adolescents' world of meaning, and second, that this ideal is often disappointed, probably because it is greatly inflated beyond realistic expectations.

Of course, in some cases the anguish our adolescents reported in love may reflect transformations of other psychodynamic issues—inadequate parenting, identity crises, failed relations with friends. But the projection of these inner issues onto the lightening board of romance, fueled by new cognitive capabilities for abstraction, makes for a more explosive situation. It is in this tinderbox of inflated ideals and unpredictable behavior that they attempt to negotiate an autonomous sense of self. Based on our findings, we would argue that disappointments in love represent one of the major sources of distress, strain, and perhaps psychiatric disorder in adolescence.

Here we think that novelists and writers have more accurately described adolescence than have social scientists. In works from *Romeo and Juliet* to Mishima's *White Snow*, the principal cause of anguish, distress, and suicide is frustrated ideals of love. Margaret Mead (1928) also deserves credit for identifying the absence of our notions of romantic love for the relatively less emotional and less tumultuous lives of traditional Samoan girls. Although a measured amount of stress may be a stimulus to growth, a "developmental challenge," we also think one could do no better in minimizing adolescents' stress than to replace their culture of love and romance with more realistic, and realizable expectations. Unable to do this, we might at least attempt to provide adolescents more support for the pain they experience in relationships.

In concluding, we should also emphasize the gender differences in our findings. Girls emotions are more social in preadolescence, and become more social in early adolescence. Their negative emotions are more often caused by breaches in the increasingly complex norms of expected behavior among friends and family. Apparently their emotional equilibrium is more strongly defined by the web of solidarity they desire with friends, lovers, and parents. Attempts at intervention with girls, therefore, should recognize that the cause and cure of strain for them is more likely to be interpersonal.

Preadolescent boys' negative emotions, by comparison, are more activity based, and remain more actively based in early adolescence. For boys the social network is less likely to be the cause, at least consciously, of their negative emotions. We might therefore be more cautious about assuming that increased social support of other social network intervention will be as influential in buffering them from or reducing their stress.

Acknowledgments

This research was supported by NIMH Grant 1 RO1 MH38324, "Stress in Daily Life During Early Adolescence," awarded to the first author.

Notes

1.   In fairness to real ethnographers, we should acknowledge that contemporary research on adolescence rarely involves the diligent, painstaking observation associated with this approach. We would also like to note that we do not do justice

to Lutz's conception of emotion, which recognizes that affective states are often negotiated with others—an idea that would be worth following through on in the study of adolescent–parent and adolescent–peer relationships.

2. The significance tests presented in this and subsequent tables use the individual emotion as the unit of analysis, an approach that could be critized for failing to recognize the non-independence of reports (see Larson & Delespaul, 1990). Separate analyses, which used the person as the unit of analysis, indicate nearly identical patterns of significance.

References

Bowerman, C. E., & Kinch, J. W. (1959). Changes in family and peer orientation of children between the fourth and tenth grades. *Social Forces, 37*, 206–211.

Brooks-Gunn, J., & Warren, M. P. (1989). Biological and social contributions to negative affect in young adolescent girls. *Child Development, 60*(1), 40–55.

Cohen, L. H., Burt, C. E., & Bjorck, J. (1987). Life stress and adjustment: Effects of life events experienced by young adolescents and their parents. *Developmental Psychology, 23*(4), 583–592.

Compas, B. E., Wagner, B. M., Slavin, L. A., & Vannatta, K. (1986). A prospective study of life events, social support, and psychological symptomatology during the transition from high school to college. *American Journal of Community Psychology, 14*(3), 241–257.

Csikszentmihalyi, M., & Larson, R. (1987). Validity and reliability of the experience-sampling method. *The Journal of Nervous and Mental Disease, 175*(9), 526–536.

DeRougemount, D. (1956). *Love in the western world.* Greenwich, CT: Fawcett Publications.

Elkind, D. (1980). Strategic interactions in early adolescence. In J. Adelson (Ed.), *Handbook of adolescent psychology* (pp. 432–444). New York: John Wiley.

Epstein, S. (1984). Controversial issues in emotion theory. In P. Shaver (Ed.), *Review of personality and social psychology: emotions, relationships, and health* (pp. 64–88). Beverly Hills, CA: Sage Publications.

Fischer, C. T., & Alapack, R. J. (1987). A phenomenological approach to adolescence. In V. Van Hasselt & J. M. Herson (Eds.), *Handbook of adolescent psychology* (pp. 91–99). New York: Pergamon.

Freud, A. (1946). *The ego and the mechanisms of defense.* (trans. by C. Baines). New York: International Universities Press.

Greene, A. L., & Larson, R. W. (1991). Variation in stress reactivity during adolescence. In A. Greene, E. M. Cumminmgs, & K. Karraker (Eds.), *Life span developmental psychology.* New York: Academic Press.

Harré, R. (1986). *The social construction of emotions* (pp. 3–14). New York: Basal Blackwell.

Harris, P. L., Olthof, T., & Terwogt, M. M. (1981). Children's knowledge of emotion. *Journal of Child Psychology and Psychiatry, 22*(3), 247–261.

Hoffman, M. L. (1980). Moral development in adolescence. In J. Adelson (Ed.), *Handbook of adolescent psychology* (pp. 295–343). New York: John Wiley.

Inhelder, B., & Piaget, J. (1958). *The growth of logical thinking: from childhood to adolescence.* Basic Books.

Larson, R. (1989). Beeping children and adolescents: A method for studying time use and daily experience. *The Journal of Youth and Adolescence, 18,* 511–553.

Larson, R. (1990). The solitary side of life: An examination of the time people spend alone from childhood to old age. *Developmental Review, 10,* 155–183.

Larson, R., Csikszentimihalyi, M., & Graef, R. (1980). Mood variability and the psychosocial adjustment of adolescents. *Journal of Youth and Adolescents, 9*(6), 469–490.

Larson, R., & Delespaul, P. (1990). Analyzing experience sampling data: A guidebook for the perplexed. In M. deVries (Ed.), *The experience of psychopathology.* Cambridge: Cambridge Press.

Larson, R., & Ham, M. (1989). *Stressful events and adolescents' mood states.* Paper presented at the Biannual Meetings of the Society for Research on Child Development.

Larson, R., & Lampman-Petraitis, C. (1989). Daily emotional stress as reported by children and adolescents. *Child Development, 60,* 1250–1260.

Larson, R., Raffaelli, M., Richards, M. H., Ham, M., & Jewell, L. (1990). The ecology of depression in early adolescence. *Journal of Abnormal Psychology, 99,* 92–102.

Larson, R., & Richards, M. H. (1991) Daily companionship in childhood and adolescence: changing developmental contexts. *Child Development,* In press.

Laursen, B., & Collins, W. A. (1988). Conceptual changes during adolescence and effects upon parent-child relationships. *Journal of Adolescent Research, 3*(2), 119–139.

Lazarus, R. S., Kanner, A. D., & Folkman, S. (1980). Emotions: A cognitive-phenomenological analysis. In R. Plutchik & H. Kellerman (Eds.), *Emotion: theory, research, and experience: Vol. 1. Theories of emotion* (pp. 189–217). New York: Academic Press.

Leone, C. (1989). *The influence of family relationships and mood states on academic achievement.* Unpublished Ph.D. Dissertation, Loyola University of Chicago.

Lewis, M., & Michalson, L. (1983). *Children's emotions and moods: Developmental theory and measurement.* New York: Plenum.

Lutz, C. A. (1988). *Unnatural emotions: everyday sentiments on a micronesian atoll and their challenge to western theory.* Chicago: The University of Chicago Press.

Mandler, G. (1980). The generation of emotion: A psychological theory. In R. Plutchik & H. Kellerman (Eds.), *Emotion: theory, research, and experience: Vol. 1. Theories of emotion* (pp. 219–243). New York: Academic Press.

Mead, M. (1928). *Coming of age in Samoa.* New York: William Morrow.

Nannis, E. D., & Cowan, P. A. (1987). Emotional understanding: A matter of age, dimension, and point of view. *Journal of Applied Developmental Psychology, 8,* 289–304.

Petersen, A. C., & Taylor, B. (1980). The biological approach to adolescence. In J. Adelson (Ed.), *Handbook of adolescent psychology* (pp. 117–155). New York: John Wiley.

Richards, M. H., Casper, R., & Larson, R. (1990). Weight and eating concerns among pre- and young adolescent boys and girls. *Journal of Adolescent Health, 11,* 203–209.

Richards, M. H., & Larson, R. (1990). Pubertal development and the daily emotional well-being in young adolescents. Submitted.

Rorty, A. O. (1980). Explaining emotions. In A. O. Rorty (Ed.), *Explaining emotions* (pp. 103–126). Berkeley and Los Angeles, CA: University of California Press.

Roseman, I. J. (1984). Cognitive determinants of emotion: A structural theory. In P. Shaver (Ed.), *Review of personality and social psychology: emotions, relationships, and health* (pp. 11–36). Beverly Hills, CA: Sage Publications.

Scherer, K. R. (1984). Emotion as a multicomponent process: A model and some cross-cultural data. In P. Shaver (Ed.), *Review of personality and social psychology: emotions, relationships, and health* (pp. 37–63). Beverly Hills, CA: Sage Publications.

Selman, R. (1980). *The growth of interpersonal understanding.* New York: Academic Press.

Simmons, R., Rosenberg, F., & Rosenberg, M. (1973). Disturbance in the self-image at adolescence. *American Sociological Review, 38,* 553–568.

Solomon, R. C. (1976). *The passions: The myth and nature of human emotion.* Notre Dame, IN: University of Notre Dame Press.

Steinberg, L. (1987). The impact of puberty on family relations: Effects of pubertal status and pubertal timing. *Developmental Psychology, 23,* 451–460.

Steinberg, L., & Silverberg, S. B. (1986). The vicissitudes of autonomy in early adolescence. *Child Development, 57,* 1–10.

Weiner, B., & Graham, S. (1984). An attributional approach to emotional development. In C. E. Izard, J. Kagan, & R. B. Zajonc (Eds.), *Emotions, cognition, and behavior,* (pp. 167–191). New York: Cambridge University Press.

3

Conflict and Adaptation in Adolescence: Adolescent-Parent Conflict

**Judith G. Smetana, Jenny Yau,
Angela Restrepo, and Judith L. Braeges**

Introduction

Developmental transitions can be stressful—not only for the developing child, but for parents as well. Consider the transition to adolescence. Adolescence is characterized by more rapid changes than any other period of the life cycle with the exception of infancy. The physical changes associated with puberty (Hill, 1988), the development of formal logic (Inhelder & Piaget, 1958), and the emergence of new social-cognitive abilities (Shantz, 1983) all may cooccur with alterations in peer networks, role expectations, transitions in schooling, and changes in family relationships. Several studies have indicated that the adolescent years are more stressful to parents than any other phase of the family life cycle (Offer, 1969; Olson, McCubbin, Barnes, Larson, Muxen, & Wilson, 1983). As compared to parents of children at other ages, parents of adolescents report some of the lowest levels of life satisfaction (Hoffman & Mannis, 1978), highest levels of distress (Pearlin & Lieberman, 1979), and greatest feelings of inadequacy (Veroff & Feld, 1970). This chapter focuses on one significant source of stress for both parents and adolescents—realignments in family relationships. Although we now know that adolescence does not typically entail storm and stress, rebellion against parents, or a generation gap, as was once thought (e.g., Freud, 1937), parent–child

43

relations in the transition to adolescence are typically characterized by disagreements and minor conflicts with parents over the everyday details of family life, such as doing the chores, doing schoolwork, choice of clothes and appearances, sibling relations, and so on (see Hill, 1988; Montemayor, 1986; Powers, Hauser, & Kilner, 1989; Steinberg, in press, for reviews of this research). Some researchers have asserted that conflict over such mundane issues must itself be insignificant. Consider this quote from Douvan and Adelson (1966): there is a "great hue and cry of conflict between the child and his parents over 'values' and 'norms' which are in fact trivial. The so-called adolescent rebellion in these cases exhausts itself on issues of manners and tastes" (p. 81).

In contrast, our data, as well as others', suggest that although rancorous, open conflict is infrequent, squabbling, emotional tensions, and disagreements are common. Thus, parent–child disagreement appears to be a normative and adaptive aspect of the transition to adolescence, although the form and tenor may vary in different families. Furthermore, we assert that conflict over everyday, mundane issues provides a context for adolescents' developing autonomy.

This chapter presents the results of recent research on adolescent–parent conflict. In this research, alterations in adolescent–parent relationships are examined within a social-cognitive framework that takes into consideration the multifaceted ways that adolescents and parents interpret their social worlds. In the first part of this chapter, we discuss the conceptual framework that informs our research. Next, we present results from a study of two-parent families with adolescents, focusing first on adolescents' and parents' interpretations of conflictual issues and then on relationships between reasoning, conflict, and family social interaction. Then, we present the results of research on adolescent–parent conflict in divorced, mother-custody families and discuss relationships between changes in family structure and normative changes in family relations during adolescence. Implications of our findings are discussed in a final section.

Conceptual Framework: Domains of Social Judgment and Adolescent–Parent Conflict

In the research presented in this chapter and elsewhere (Smetana, 1988b, 1989; Smetana, Yau, & Braeges, 1989), we conceptualize adolescent–parent conflict in terms of adolescents' and parents' attempts to coordinate conflicting social-cognitive perspectives. Our description of these perspectives is derived from a domain model of social-cognitive development that describes social knowledge as developing within three developmentally and conceptually distinct domains (Smetana, 1983; Turiel,

1983). Before describing the study itself, we outline this model of social development and its relevance to adolescent–parent relationships.

In the research presented in this chapter, the family is viewed as a constituted social system with a social organization entailing hierarchical structures, patterns of authority, rules, and conventions. We hypothesized that adolescent–parent conflict may arise when adolescents and parents have different interpretations of those rules and expectations. For instance, parents may justify their expectations that adolescents clean up their rooms on the basis of conventional concerns (for instance, with the need for order or for family members to coordinate their activities), whereas adolescents might view cleaning their room as an issue that is legitimately under their personal jurisdiction. Concepts of social convention and personal jurisdiction, as well as concepts of morality, have each been described in the domain specificity model.

According to this model, concepts of convention are defined as the arbitrary and agreed-on behavioral uniformities that coordinate the interactions of individuals within different social systems. Examples are modes of address, dress, sex roles, manners, or mores regarding sexuality. A great deal of empirical research (Davidson, Turiel, & Black, 1983; Nucci, 1981; Smetana, 1981, 1983, 1985; Turiel, 1983; Weston & Turiel, 1980) indicates that concepts of convention can be separated both analytically and empirically from moral judgments, or judgments regarding how individuals ought to relate to one another. Judgments regarding social conventions serve social-organizational ends by providing individuals with a set of expectations regarding appropriate behavior. Moral judgments, however, are prescriptive, categorical judgments, structured by justice, that pertain to issues such as others' welfare, trust, or the equitable distribution of resources. In contrast to conventions, moral acts are not arbitrary; although moral prescriptions are an aspect of social organization, they are determined by factors inherent in social interactions (i.e., their intrinsic effects on others) rather than by their function in maintaining the social system.

We distinguish further between concepts of convention and social organization and children's understanding of themselves and others as psychological systems (Nucci, 1981; Smetana, 1982; Turiel, 1983). The psychological domain pertains to children's understanding of self, identity, and personality and their attributions regarding their own and others' thoughts and behavior. In particular, concepts of convention have been empirically distinguished from personal issues, which are one aspect of the psychological domain. Personal issues are issues that have consequences that pertain only to the actor, and, thus, are viewed as beyond societal regulation and moral concern. They include issues such as choice of one's friends, the content of one's correspondence, one's recreational activities, and actions which focus on the state of one's body, such as aspects of physical appearance or smoking (Nucci, 1981). Developing notions of personal choice have been hypothesized to represent an important aspect of the individual's autonomy or distinctiveness from others (Nucci, 1981).

It has been proposed that social conventions, morality, and personal issues constitute conceptually and developmentally distinct domains of social judgment (Smetana, 1983; Turiel, 1983). That is, although there may be overlap or intersections among the domains, concepts within each domain form separate, self-regulating developmental systems. Research indicates that children across a wide age range distinguish the domains using distinctive criteria (for more detail on this research, see Turiel, Killen, & Helwig, 1987) and that different types of social orientations coexist in children's social judgments (see Turiel & Davidson, 1986 for further discussion of the epistemological basis for these domain distinctions).

Although most research from this perspective has focused on children's judgments about events that are prototypical of each domain, recent research has examined how children evaluate and coordinate issues that entail overlap, conflict, or ambiguity between the domains. We conceptualized adolescent–parent conflict in terms of such domain conflicts. That is, children's and parents' competing goals in family situations may result in different interpretations of events, which, in turn, may lead to conflict and disagreement in parent–child relationships.

Adolescent–Parent Conflict: An Empirical Investigation

This framework had at least two methodological implications for the study of conflict and transitions in adolescent–parent relationships. First, since it was hypothesized that conflict and tensions arise from parents' and children's different interpretations of family expectations, it was necessary to examine parents', as well as children's views of family conflict. As conflict, by definition, presupposes at least two opposing perspectives (Shantz, 1987), this may seem to be a necessary—indeed self-evident—component of studying adolescent–parent conflict. However, few studies have specifically focused on the coordination (or lack of coordination) of perspectives that may underlie conflict. Most interview studies have focused on children's perspectives on these issues, and parents' views typically have not been obtained. Furthermore, the focus on the match or mismatch between parents' and children's interpretations of everyday situations required that parents and children be interviewed about actual conflicts. Most interview studies have assessed conflict on responses to a small set of issues, predetermined by the investigator, that may be of varying relevance to individual families. Subjects rarely have been asked about real-life conflicts of relevance to their families. In this study, both parents and adolescents were considered integral to the research, and conflict was assessed on issues raised by the subjects themselves.

Study Design and Methods

The results discussed here are based on interviews with 102 children from two-parent families. The children were approximately evenly divided into boys and girls at four ages: preadolescents (fifth and sixth graders; $n = 26$), early adolescents (seventh and eighth graders; $n = 26$), mid-adolescents (ninth and tenth graders; $n = 26$), and late adolescents (eleventh and twelfth graders; $n = 24$). Both parents also participated in the research. The sample was primarily Caucasian, middle- to upper-middle class, and well educated. Families were recruited with the cooperation of a local school district and invited to participate in a 2½- to 3-hour session at the University. Family members were interviewed individually and then videotaped during a Family Social Interaction Task (described in a subsequent section).

Family members were interviewed about rules, authority, and relationships with parents (or adolescents) in general and then about self-generated issues of conflict. To assess conflict on the issues deemed salient by each participant, conflict was first operationally defined. The definition included disagreements between parents and children over what family members might perceive as minor issues (like feeding the pets or doing the chores), as well as more major issues (such as drugs and sex). However, we did not specify the extent to which these disagreements had to be explicit, verbal, or resolvable. Subjects were asked to generate exhaustive lists of the disagreements and conflicts they had with parents (or children); these issues then became the focus of the subsequent interview. Participants were interviewed extensively to obtain their interpretations and ratings (on several dimensions) of each conflict.

For each issue of conflict, two types of interpretations were obtained. First, family members reasoned about, or justified, the wrongness or permissibility of the event from their own perspective. Then they reasoned about the issue from the other's perspective. The former are referred to as *justifications*, and the latter are referred to as *counterarguments*. Justifications and counterarguments were scored in 19 justification categories expanded from previous research on social-cognitive domain distinctions (Davidson et al., 1983; Nucci, 1981; Smetana, 1985). For purposes of analysis and on the basis of previous research, justifications were collapsed into social-cognitive domains. The moral category included justifications pertaining to appeals to fairness ("You always ask me to do it; you never ask her"), others' welfare ("You'll hurt him," "We worry that someone will hurt you") and obligation ("You have a duty to your parents").

Social-conventional justifications pertained to social coordination ("We're all part of the family, so we all have to chip in and help"; "With your mother working, we all have to do our jobs so that things will get done around here"), customs and social norms ("That's the way all my friends look"; "No one dresses like that anymore"), politeness ("It's rude to talk to your mother like that"), appeals to authority ("I'm your mother and I told you to do it"; "That's against the law"), responsibility ("You need to learn some responsibility"), punishment avoidance ("You'll get grounded"), and social nonconformity ("I'd be embarrassed if my friends saw you looking like that"; "People will think I'm weird").

The psychological category included justifications pertaining to adolescents' psychological or dispositional characteristics ("You're just lazy"), interpersonal relations ("You should love your brother"), developmental appropriateness ("You're too young to make that decision"), egoistic reasons ("I know it's wrong, but I want to do it anyway"), and justifications that the acts are unintentional ("I forgot"; "I didn't mean to hurt him").

Because of their frequency and their hypothesized relevance here, personal choice justifications ("It's my room and I should be able to decide how it looks"; "It's no big deal—it doesn't hurt anybody else") and justifications pertaining to autonomy and individuation ("I'm just expressing who I am"), both aspects of the psychological domain, were combined and examined separately from other psychological justifications. Prudential justifications ("You'll catch a cold") and pragmatic justifications ("I can't do it—I have basketball practice") were also combined into a separate category. (For more detailed description of the methods and of these justification categories, see Smetana, 1988a,b, 1989.)

Interview Findings

Types of Conflicts. Conflicts were seen to occur primarily over chores (18%), interpersonal relationships (16%), regulating the child's activities (12%), personality characteristics (11%), homework (9%), bedtime and curfew (9%), regulating social relations (8%), and appearance (8%). With only a few exceptions, there was strong agreement between parents and adolescents over the types of issues that cause conflict. These issues were not seen to vary in frequency from preadolescence to late adolescence, nor were there significant differences in the issues raised by parents and children.

Justifications. Although adolescents and parents agreed on the issues that cause conflict in their relationship, their interpretations of these issues differed. The percentages of different justifications used by parents and adolescents are depicted in Figure 1. Adolescents most frequently viewed conflicts as occurring over issues of exercising or maintaining personal jurisdiction; these justifications accounted for 50% of their responses. As hypothesized, parents' interpretations of these issues differed markedly, with adolescents and parents constructing the issues in conceptually different domains. As can be seen, mothers' and fathers' orientation to these issues was primarily social-conventional (constituting 48 and 44% of their responses, respectively), but this perspective was infrequent among children and adolescents (13%). As the figure indicates, parents and adolescents differed in their moral, pragmatic and prudential, and psychological interpretations of conflicts as well.

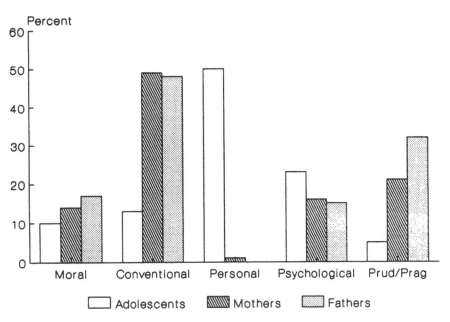

Figure 1.

Counterarguments. As depicted in Figure 2, the same mismatches, indeed in nearly the inverse pattern, were also found in adolescents' and parents' counterarguments. When asked to take their parents' perspective on the conflict under consideration, adolescents' reasoning was most frequently conventional in nature. Similarly, when asked to take their children's perspective, parents understood and articulated adolescents' personal orientation, although they themselves never viewed the issues as under adolescents' personal jurisdiction. Reflecting this, adolescents' counterarguments were never personal. Mirroring parents' justifications, adolescents also gave more prudential or pragmatic and moral counterarguments than parents did. Parents, in contrast, gave more psychological attributions than adolescents did. Thus, preadolescents and adolescents understood but rejected or subordinated their parents' conventional interpretations of conflictual issues and reinterpreted them as issues of personal jurisdiction. Parents similarly understood but rejected or subordinated their adolescents' claims to personal jurisdiction, restating the issues instead in conventional terms.

There were few age differences in justifications and counterarguments. There was, however, a statistically significant interaction between

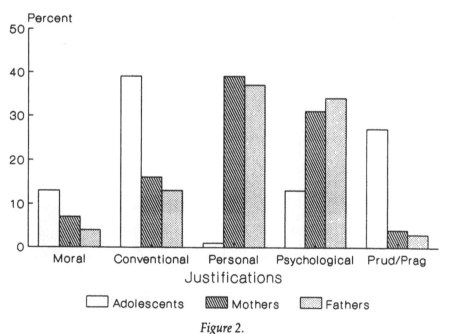

Figure 2.

age, sex, and family member in conventional counterarguments. Eleventh and twelfth grade boys evidenced more conventional counterarguments than fifth through eighth grade boys (65 vs. 34%). Thus, the findings for boys suggest an increasing ability with age to take their parents' perspectives and view conflicts within a conventional framework.

Early adolescent girls, however, offered significantly fewer conventional counterarguments than girls in either preadolescence or late adolescence (22 vs. 56 and 39%). It is possible that declines in girls' ability or willingness to take their parents' conventional perspectives in early adolescence are perceived by parents as a signal of rebellion, which then leads to conflict. Researchers have typically tied increases in conflict between mothers and daughters in early adolescence to girls' pubertal development (e.g., Hill, 1988). These findings suggest an alternative, social-cognitive explanation for the pervasive finding of difficult mother–daughter relationships in early adolescence. It is interesting to note that Maccoby (1983) has hypothesized that the move toward self-regulation in early adolescence, which includes questioning the limits of authority, is stressful for children. Furthermore, others have found that mothers find early adolescents' autonomy demands particularly stressful (Small, Eastman, & Cornelius, 1988).

Family Social Interactions

These findings raise a number of issues. First, if adolescents' personal reasoning reflects a social-cognitive aspect of the individuation process, it would be useful to know more about the types of family social interactions that facilitate or inhibit personal reasoning. In addition, researchers have disagreed as to whether adolescents' emotional autonomy from parents reflects a healthy developmental process or whether it reflects detachment and distancing from unsupportive parents (Ryan & Lynch, 1989). An examination of family social interactions related to adolescents' appeals to personal jurisdiction may shed some light on this issue.

Furthermore, there is some disagreement as to whether adolescent–parent conflict is adaptive. Traditionally, family researchers have asserted that healthy families disagree less and agree more (e.g., Jacob, 1974). However, this question has seldom been addressed in nonclinical populations of families with adolescents. More recently, Cooper, Grotevant, and Condon (1983) have found that open disagreement may facilitate the development of perspective taking and identity, suggesting a more adaptive view of parent–adolescent conflict. We addressed this issue by examining relationships among family social interactions, reasoning about conflicts, and family members' perceptions of the severity and frequency of conflict.

In addition to the individual interviews, families also participated in a videotaped 26-minute Family Social Interaction Task. Families spent 5 minutes selecting and agreeing on three issues of family conflict to discuss and then spent 7 minutes discussing each issue. The task was based on procedures used elsewhere (Zahaykevich, Sirey, & Brooks-Gunn, 1988). The videotaped family social interactions were scored using coding systems at two different levels of analysis. The Constraining and Enabling Coding System for coding adolescent–parent interaction (Hauser, Powers, Weiss-Perry, Follansbee, & Rajanpark, 1985) provided a microanalytic view of family social interaction through an analysis of family discourse; summary ratings, described in a subsequent section, provided a more molar view.

Constraining and Enabling Coding. The videotapes were transcribed, and the protocols were divided into speech units based on previous research (Condon et al., 1983) and coded using the Constraining and Enabling Coding System (referred to as the CECS). The CECS codes two descriptive types of family interactions: cognitive/attentional and affective/relational. Within each are interaction styles that are seen to facilitate or encourage expression of more independent thoughts and perceptions, and those that are seen to inhibit or undermine development by resisting adolescents' separation or differentation from parents. The first style is referred to as enabling and includes *cognitive enabling* (focussing, problem-solving, curiousity, and explaining/declaring) and *affective enabling* (acceptance and empathy). The second style is referred to as constraining and includes *cognitive constraining* (distracting, withholding, indifference) and *affective constraining* (excessive gratifying, judging, and devaluing). Enabling interactions in both parents and children have been found to facilitate adolescents' ego and moral development (Powers, 1988; Powers, Hauser, Schwartz, Noam, & Jacobson, 1983; Hauser, Powers, Noam, Jacobson, Weiss, Follansbee, & Rajanpark, 1984). To control for differences in the number of utterances across and within families, scores for each of the interaction types were expressed as proportions, based on the total number of utterances per family member.

Summary Ratings. The Family Social Interaction videotapes were also rated by trained coders, one with training in clinical psychology (A.R.), on a series of five-point summary scales assessing affect, communication, conflict, and power based on a detailed coding manual developed for these ratings (described in more detail in Restrepo, 1986). The 59 items pertaining to mothers, fathers, adolescents, and the family as a whole were then factor analyzed using principal components analysis. The analysis yielded seven factors. Three factors pertained to communication (Maternal Communication, Paternal Communication, and Adolescent Communication), with similar items loading on each factor [for instance, teen (or mother or father) expresses ideas clearly; teen (or mother or father) listens to others' thoughts and feelings; and teen (or mother or father) engages others in the task]. The remaining factors were labeled Unconflicted Family Relations (for example, teen acknowledges differences and disagreements; mother–teen dyad is not at all conflictual; family is warm, open, and comfortable), Family Uses Humor (for example, teen jokes, laughs, and uses humor), Family is Enmeshed (family is overly close and concerned with each other; teen is very powerful), and Family Resolves Conflict (e.g., teen attempts to resolve issues). Except for the Family is Enmeshed factor ($\alpha = .65$), Cronbach αs for the factors were high, ranging from .86 to .96 ($M = .92$).

The analyses reported in the following sections examined family social interactions that predicted adolescents' personal reasoning about conflicts and families' ratings of the severity and frequency of conflict. Since the two sets of family social interaction variables were uncorrelated, the seven factors emerging from the factor analyses of the summary ratings and enabling and constraining interactions for each family member, as well as sociodemographic variables (adolescents' age and sex, mother's age, father's age, and SES) were regressed on each dependent measure using stepwise multiple regression. (To reduce problems with multicolinearity, cognitive enabling was omitted from the analyses due to its high negative correlations with cognitive constraining and affective enabling.) Because previous research has demonstrated powerful sex differences during adolescence, all analyses were performed separately for families with boys and girls; there was a total of 153 subjects for each analysis.

Family Social Interactions and Personal Reasoning about Conflict. Low scores on independent observers' ratings of Adolescent Communication accounted for the largest proportion of the variance in boys' personal reasoning (17%; total $R^2 = .51$). Affective constraining in both mothers and fathers was positively related to boys' personal reasoning, and adolescent boys' affective enabling was negatively related to their personal reasoning ($r = .38, .18, -.11, p < .001, .05, .05$, respectively), with all three variables contributing significantly to the regression. These findings are consistent with the view that adolescents' expression of autonomy from parents reflects a negative detachment from rejecting and unsupportive parents (Hill & Holmbeck, 1987; Ryan & Lynch, 1989). Age contributed significantly to the regression and was negatively correlated with personal reasoning. This finding is consistent with previous findings that autonomy is a particularly salient issue in early adolescence (Steinberg & Silverberg, 1986).

A different pattern emerged for girls. Mothers' and fathers' affective constraining significantly predicted personal reasoning, but unlike the findings for boys, the relationships were negative: parents who were low in affective constraining had daughters who appealed more to personal jurisdiction. In addition, reasoning about personal jurisdiction was greater in girls who were low in affective constraining and high in affective enabling. These findings suggest that personal reasoning is a more positive manifestation of autonomy for girls than for boys. The other findings are consistent with this speculation. Girls' personal reasoning was also significantly predicted by low scores on Family is Enmeshed and high scores on Family Resolves Conflicts, Family Uses Humor, and Father Communication. Overall, 50% of the variance in girls' personal reasoning was accounted for by these variables. Thus, these findings are consistent with Steinberg and Silverberg's (1986) conjecture that self-reliance in girls (but not boys) is facilitated by close family relationships and that autonomy may be a more salient psychological concern for adolescent boys. Further, these authors claim that autonomy in boys is expressed through many types of "quasi-independent" behavior, because boys have so much trouble establishing genuine autonomy.

Family Social Interactions and Ratings of Conflict Severity.   In families with boys, more serious conflicts (as rated by family members) were predicted by high cognitive constraining in mothers and sons, high affective enabling in fathers, and low ratings on Family Uses Humor, Unconflicted Family Relations, and Family is Enmeshed. The latter three variables, which accounted for 26% of the variance, provide independent validation for families' self-report of the severity of conflict. Not surprising, more serious conflicts were also more frequent ($r = .23$, $p < .05$). Finally, age also significantly predicted the severity of conflict, with conflicts rated as more serious in families with mid-adolescents than in other families (total $R^2 = .53$ for families with boys). The literature has presented a conflicting picture of age trends in parent–adolescent conflict, perhaps because researchers have studied narrow age ranges and focused primarily on early adolescence. These findings suggest that this focus has been misplaced.

Parental constraining also predicted conflict severity in families with girls, although the constraining was affective (excessive gratifying, judging, and devaluing; $r = .31$, $.44$, $p < .001$ for mothers and fathers, respectively) rather than cognitive. Parental affective constraining accounted for 27% of the variance in conflict severity in families with girls. Girls in families with more serious conflicts were less affectively enabling, and the families were rated as being more enmeshed. Together these variables accounted for 44% of the variance in the severity of conflicts among families with girls.

Family Social Interactions and Ratings of Conflict Frequency. In both families with boys and girls, age was the strongest predictor of conflict frequency, accounting for 17 and 16% of the variance, respectively (total $R^2 = .63$ for families with boys; $R^2 = .56$ for families with girls). Although the previous analyses revealed that conflicts were more serious in families with mid-adolescent boys, the results of these analyses indicated that conflict frequency was negatively correlated with age for both boys and girls ($r = -.42, -.28, p < .001$, respectively). These findings suggest that one source of the inconsistencies in age trends found in parent–adolescent conflict may be the different indices of conflict used.

High affective constraining in mothers and low scores on observers' ratings that Family is Enmeshed significantly predicted the frequency of conflicts in families with boys and girls. In addition, low affective enabling in mothers, high cognitive constraining in adolescent girls, and low scores on observers' ratings of Adolescent Communication and Family Uses Humor predicted conflict frequency in families with girls. For families with boys, conflict frequency was also predicted by high ratings on Family Resolves Conflicts. In addition, more frequent conflict in families with boys was positively associated with fathers' conventional justifications and negatively associated with adolescent boys' prudential/pragmatic justifications. However, reasoning did not predict conflict frequency in families with girls.

These results are consistent with Jacob's (1974) view that healthy families disagree less, although the specific patterns of social interactions differed somewhat for families with boys and girls. Parental constraining interactions, and particularly affective constraining, including excessive gratifying, judging, and devaluing, were related to greater adolescent–parent conflict. We do not know, however, whether parents' attempts to inhibit adolescents' separation or differentiation actually cause greater parent–child conflict, or whether parents become more constraining in response to more conflictual parent–child relations. Longitudinal research would be necessary to answer this question. However, other investigators (Hauser et al., 1984; Powers et al., 1983) have reported that parental enabling is related to subsequent adolescent ego development, lending some credence to the interpretation that parental (and adolescent) interaction styles that are seen to facilitate the expression of more independent thoughts and perceptions (e.g., enabling interactions) are also predictive of less conflictual parent–child relations during adolescence.

The findings discussed thus far pertain only to intact, two-parent families. However, fewer and fewer children are growing up in such families. Thus, it is important to determine whether the findings can be generalized to single-parent, divorced families. Adolescents growing up in single-parent families experience a fundamentally different family social system, and the different balances of authority, patterns of relationships, rules, and conventions in single-parent than two-parent families all may impact the way adolescents and parents conceptualize (and experience) the normative conflicts that emerge in adolescence. In the research discussed in the following section, adolescent–parent conflict in two-parent, married families and single-parent, mother-custodial families is compared.

Adolescent–Parent Conflict in Divorced, Single-Parent Families

The research discussed previously suggests that adolescent–parent conflict occurs when childrens' attempts to assert their autonomy competes with parents' conventional goals of regulating the household, maintaining authority, and upholding conventional standards. However, married families have been characterized as being more hierarchical and having more of an "echelon" structure than divorced families (Hetherington, 1989; Weiss, 1979). Thus, the desires for independence and autonomy that typically emerge in early adolescence may elicit more conflict in families where there are two adults who reinforce each others' decisions and roles as parents than in single-parent families, where children already have been granted considerable independence, power, and responsibility in family decisionmaking (Dornbusch, Carlsmith, Bushwall, Ritter, Leiderman, Hastorf, & Gross, 1985; Hetherington, 1989). The comparative analyses reported in this section examine the hypothesis that adolescent–parent conflict is greater in married than divorced families. Although this hypothesis may appear counterintuitive, it is consistent with a growing body of literature that suggests that successfully controlling or dealing with a series of stressful life events may increase competence and resilience (Hetherington, 1984).

Divorce is a multistage process of radically changing family relationships (Wallerstein, 1983). The first 2 years following divorce may be considered an acute phase; children and parents experience a variety of problems, including emotional distress, behavior problems, and disruptions of family functioning (Hetherington, 1989). However, most of the behavioral effects of divorce are ameliorated over time (Hetherington &

Camara, 1984; Wallerstein & Kelly, 1980), resulting in the establishment of a postdivorce family. The results reported here focused on postdivorce families to examine adolescent–parent conflict in stable, single-parent families.

Overview of Methods

The results are based on interviews with 28 single-parent families with children ranging from sixth to eleventh grades and a subset of 66 two-parent families with same-age children. Divorced and married families were evenly divided into two ages: families with sixth through eighth graders (referred to here as early adolescent families) and families with ninth through eleventh graders (referred to here as mid-adolescent families). Divorced mothers had been divorced prior to their child's adolescence (children were, on average, 7 years of age at the time of divorce), had not remarried, and according to their report, were not currently cohabiting. Thus, the divorced sample consisted of "stable" divorced families (Hetherington, 1989; Wallerstein, 1983). The two-parent comparison sample was selected from the larger two-parent sample using the two criteria: the adolescents were in the sixth through eleventh grades, and only natural parents and their adolescent were included.

Divorced mothers and their adolescents were administered the same interviews as parents and children in two-parent families. Individually interviewed mothers and adolescents were asked to generate actual issues of conflict—for adolescents from divorced families, the conflicts were with the custodial mother only—and then were interviewed about each issue. They justified their perspectives on the disputes and rated each issue for the frequency and severity of conflicts. On completion of the interviews, divorced families also participated in the Family Social Interaction Task. (In the analyses present below, socioeconomic status was controlled, as divorced families were lower in SES than married families.)

Ratings of Conflict

As hypothesized, adolescent–parent conflict was greater in married than divorced families, particularly in early adolescence. Married parents of early adolescents generated a greater number of conflicts (an average of 4.0 as compared to 2.87) and reported having more frequent conflicts ($M = 3.82$ and 3.52 on a 5-point scale, where $5 = $ most frequent) than divorced mothers of early adolescents, and early adolescents from two-parent families reported more serious conflicts than early adolescents from divorced families ($M = 2.25$ and 2.03 on a 5-point scale, where 5 = most serious). The results indicate that although parent–child conflict may be a normative aspect of changing family relations in the transition to adolescence, its course may be exacerbated or attenuated in different family structures.

Types of Conflicts

There were few differences between divorced and intact families in the types of conflicts they experienced. However, divorced families with boys reported fewer conflicts over regulating the child's activities than other families. This is consistent with reports that sons in single-parent families have greater independence over decision making (Dornbusch et al., 1985), spend less time at home with their parents (Hetherington, 1989; Wallerstein & Kelly, 1980; Weiss, 1979), and receive less chaperonage than other adolescents (Flanagan, 1987; Hetherington, 1989; Santrock, Warshak, Lindbergh, & Meadows, 1982). Furthermore, divorced mothers of boys reported more conflict over their sons' personality characteristics and behavioral style than did divorced mothers of girls. Independence may have its costs! Divorced mothers may find their sons' independence irritating and itself a source of conflict.

Divorced and married families did not differ in the frequency of conflicts over chores and household duties, even though the absence of a father in the home usually means less help for the mother in childrearing and household tasks (Hetherington & Camara, 1984). In addition, although girls from single-parent families have more problems over heterosexual relationships in adolescence than girls from intact families (Hetherington, 1972), divorced families with girls and boys did not differ in the frequency of conflicts over this issue.

Reasoning about Conflict

Because parent–child relations are more hierarchical in married as compared to divorced families (Hetherington, 1989; Weiss, 1979), we expected that married parents would be more conventional in their orientation to conflicts than divorced parents. This hypothesis was confirmed: Married families offered more conventional justifications for disputes than divorced families (31% of responses, as compared to 22% of responses). Their greater reliance on justifications pertaining to authority and social coordination supports the notion that differences in conventional reasoning stem from structural differences in married and divorced families, since such justifications can be seen as pertaining to maintaining hierarchical social systems. It is also possible, however, that parents who are less conventional in their orientation to these issues are more likely to divorce!

Single-parent families also offered more psychological justifications for conflicts than did intact, two-parent families (31% of responses, as compared to 18%). Further analyses indicated that divorced families were more likely to reason about interpersonal issues and friendships. Justifications coded in this category most frequently pertained to sibling relationships, but they also pertained to choice of friends and dating. Thus, although divorced and married families did not differ in the frequency of conflicts over heterosexual relationships, as Hetherington's (1972) findings might predict, these issues may have emerged in divorced than married families' greater use of interpersonal justifications. Divorced families also were more likely than married families to reason that the acts causing conflict were unintentional. This is consistent with the finding that conflicts were less serious in single-parent families than in married families.

Early adolescents from married families also appealed to exercising or maintaining personal jurisdiction more than early adolescents in single-parent families. Indeed, the differences were rather striking; appeals to personal jurisdiction comprised 60% of the justifications given by early adolescents from married families, whereas only 35% of the explanations for conflicts among early adolescents from divorced families pertained to personal choice. These findings are consistent with the results of other studies, which indicate that adolescents in divorced families are more independent in their decision making than adolescents in married families (Dornbusch et al., 1985) and that divorced mothers are more permissive and less controlling than mothers in intact families (Flanagan, 1987; Hetherington, 1989; Santrock et al., 1982). Thus, the greater frequency of reasoning about personal jurisdiction among adolescents in intact than divorced families may reflect the greater pressure for autonomy in these families. As expected, these differences were found only in early adolescence, when autonomy issues are most salient (Steinberg & Silverberg, 1986). Since it is these autonomy demands that mothers find stressful (Small et al., 1988), a further implication of these findings is that divorced mothers may find parenting an adolescent less stressful than married mothers do!

Are stably divorced, mother-custody families merely denying the existence of conflict in their families, or are they really less conflictual than married families? Analyses of these family social interactions, described in the next section, were conducted to address this issue.

Family Social Interactions

Overall, divorced mothers and their adolescents were found to function in ways that facilitate adolescent development (Powers, 1988;

Powers et al., 1983; Hauser et al., 1984). Divorced families showed higher levels of affective responsiveness (acceptance and empathy) than intact families, and divorced mothers were less cognitively constraining than married parents. Furthermore, adolescents from divorced families evidenced more affective enabling than adolescents from married families. Divorced families with mid-adolescents were both more affectively responsive and less affectively constraining than married families with mid-adolescents. These findings (presented in Table 1) are consistent with research indicating that divorced mothers expect greater maturity from their children than do married parents (Hetherington, 1989; Weiss, 1979). The results of these analyses suggest that the lower level of conflict reported among adolescents in divorced than married families may reflect positive styles of interaction and adaptation.

Thus, this research suggests that successful adaptation to parental divorce and life in a single-parent family can attenuate the parent–child conflict that typically accompanies the transition from childhood to adolescence. Although the social interaction data can be seen as supporting the findings from the individual interviews, caution is necessary in interpreting the results from the social interaction task, since others have found differences between dyadic and triadic social interactions in families with adolescents (Gjerde, 1986). However, these differences were in the opposite direction from those found here; Gjerde found, for instance, that the presence of the father enhanced the quality of mother–son relations. Thus, although further research comparing mother–child relations in single-parent and two-parent families would be necessary to address this issue more definitively, there appears to be some support for the conclusions drawn here.

It is likely that the timing of divorce determines whether divorce will have a salutory or negative effect on parent–child relations. If the separation or divorce occurs as the child enters adolescence, the increases in stress and conflict between parents that occurs immediately following

Table 1. Constraining and Enabling Interactions (in %)

| | Married families | | | | Divorced families | | | |
| | Adolescents | | Parents | | Adolescents | | Mothers | |
	Early	Mid	Early	Mid	Early	Mid	Early	Mid
Cognitive constraining	8	7	5	5	12	4	2	1
Cognitive enabling	78	81	86	84	72	84	87	90
Affective constraining	6	6	3	4	7	1	4	1
Affective enabling	8	6	6	7	10	11	7	7

parental separation and divorce (Hetherington, 1989; Wallerstein & Kelly, 1980) may exacerbate the conflict that typifies parent–child relations during this developmental period. However, if the family has been divorced prior to the child's adolescence, giving the family system more time to stabilize, conflict may be attenuated. A similar proposition has been advanced by Simmons, Burgeson, and Reef (1988), who found that adaptation to the multiple changes of adolescence is more successful if the changes occur cumulatively rather than simultaneously. The findings presented here suggest that successful adjustment to life in a single-parent family may help families deal more competently and with greater resilience to the realignments in family relationships that occur during early adolescence.

Conclusions

The results of this research demonstrate the utility of using adolescent–parent conflict as context for studying social-cognitive processes during adolescence. They also point to the importance of examining the coordination between adolescents' and parents' reasoning and between adolescents' and parents' reasoning and social interactions. We began by asserting that conflict provides a context for debates over the extent of adolescents' developing autonomy; in this respect, conflict can be seen as having an adaptive function during adolescence. However, the results of analyses reported here also indicate that conflict is related to more negative styles of parental and adolescent social interactions, styles that have been found in other research to inhibit adolescent development (Hauser et al., 1984; Powers, 1988; Powers et al., 1983). More research is needed to understand the role of conflict in facilitating both separation from and maintenance of mutually supportive relations with parents. Especially intriguing are the sex-differentiated patterns of social interaction associated with adolescents' reasoning about personal jurisdiction. These findings suggest that autonomy may have a different meaning in the development of adolescent boys and girls. The findings reported here call for more longitudinal research on the social contexts of adolescent development.

Acknowledgments

We thank Beth Arcuri, Lisa Elliot, Dave Farrokh, Mario Kelly, Jeffrey Lamineaux, Cynthia Rohrbeck, Rubina Saigol, Mark Strubel, and Michelle Ward for their assistance with data collection, coding, and data entry, Rusti Berent for her help with statistical analyses, and Melanie

Killen for her comments on an earlier version of this manuscript. We are also very grateful to the principals and teachers of the Brighton School District for their help in recruiting families and the families who participated in this research. This project was supported by NIMH Grant RO1-MH39142 to J.G.S. Portions of the research findings presented in this chapter were presented at the Biennial Meetings of the Society for Research in Child Development, Baltimore, MD, April, 1987 and the Biennial Meetings of the Society for Research on Adolescence, Alexandria, VA, March 1988.

References

Condon, S.M., Cooper, C.R., & Grotevant, H.D. (1983). *Manual for the analysis of family discourse*. Unpublished manuscript, University of Texas.

Cooper, C.R., Grotevant, H.D., & Condon, S.M. (1983). Individuality and connectedness in the family as a context for adolescent identity formation and role-taking skill. In H.D. Grotevant & C.R. Cooper (Eds.), *New directions for child development: Adolescent development in the family* (pp. 43–59). San Francisco: Jossey-Bass.

Davidson, P., Turiel, E., & Black, A. (1983). The effect of stimulus familiarity on the use of criteria and justifications in children's social reasoning. *British Journal of Developmental Psychology, 1*, 49–65.

Dornbusch, S.M., Carlsmith, J.M., Bushwall, S.J., Ritter, P.L., Leiderman, H., Hastorf, A.H., & Gross, R.T. (1985). Single-parents, extended households, and control of adolescents. *Child Development, 56*, 326–341.

Douvan, E., & Adelson, J. (1966). *The adolescent experience*. New York: John Wiley.

Dworkin, R. (1978). *Taking rights seriously*. Cambridge, MA: Harvard University Press.

Flanagan, C. (1987). *Parent-child decision-making, curfew, and closeness in single-parent, married, and remarried families*. Paper presented at the biennial meetings of the Society for Research on Child Development, Baltimore, MD.

Freud, A. (1937/1958). *The ego and the mechanisms of defense*. London: Hogarth Press.

Gjerde, P.F. (1986). The interpersonal structure of family interaction settings: Parent-adolescent relations in dyads and triads. *Developmental Psychology, 22*, 297–304.

Hauser, S.T., Powers, S.I., Noam, G.G., Jacobson, A.M., Weiss-Perry, B., Follansbee, D.J., & Rajanpark, D.C. (1984). Familial contexts of adolescent ego development. *Child Development, 55*, 195–213.

Hauser, S.T., Powers, S.I., Weiss-Perry, B., Follansbee, D.J., & Rajanpark, D.C. (1985). *Constraining and enabling family coding system*. Unpublished manuscript, Harvard Medical School.

Hetherington, E.M. (1972). Effects of father absence on personality development in adolescent daughters. *Developmental Psychology, 7*, 313–326.

Hetherington, E.M. (1984). Stress and coping in children and families. In A. Doyle, D. Gold, & D.S. Moskowitz (Eds.), *Children in Families Under Stress:*

New Directions in Child Development (Vol. 24, pp. 7–33). San Francisco: Jossey-Bass.

Hetherington, E.M. (1989). Coping with family transitions: Winners, losers, and survivors. *Child Development, 60,* 1–14.

Hetherington, E.M., & Camara, K.A. (1984). Families in transition: The processes of dissolution and reconstitution. In R. Parke (Ed.), *Review of Child Development Research, Vol. 7: The Family* (pp. 398–439). Chicago: University of Chicago Press.

Hill, J.P. (1988). Adapting to menarche: Familial control and conflict. In M.R. Gunnar and W.A. Collins (Eds.), *21st Minnesota Symposium on Child Psychology: Development in the transition to adolescence* (pp. 43–78). Hillsdale, NJ: Erlbaum.

Hill, J.P., & Holmbeck, G.N. (1987). Familial adaptation to biological change during adolescence. In R.M. Lerner & T. Foch (Eds.), *Biological-Psychosocial interactions in early adolescence: A life-span perspective* (pp. 207–223). Hillsdale, NJ: Erlbaum.

Hoffman, L., & Manis, J. (1978). Influences of children on marital interaction and parental satisfaction and dissatisfaction. In R.M. Lerner & G.B. Spanier (Eds.), *Child Influences on Marital and Family Interaction.* New York: Academic Press.

Inhelder, B., & Piaget, J. (1958). *The growth of logical thinking from childhood to adolescence.* New York: Basic Books.

Jacob, T. (1974). Patterns of family conflict and dominance as a function of child age and social class. *Developmental Psychology, 10,* 1–12.

Maccoby, E.E. (1983). Social-emotional development and responses to stressors. In N. Garmezy & M. Rutter (Eds.), *Stress, Coping, and Development in Children* (pp. 217–234). New York: McGraw-Hill.

Montemayor, R. (1986). Family variation in parent-adolescent storm and stress. *Journal of Adolescent Research, 1,* 15–31.

Nucci, L.P. (1981). The development of personal concepts: A domain distinct from moral or societal concepts. *Child Development, 52,* 114–121.

Offer, D. (1969). *The psychological world of the teenager.* New York: Basic Books.

Olson, D., McCubbin, H., Barnes, H., Larson, A., Muxen, M., & Wilson, M. (1983). *Families, what makes them work.* Beverly Hills, CA.: Sage.

Pearlin, L., & Lieberman, M. (1979). Sources of emotional distress. *Resources in Community Mental Health, 1,* 217–248.

Powers, S.I. (1988). Moral judgment development in the family. *Journal of Moral Education, 17,* 209–219.

Powers, S.I., Hauser, S.T., & Kilner, L.A. (1989). Adolescent mental health. *American Psychologist, 44,* 200–208.

Powers, S.I., Hauser, S.T., Schwartz, J.M., Noam, G.G., & Jacobson, A.M. (1983). Adolescent ego development and family interaction: A structural-developmental perspective. In H.D. Grotevant & C.R. Cooper (Eds.), *New directions for child development: Adolescent development in the family* (pp. 5–26). San Francisco, Jossey-Bass.

Restrepo, A. (1986). *Gender and age differences in parent-adolescent conflict.* Unpublished Master's of Science Thesis, University of Rochester.

Ryan, R.M., & Lynch, J.H. (1989). Emotional autonomy versus detachment:

Revisiting the vicissitudes of adolescence and young adulthood. *Child Development, 60,* 340–356.

Santrock, J.W., Warshak, R., Lindbergh, C., & Meadows, L. (1982). Children's and parents' observed social behavior in stepfather families. *Child Development, 53,* 472–480.

Simmons, R.G., Burgeson, R., & Reef, M.J. (1988). Cumulative change at entry to adolescence. In M.R. Gunnar & W.A. Collins (Eds.), *21st Minnesota Symposium on Child Psychology: Development during the transition to adolescence* (pp. 122–150). Hillsdale, NJ: Erlbaum.

Shantz, C.U. (1983). Social cognition. In J.H. Flavell & E.M. Markman (Eds.), *Handbook of child psychology: Vol. 3. Cognitive development* (pp. 495–555). New York: Wiley.

Shantz, C.U. (1987). Conflicts between children. *Child Development, 58,* 283–305.

Small, S.A., Eastman, G., & Cornelius, S. (1988). Adolescent autonomy and parental stress. *Journal of Youth and Adolescence, 17,* 377–391.

Smetana, J.G. (1981). Preschool children's conceptions of moral and social rules. *Child Development, 52,* 1333–1336.

Smetana, J.G. (1982). *Concepts of self and morality: Women's reasoning about abortion.* New York: Praeger.

Smetana, J.G. (1983). Social-cognitive development: Domain distinctions and coordinations. *Developmental Review, 3,* 131–147.

Smetana, J.G. (1985). Preschool children's conceptions of transgressions: The effects of varying moral and conventional domain-related attributes. *Developmental Psychology, 21,* 18–29.

Smetana, J.G. (1988a). Adolescents' and parents' conceptions of parental authority. *Child Development, 59,* 321–335.

Smetana, J.G. (1988b). Concepts of self and social convention: Adolescents' and parents' reasoning about hypothetical and actual family conflicts. In M.R. Gunnar & W.A. Collins (Eds.), *21st Minnesota Symposium on Child Psychology: Development during the transition to adolescence* (pp. 79–122). Hillsdale, NJ: Erlbaum.

Smetana, J.G. (1989). Adolescents' and parents' reasoning about actual family conflict. *Child Development, 60,* 1052–1067.

Smetana, J.G., Yau, J., & Braeges, J.L. (1989). *Adolescent-parent conflict in married and divorced families.* Unpublished manuscript, University of Rochester.

Steinberg, L. (In press). Interdependency in the family: Autonomy, conflict, and harmony in the parent-adolescent relationship. In S.S. Feldman & G.R. Elliot (Eds.), *At the threshhold: The developing adolescent.* Cambridge, MA: Harvard University Press.

Steinberg, L., & Silverberg, S.B. (1986). The vicissitudes of autonomy in early adolescence. *Child Development, 57,* 841–851.

Turiel, E. (1983). *The development of social knowledge: Morality and convention.* Cambridge: Cambridge University Press.

Turiel, E., & Davidson, P. (1986). Heterogeneity, inconsistency, and asynchrony in the development of cognitive structures. In I. Levin (Ed.), *Stage and structure: Reopening the debate* (pp. 106–143). Norwood, N.J.: Ablex.

Turiel, E., Killen, M., & Helwig, C.C. (1987). Morality: Its structure, functions, and vagaries. In J. Kagan and S. Lamb (Eds.), *The emergence of moral concepts in young children* (pp. 155–244). Chicago: University of Chicago Press.

Veroff, J., & Feld, S. (1970). *Marriage and work in America.* New York: Von Nostrand Reinhold.

Wallerstein, J.S. (1983). Children of divorce: Stress and developmental tasks. In N. Garmezy & M. Rutter (Eds.), *Stress, coping, and development in children* (pp. 265–302). New York: McGraw-Hill.

Wallerstein, J.S., & Kelly, J.B. (1980). *Surviving the breakup.* New York: Basic Books.

Weiss, R.S. (1979). Growing up a little faster: The experience of growing up in a single-parent household. *Journal of Social Issues, 35,* 97–111.

Weston, D., & Turiel, E. (1980). Act-rule relations: Children's concepts of social rules. *Developmental Psychology, 16,* 417–424.

Zahaykevich, M., Sirey, J.A., & Brooks-Gunn, J. (1988). *Mother-daughter individuation during early adolescence.* Unpublished manuscript, University of Rochester.

4

Psychosocial Stress during Adolescence: Intrapersonal and Interpersonal Processes

Bruce E. Compas and Barry M. Wagner

More than any other developmental period, adolescence has been characterized in the psychological and sociological literatures as fraught with struggles that are both intrapersonal and interpersonal in nature. In the intrapersonal domain, adolescence has been described as a period in which identity formation is a central developmental task. Achieving a sense of personal autonomy and an identity that is separate from the family is of utmost importance. Significant interpersonal tasks during adolescence are thought to include increased involvement with the peer group balanced against continued attachment to the family.

Both the intrapersonal and interpersonal domains serve as sources of psychosocial stress during adolescence. Stressful events encountered by adolescents in both domains have been shown to be associated with maladjustment and psychopathology in this age group (Compas, 1987; Johnson, 1986). However, these personally experienced events may have consequences not only for the individual adolescent who encounters them but for others in her or his social environment as well. Further, adolescents do not live in an insular world in which the only threat to their well being comes from adverse circumstances and events that they encounter personally. On the contrary, adolescents are part of a network of close interpersonal relationships with peers and families, as shown by studies of adolescents in the context of the family (see Smetana et al., this volume). As a result, adolescents are potentially vulnerable to the effects of stressful events experienced by others in these social networks.

Building on the theme of the importance of intrapersonal and interpersonal processes in adolescence, we will make two basic points: (1) interpersonal stressors during adolescence have personal meaning and consequences, and (2) personal stressors experienced by adolescents and others in their social environment have interpersonal meaning and consequences. In addressing these two points, we will highlight important age and gender differences in stress during adolescence. We will first review studies that provide evidence for the impact of interpersonal stressors, including "network stress," on the adjustment of adolescents. Next, we will review evidence indicating that stressful events experienced by adolescents and their parents have direct and indirect effects on one another's well being, and we will describe the types of person to person processes that are involved in the transmission of stress and distress. Finally, we will highlight the need for an integrative framework of intrapersonal and interpersonal processes in adolescent stress and adjustment to serve as a model of the mechanisms through which personal and interpersonal stressors exert their impact on adjustment.

The Personal Ramifications of Interpersonal Stress

Adolescence is a period in which relationships outside of the family multiply, take on new meanings, and deepen in intensity. These new bonds broaden and enrich the world of the adolescent, but also carry with them the increased possibility for loss, rejection, and conflict. Adolescents tend to become acutely aware of their status in the peer society, and pressures to conform to the norms of the peer group peak in mid-adolescence (Berndt, 1979). The emotional intensity of friendships increases over earlier years; adolescents may entrust their friends with their deepest secrets, expecting that the trust will be upheld (Selman, 1980; Youniss, 1980). Because of the increased intensity of friendships, adolescents may suffer more than younger children when there is a break in a relationship, for example, when a friend moves away or they move away from a friend. Further, adolescents gradually begin to explore intimate, sexual relationships, and with these may come new found fears as well as a heightened risk of emotional rejection.

At the same time that adolescents are opening up new possibilities in the world of friendships and intimate relationships, family relationships generally retain their importance as sources of both support and stress. Although adolescence has been conceptualized as a stormy period for family relationships, research has now documented that in fact family relationships during this period tend not to be conflict-ridden overall

(Offer et al., 1981). In the course of developing increased autonomy and breaking old dependencies on parents, adolescents increasingly assert their own opinions and desires, and in most families there is movement toward increased mutuality in relationships with parents (Grotevant & Cooper, 1985; Hauser, Powers, Noam, Jacobson, Weiss, & Follansbee, 1984; White, Speisman, & Costos, 1983). The change within families toward a new balance of power can bring with it increased conflict, particularly between the mother and the adolescent (Silverberg & Steinberg, 1987). In many cases, this is undoubtedly experienced by the family members as stressful, even though mild conflict might in fact be a healthy sign of increased adolescent individuation (Montemayor, 1983).

Although it has long been acknowledged that interpersonal relationships during adolescence are potentially quite stressful, and might exact a toll on adolescents' psychological well-being, surprisingly little research has focused on specific types of interpersonal relationships as sources of stress and whether they are linked to psychological distress. Thus it remains unclear whether family, peer, or intimate relationships might constitute greater sources of stress for some adolescents compared with others. Based on the few existing studies in this area, which have used relatively brief checklists of major life events, it does appear that there may be sex differences both in reports of numbers of stressful events experienced and in the association of stressful interpersonal events with psychological symptoms. For example, Burke and Weir (1978) found that adolescent females ages 13–20 reported more stressful concerns regarding acceptance by peers and relationships with the opposite sex than males, and Compas, Slavin, Wagner, and Vannatta (1986) found that female high school students reported more major negative events concerning family/parents and sexuality than did males. Siddique and D'Arcy (1984) found greater correlations of family stress and peer stress with psychological symptoms for females than for males. Thus, adolescent females appear to report more major interpersonal stress than males, and the relationship of major life stress with psychological symptoms may be stronger for adolescent females than males. This pattern of greater vulnerability to stress in adolescent females than males is in contrast to other findings that indicate that boys may be more vulnerable to psychopathology than are girls (e.g., Rutter, 1983). This suggests that there may be differences in vulnerability to stress during preadolescence and adolescence.

In a recent study, we reasoned that many of the interpersonal stresses that might have an impact on adolescents are common, everyday occurrences rather than major events (Wagner & Compas, 1990). That is, adolescents may experience as much stress in facing such everyday occurrences as disagreements with parents, friends, or boyfriends or girlfriends as they would if faced with major, infrequent events such as being turned down for membership in an organization, starting a new intimate relationship, etc. We asked samples of junior high students ($N = 93$), high school students ($N = 140$), and college students ($N = 145$) to complete the age-appropriate version of the Adolescent Perceived Events Scale (APES; Compas, Davis, Forsythe, & Wagner, 1987), in order to investigate the degree to which adolescents reported having experienced a wide variety of both everyday interpersonal stresses as well as major stresses of adolescence during the prior three months. On the APES, respondents check from a list of possible events those events that have occurred, and rate each event that has occurred on three scales: desirability, impact, and frequency of occurrence. The APES includes both normative and atypical events that are of major and minor magnitude, and represent both positive and negative experiences of adolescents. In this discussion, we will be concerned only with counts of events rated as undesirable (i.e., negative) by the respondent. In addition, junior high students in the study completed the Youth Self-Report version of the Child Behavior Checklist (YSR; Achenbach & Edelbrock, 1987), and senior high and college students completed the Symptom Checklist 90 Revised (SCL-90R; Derogatis, 1983). Both of these psychological symptom scales were administered to allow for testing of the relations between interpersonal stresses and psychological symptoms.

One of the important questions that we were interested in with regard to interpersonal stresses was whether or not adolescents are affected by stressful events occurring in the lives of others in their social networks. Kessler and McLeod (1984) coined the term "network event" to describe events that might be experienced as stressful by the respondent but that have occurred to others, not to the respondent. Kessler and McLeod found that adult women both report more stress occurring in the lives of others than males, and show a greater relation than males between these network events and psychological symptoms. Kessler and McLeod speculated that adult women may be more emotionally involved and concerned with the needs of a wider range of people than men, and may provide more social support than men. Ultimately this involvement and support overload can be draining, leading to the development of psychological symptoms.

Stressful network events have not been previously investigated among adolescents, although there is some reason to speculate that adolescent females, like adult females, might be more subject to network events and their deleterious effects. Gilligan (1982) reported that throughout the adolescent period, girls' emphasis on their relationships and connections with others tends to evolve into an ethnic of responsibility for seeing to the needs of others; this might in fact place them at higher risk for experiencing distress associated with the stress of others. Further, Thorbecke and Grotevant (1982) reported a positive correlation between competitiveness and commitment to friendships among adolescent males, and a negative correlation between competitiveness and commitment to friendships among adolescent females. They interpreted these findings as indicating that separateness and autonomy are inherent to adolescent males' self-definition with regard to interpersonal relationships, while mutual concern may be central to relationships for adolescent females. Further, competitiveness may be potentially disruptive for girls' friendships. Again, this could help to explain why females may be more likely than males to respond with concern to the stress of others.

We analyzed the numbers of stressful interpersonal events reported on the APES by male and female adolescents in several event subcategories, including network events involving friends or family members (e.g., "Something bad happens to a friend"), family events (e.g., "Problems or arguments with parents, siblings, or family members"), peer events (e.g., "Friend moves away from you, or you move away from friend"), intimacy events (e.g., "Breaking up with or being rejected by a boyfriend or girlfriend"), and, as a contrast, stressful academic events, which are less interpersonal in content than the others (e.g., "Doing poorly on an exam or paper"). Family, peer, intimacy, and academic events all directly involved the respondent, while network events occurred in the lives of others but did not directly involve the respondent. The number of events reported in each of the event subcategories as a function of gender and age is shown in Table 1. Separate multivariate analyses of variance (MANOVAs) for each of the three samples were performed in order to test whether males or females reported more of any of the event subcategories. In each case, the multivariate dependent variable consisted of the number of negative events reported in five stressful event categories (network, intimacy, family, peer, and academic stresses). In

Table 1. Mean Number of Negative Events and Psychological Symptoms (Standard Deviations in Parentheses)

Variable	Junior High		High School		College	
	Males	Females	Males	Females	Males	Females
Negative events						
Network	2.16(2.06)	3.74(3.06)	1.54(2.06)	3.51(2.76)	2.49(1.99)	3.81(2.34)
Family	1.42(1.35)	2.80(1.97)	1.92(1.96)	2.81(2.21)	1.61(1.47)	1.86(1.45)
Intimacy	0.74(1.03)	1.60(1.26)	0.98(1.06)	1.42(1.21)	1.43(1.17)	1.51(1.24)
Peer	1.44(1.65)	2.26(2.04)	2.24(1.92)	3.03(2.06)	2.78(1.99)	3.27(1.76)
Academic	1.70(1.75)	2.04(1.77)	2.88(1.95)	2.96(1.80)	3.33(2.09)	3.31(1.82)
Total behavior problems (junior high) or global severity index						
	43.60(21.62)	52.28(22.38)	0.87(0.51)	1.17(0.58)	0.83(0.57)	0.98(0.49)

the junior high sample, the multivariate main effect for sex was significant, and univariate analyses revealed that females reported more of each of the interpersonal stresses—i.e., more negative network, intimacy, peer, and family events—but did not differ from males on academic events. In the senior high sample, there again was a main effect for sex, with females reporting more negative network and intimacy events than males. In the college sample, the multivariate main effect was not significant, although univariate tests indicated that females did report more negative network events than males.

Thus, with regard to reports of interpersonal stresses, the results were broadly consistent with prior findings. That is, adolescent females reported more negative interpersonal stresses than males. This suggests either that they experience more interpersonal stress than males, or that they are more willing to admit to the experience of interpersonal stress than males. Regarding the absence of significant findings in the college sample, there appears on Table 1 to be a tendency for college males to report more stresses than younger males (note particularly the increase in intimacy stress among college males in Table 1), and also a tendency for college females to report fewer family stresses than their younger counterparts. However, any comparisons across the three samples in this study are suggestive only, because there were variations from sample to sample in the APES events comprising the stress subcategories, and because there also were variations across samples in the measures used to assess psychological symptoms, in the sampling procedures, and in the socioeconomic status (SES) of the three samples (the junior high SES was lower than the high school SES, which in turn was lower than the college student sample SES).

The finding that females in all three samples reported more negative network events than males suggests that females much younger than those studied by Kessler and McLeod (1984) experience more stress than males in the lives of others. Adolescent females may be more sensitive to, or perhaps more aware of, the stresses and well-being of others than adolescent males. As Gilligan (1982) suggested, adolescent females' experience of network events may be rooted in their orientation to care for the needs of others. Further, adolescent females may be more dependent upon others for development of personal identity. Thus, stress within their social network is potentially a source of greater disruption to self-esteem.

Table 2 presents the correlations of each of the various event subcategories with psychological symptoms for the three samples of adolescents. SES was unrelated to either number of stressful events or psychological symptoms. The results indicate that each of the stress subcategories is related to psychological symptoms in the junior high and senior high

Table 2. Pearson Correlation Coefficients of Number of Negative Events with Psychological Symptoms

	Junior High (N = 93)	Senior High (N = 140)	College (N = 145)
1. Network events	.378	.312	.126[a]
2. Family events	.680	.276	.089[a]
3. Intimacy events	.475	.241	.137[a]
4. Peer events	.395	.402	.225
5. Academic events	.270	.248	.262

[a]Not significant at $p < .004$. An ordered Bonferroni procedure was used to control for Type I error rate.

samples, but in the college sample only academic and peer stresses were significantly related to psychological symptoms. Regression analyses in which psychological symptoms were regressed on the stressful event subcategories and sex indicated that there were no significant interactions between sex and stressful events in predicting psychological symptoms in any of the three samples. Thus, unlike the earlier noted report of Siddique and D'Arcy (1984), there was no evidence from these findings that the greater numbers of interpersonal stresses reported by females were taking their toll in the way of greater psychological symptoms.

There was also an interesting suggestion of a developmental patterning of the relations between interpersonal stresses and psychological symptoms. Stepwise regression analyses were performed, in which either the SCL-90R scores or the Youth Self-Report scores (as appropriate to the sample) were regressed on each of the stressful event subcategories. In the junior high sample, negative family events were entered first into the equation by the stepwise regression program, accounting for 46% of the variance in total behavior problems; negative intimacy events accounted for an additional 2% of the variance in the second step, and no further variance was accounted for by other stressors. In the high school sample, the regression program entered peer events in the equation first, accounting for 15.58% of the variance in SCL-90R scores; no other variables accounted for additional variance. In the college sample, only negative academic events entered into the equation, accounting for 6.23% of the variance. As a further test of this patterning, the unique predictive power of each of the event subcategories was examined by testing the significance of the percent of variance in psychological symptoms accounted for by each event subcategory when it was entered last in the regression equation, after controlling for each of the other stress subcategories (i.e., a test of the squared semipartial correlation). The results were consistent with the stepwise analyses; only negative family events in the junior high sample ($sr^2 = .20$), negative peer events in the high school sample ($sr^2 = .05$), and negative academic events in the college sample ($sr^2 = .04$) had unique predictive power.

These findings may be understood within a developmental framework. That is, as the adolescent matures, he or she becomes invested and concerned with occurrences in the peer network, and begins to separate somewhat from involvement in the family (Offer et al., 1981; Silverberg & Steinberg, 1987). As noted earlier, conformity and concerns about acceptance by the peer group seem to peak during mid-adolescence (Berndt, 1979), which may in part explain the magnitude of the association between peer stresses and psychological symptoms in the senior high sample. By older adolescence, dependency on the peer group has subsided. Not surprisingly, academic occurrences represented the domain of greatest psychological cost for those older adolescents attending college, as these students presumably are quite invested in academic achievement. It is striking that the correlation of negative family events with psychological symptoms was only .09 among the college students, and the correlation in the junior high sample was .68. This suggests a powerful disconnection from family stresses over the course of adolescence, perhaps culminating at the point when the adolescent is physically removed from the home. However, in light of the SES differences between samples, an alternative explanation is that family stresses are more related to psychological symptoms among lower SES families. A long-term longitudinal study of stress and symptoms would be necessary to better understand the developmental changes in the stress process during adolescence.

The Interpersonal Ramifications of Personal Stress

The studies reviewed above indicate that stressful events of an interpersonal nature have a strong association with adolescent maladjustment. However, to gain a more complete understanding of the interpersonal nature of stress and psychopathology during adolescence, an examination of the process of the transmission of the effects of stress from person to person needs to be considered. That is, the effects of personally relevant stressful events on others in an individual's social network must be examined. Events that occur to an adolescent may have an impact on family members and peers whether or not the events are perceived as stressful by the adolescent. Similarly, stressors encountered by parents, siblings, and peers may hold meaning for an adolescent even when these events do not directly involve the adolescent. However, the mechanisms through which stress is transmitted from others to the adolescent and from the adolescent to others may differ.

Consider, for example, a young adolescent who has encountered a number of school-related stressors, including classes or teachers that she does not like, hassles completing homework, and receiving poor grades. Because she is not strongly invested in succeeding academically, she does not experience any noticeable degree of emotional upset in response to these stressors. However, even though these events are not directly experienced by her parents, the events may have a direct relation to the distress of her parents because they hold particular meaning or significance for them. This would be especially true for parents who are highly invested in academic achievement and who hold high aspirations for their children's academic success. Minor school problems may imply the possibility of more major school difficulties for their daughter in the future, including continued poor grades and difficulties in being admitted to college. Events such as these may be a source of distress for parents independent of the adolescent's reaction to them. Stressful events in adolescents' lives may thus be *directly* related to others in their social networks, especially their parents.

The processes by which adolescents are affected by the stress of others may be somewhat different. Imagine that the parents of this same young adolescent both have experienced a number of recent job-related stressors. In her work, her mother has been struggling with a chronic poor relationship with her supervisor and frequently considers quitting her current job. Her father has been faced with economic stress at work, as his company has been hit with a slump in sales, resulting in lower pay raises and numerous layoffs of his co-workers. Unlike her parents, however, this young adolescent may not be directly affected by these stressors. Instead, the meaning of parents' stress may be communicated to their children through the distress and psychological symptoms that parents display. If mother or father display substantial increases in symptoms of depression, anxiety, hostility, or other forms of distress in association with the occurrence of these stressors, then the adolescent may infer that these events are a source of threat to the well being of her parents and potentially to the family as a whole. If, however, mother or father respond benignly to these stressors, their occurrence may not be perceived as a threat by the young adolescent. This may be particularly likely if the stressor is one with which the adolescent has little or no personal experience, such as work and financial-related stressors. This would suggest that adolescents may be *indirectly* affected by stress in the lives of family members and friends.

Studies that have examined the direct relations between adolescent stress and parents' psychological symptoms, and between parents' stress and adolescents' symptoms have produced mixed results (e.g., Cohen, Burt, & Bjork, 1987; Fergusson, Horwood, Gretton, & Shannon, 1985; Hammen, Adrian, Gordon, Burge, Jaenicke, & Hiroto, 1987; Holahan &

Moos, 1987; Thomson & Vaux, 1986). Holahan and Moos (1987) and Fergusson et al. (1985) found that major life events reported (experienced) by parents were significantly related to mothers' reports of their children's behavior problems. In contrast, Cohen et al. (1987) did not find significant relations between either maternal or paternal major life events and their young adolescent children's self-reports of depression, anxiety, or self-esteem. Thomson and Vaux (1986) found a significant relation between paternal major life events and their children's self-reports of "affective balance" but no relation between fathers' major life events and their children's self-reports of depression, nor between mothers' major life events and their children's self-reported depression or affective balance. Furthermore, Thomson and Vaux failed to find an association between parents' reports of daily stressors and their children's depression or affect. Adolescents' self-reported major and daily stressors were related to mothers' self-reports of depression and affective balance and to fathers' self-reports of affective balance. Finally, Hammen et al. (1987), in a study of mothers with unipolar depression, bipolar depression, medical disorders, or no medical or psychological disturbance, found that mothers' chronic stressful conditions (or strains) were associated with diagnoses of depression in their children, as well as with mothers' reports of their children's behavior problems and children's self-reports of depression.

The mixed findings of these studies suggest two things. First, as discussed above, the association between child or adolescent stress and parents' psychological symptoms may be direct, while there may not be a comparable direct link between parents' stress and adolescents' psychological symptoms. Second, the associations among parent and child stress and symptoms may be affected by the source of information for these variables. Specifically, parents' stressful events appear more closely associated to their children's maladjustment when parent reports are used to measure both variables (e.g., Fergusson et al., 1985; Holahan & Moos, 1987) than when they are assessed by different informants (e.g., Cohen et al., 1987).

To address these issues we assessed major and daily stressful events and psychological symptoms in a sample of young adolescents, their mothers, and their fathers (Compas, Howell, Phares, Williams, & Ledoux, 1989). In this study we utilized parents' and adolescents' self-reports of each of these variables and analyzed the families of adolescent boys and girls separately. Structural equation causal modeling (LISREL; Joreskog & Sorbom, 1986) was used to examine the relations of stress and psychological symptoms between parents' and their children and between spouses. As we hypothesized, there was not a direct path from parents' major or daily stressful events to emotional/behavioral problems reported by their young adolescent children. Partial support was found for the hypothesis that the effects of parents' stress would be mediated by their psychological symptoms. Specifically, there were significant paths from both fathers' and mothers' daily hassles to their own psychological symptoms. Further, fathers' but not mothers' psychological symptoms were related to their sons' and daughters' emotional/behavioral problems. That is, the effects of fathers' daily stress on their young adolescent children were mediated by the psychological symptoms that fathers experienced in association with these stressors. The absence of a similar effect for mothers' symptoms was unexpected. These findings suggest that fathers' symptoms may hold considerably greater emotional meaning for their young adolescent children than do symptoms of psychological distress experienced by their mothers. This pattern of findings is even more striking in light of the higher base rate of symptoms reported by mothers in this sample, indicating that fathers' symptoms may be more salient and have greater impact because they occur less often. An alternative explanation for this pattern is that fathers may exert greater influence on their young adolescent children because of imbalances in the power relationships of mothers and fathers in these families, with mothers' distress being discounted because of her lower status in the family. These possibilities warrant direct investigation in future research.

Because of the unexpected nature of the stronger association of fathers' as opposed to mothers' symptoms with their children's maladjustment, these findings warranted replication. We had an opportunity to examine the stability of the findings in follow-up data obtained on this sample nine months later. Using multiple regression analyses to examine risk factors for young adolescents emotional/behavioral problems, we found that fathers' but not mothers' psychological symptoms were predictive of young adolescents' self-reported maladjustment at both points in time (Compas, Howell, Phares, Williams, & Giunta, 1990). Additionally, fathers' daily stressors were predictive of adolescents' daily stressful events in the longitudinal analyses over 9 months. The replicability of these findings strengthens our confidence that the association between fathers' stress and the emotional distress of their young adolescent children is mediated by fathers' symptoms. Further, these findings underscore the importance of understanding the contribution of fathers as well as mothers to the psychological well being of their young adolescent children.

A very different picture emerged when mothers' reports of their children's emotional/behavioral problems were used as the criterion variable in these analyses (Compas et al., 1990). In the regression analyses at both points in time, mothers' but not fathers' psychological symptoms were related to mothers' reports of their children's maladjustment. Mothers' and fathers' daily hassles were related to their own and their spouses' psychological symptoms but neither parents' hassles were related to mothers' reports of their children's problems. Once again, adolescents' emotional distress was associated with parents' psychological symptoms but this time the significant relation involved mothers' rather than fathers' symptoms. However, as suggested above, the patterns of interpersonal associations of stress and symptoms are affected by which informants are used to measure these variables. These findings suggest that some of these associations may be affected by common method variance in the measures of parent and adolescent psychological symptoms, at least in the analyses predicting mothers' ratings of their children's symptoms. Although this issue warrants further attention, we believe that it is important to keep in mind that reports of adolescents' emotional/behavioral problems by mothers, fathers, and adolescents themselves represent different perspectives on these problems (Compas & Phares, 1991; Phares, Compas, & Howell, 1989). That is, parents and children have unique views of children's distress, and these views are affected by their definitions of mental health and maladjustment and their awareness of different problems. We believe it is important to identify the predictors of each of these perspectives on adolescent maladjustment, even if the patterns of predictors vary across different informants.

Turning to the question of the possible interpersonal effects of adolescents' stressful events on others in their social networks, we examined the paths from adolescents' daily stressors to their parents' psychological symptoms to determine whether there were direct effects of adolescents' stress on their parents that were not mediated by adolescents' symptoms (Compas et al., 1989). Significant paths were found from boys' daily stressors to their mothers' and fathers' symptoms and from girls' daily stressors to their mothers' (but not fathers') symptoms. These paths remained significant even after stressful events directly involving parents were excluded from the analyses. These findings are consistent with the hypothesis that parents may be able to infer meaning, and therefore be directly affected by, stressful events experienced by their young adolescent children. The notion that adults are more likely than adolescents to infer meaning directly from stressful events in others' lives was further supported by significant paths from fathers' daily stressors to mothers' psychological symptoms in families of both boys and girls and from mothers' daily stressors to fathers' psychological symptoms in families of boys.

We believe that the significance of these data lies in their implications for the importance of interpersonal processes in the transmission of stress and psychological symptoms in the lives of young adolescents. The findings clearly indicate that young adolescents are embedded in close relationships within the family, relationships that serve as conduits for stress and emotional distress between adolescents and their parents. The fact that the transmission of stress is more direct from adolescents to their parents than from parents to adolescents indicates that there may be important developmental changes that occur in ways in which stress is transmitted through social relationships. It seems likely that these processes may change during adolescence. Young adolescents may need the information that is supplied by parents' symptoms to understand the meaning of parents' stressful experiences. However, older adolescents may have sufficient experience with a wide variety of stress to directly respond to parents' stressful encounters. Thus, adolescence may be marked by changes in the *ways* that adolescents are affected by the stress of others, with younger adolescents being particularly vulnerable to their parents' psychological symptoms.

Toward a Model of the Intrapersonal and Interpersonal Processes in Psychosocial Stress

The research described above clearly reflects the two main points we wish to make. First, stressful events of an interpersonal nature have ramifications for the personal adjustment and functioning of adolescents. Second, personal events experienced by adolescents and others in their social networks (especially family members) have consequences that eminate to one another in these networks. Throughout this research, a stressful event was considered interpersonal in nature if either another person was involved in the stressful encounter or if the event occurred in the life of another person in the individual's social network. For example, in several of these studies items on inventories of adolescent stress (e.g., the Adolescent Perceived Events Scale; Compas et al., 1987) were analyzed as sources of interpersonal stress if they involved another (e.g., fights or arguments with a friend) or if they were an example of network stress (e.g., something bad happens to a friend). Alternatively, the interpersonal effects of stress were examined through the associations between stress or psychological symptoms reported by one individual and the symptoms reported by another.

These methods represent an important first step in examining psychosocial stress as an interpersonal process and in breaking away from the tradition in stress research of studying individuals' stress and associated symptoms in isolation from others in their social environment. However, we do not believe that these methods are adequate to completely capture the psychological processes that determine whether a stressful event is interpersonal in nature. When we label an event as an interpersonal stressor because it involved another person we are making an assumption about *why* the event was stressful for the individual. However, the reason that event was stressful may be embedded in a complex set of psychological processes that determine its meaning or functional significance. That is, it is the *psychological meaning* of the event that determines whether a stressor is interpersonal.

Cognitive and transactional models of stress and coping have emphasized the role of the perceived meaning of a stressful encounter in determining its impact on the well being of the individual (e.g., Lazarus & Folkman, 1984; Taylor, 1983). For example, the process of primary appraisal of the person–environment relationship is critical in determining whether a particular situation or event is experienced as stressful. Primary appraisals of stress are defined as those that involve perceptions of harm/loss, threat and challenge. In harm/loss appraisals, some damage of a physical or psychological nature to the person has already been sustained. Threat appraisals involve physical or psychological harms or losses that have not yet taken place but are anticipated. Challenge appraisals focus on encounters that involve the potential for growth or gain. However, the meaning of the stressful event that one has encountered is determined by the aspect of the individual's life that the event represents and what the individual has at stake in that domain (Lazarus & Folkman, 1984).

Clearly the environmental context in which an event occurs is one of the central factors in determining the meaning of the event. However, related work in cognitive evaluation theory (e.g., Deci & Ryan, 1985; 1987), self-system theory (e.g., Connell, (in press), and achievement motivation theory (e.g., Dweck & Elliott, 1983; Elliott & Dweck, 1988) suggests that the meaning of a stressful event is represented in the *goal* of the individual that has been threatened, challenged, or lost. That is, these theories assume that much or most behavior that is significant in an individual's life is motivated toward a goal. For example, within cognitive evaluation theory and self-system theory these goals include competence (personally being able to produce specific outcomes, both in the sense of achieving positive ends and avoiding negative outcomes), autonomy (the experience of choice in the initiation, maintenance, and regulation of behavior, and the experience of connectedness between one's action and personal goals and values), and relatedness (to feel securely connected to the social surround and to experience oneself as worthy and capable of love). These goals represent just a few of the domains in which stressful events may have their meaning. The goal of relatedness is most relevant to the present discussion. Stressful events that involve threats or challenges to or the loss of relatedness would be expected to hold particular interpersonal meaning for the adolescent. When the pursuit of these goals is blocked or threatened or the possibility of goal attainment has been lost, a person–environment relationship has been established that fits with Lazarus and Folkman's definition of stress, i.e., "a particular relationship between the person and the environment that is appraised by the person as taxing or exceeding his or her resources and endangering his or her well-being" (1984, p. 19).

The experience of stress results when an event that holds meaning with regard to a personal goal occurs in a domain in which the individual feels incompetent or a lack of efficacy (i.e., an area of personal vulnerability). We examined this model of vulnerability by testing the interaction between two sources of stress, interpersonal events and academic achievement events, and perceptions of personal competence in these two domains in a sample of young adolescents (Compas & Banez, 1989). Psychological symptoms were related to the combination of stressful events and perceived personal inadequacy, for example, high interpersonal stress and low perceived social competence. However, this study was limited in that events were classified into the two domains based on ratings by external judges about the meaning of the event. The interaction of types of events and personal vulnerabilities needs to be examined using alternative methods to determine the meaning of the stressful events.

Identification of the specific domain of one's life that is represented in a stressful encounter is a complex task. In some cases the meaning of an event is clear to the individual. For example, when a teenager loses his girlfriend to another he is likely to be acutely aware of the interpersonal significance of this event, including the loss of feelings of relatedness, feelings of security, and being worthy of love. Thus, the context of the event is highly salient in determining its meaning. However, there may also be other levels of meaning in the loss of a girlfriend, including a loss of social self-esteem or competence in the eyes of others in the peer group. It may be possible to directly ask individuals about the meaning of stressful events, focusing on the goals that they feel have been threatened, challenged, or lost. However, the meaning or significance of a stressful encounter may not be directly within the awareness of the individual (cf. Nisbett & Ross, 1980, for an extensive discussion of levels of awareness of cognitive processes). In these instances additional information about the meaning of an event may be gained from observations or self-reports of the individual's responses to the event.

Understanding the meaning of a stressful event could involve inferences made from coping strategies used to deal with the event. For example, failure on an exam in school may appear to be an event pertaining to academic achievement. It may be stressful because the event represents a threat to the adolescent's goals of learning or performance. However, academic failure may also be stressful because it creates conflict and tension in the adolescent's relationship with her or his parents. For example, if the adolescent has failed to meet his or her parents' achievement expectations, this may result in an angry rebuke from the parents, punishment, and ensuing conflict or disengagement between the adolescent and parents. The greatest significance and meaning of the event may lie in the disrupted interpersonal relationships (i.e., harm to the goal of relatedness) rather than the failure in the achievement domain. Thus, an event that appears to be in the domain of achievement or competence may in fact be stressful because of its interpersonal meaning.

Similar processes may be involved in inferring meaning in stressful events in the lives of others. We are currently pursuing this possibility by examining the ways in which children and adolescents cope with their parents' cancer. For example, when a parent has been diagnosed with cancer, this event may hold meaning for an adolescent or child in one or more of several different domains. At the most basic level it presents the threat of an interpersonal loss of enormous magnitude, particularly if the cancer is life threatening. However, parental cancer may also threaten a child or adolescent's competence because it places a number of new demands on the child to fill roles and tasks previously fulfilled by the ill parent. For example, the ill parent may be unable to fulfill many of the roles and duties that she or he previously performed in the daily functioning of the family. Alternatively, the spouse may be unable to maintain his or her typical role because of increased demands to take care of the ill parent.

Preliminary examination of responses to our structured interviews with cancer patients, their spouses, and their children administered four times over the course of a year from the time of the diagnosis has provided examples of the range of possible meanings of cancer as a stressor for families. A portion of the interview asks the respondent to report how she or he has been coping with the illness and its treatment. One adolescent reported that she and her father had sent flowers to her mother in the hospital so that "she won't forget about me." This response poignantly reflects the threat that the cancer poses to this girl's sense of relatedness with her mother, highlighting the interpersonal nature of the stress. In contrast, a boy indicated that he coped with his mother's cancer by trying to be more helpful with work around the house. Although this has a strong interpersonal element in that it involves the provision of interpersonal support to his mother, it also reflects the new challenges to this boy's competence that his mother's illness may present. He may now need to carry out a number of new and difficult duties involving cooking of meals, cleaning, or caring for younger siblings that require the development of new skills and competencies. Thus, his mothers' illness may be stressful because it also presents challenge to his competence.

In summary, we believe that a more complete understanding of the nature and effects of interpersonal stress during adolescence will result from the use of alternative methods to identify stressors that hold interpersonal meaning for adolescents and others in their social networks. The context of the stressful event and the psychological processes involved in generating and inferring the meaning of a stressful encounter need to be assessed using a variety of methods and should not be limited to the classifications of events solely on the basis of who or what was involved in encounter. In this way, models of psychosocial stress that have emphasized intrapersonal factors and the cognitive appraisal processes of the individual can enrich and be enriched by our understanding of the social and interpersonal nature of stress.

Acknowledgments

Preparation of this chapter was supported by National Institute of Mental Health Grant MH43819, and by an NIMH Training Grant to the Consortium on Family Process and Psychopathology, T32-MHI8626.

References

Achenbach, T.M., & Edelbrock, C. (1987). *Manual for the Youth Self Report Profile.* Burlington, VT: Department of Psychiatry, University of Vermont.
Berndt, T.J. (1979). Developmental changes in conformity to peers and parents. *Developmental Psychology, 15,* 608–616.
Burke, R.J., & Weir, T. (1978). Sex differences in adolescent life stress, social support, and well being. *Journal of Psychology, 98,* 277–288.
Cohen, L.H., Burt, C.E., & Bjork, J.P. (1987). Effects of life events experienced by young adolescents and their parents. *Developmental Psychology, 23,* 583–592.
Connell, J.P. (in press). Context, self and action: A motivational analysis of self-system processes across the life-span. In D. Cicchetti (Ed.), *The self in transition: Infancy to childhood.* Chicago: University of Chicago Press. In press.
Compas, B.E. (1987). Stress and life events during childhood and adolescence. *Clinical Psychology Review, 7,* 275–302.
Compas, B.E. & Banez, G.A. (1990). *Perceived competence as a source of vulnerability and resistance to stress in young adolescents.* Unpublished manuscript, University of Vermont.
Compas, B.E., Davis, G.E., Forsythe, C.J., & Wagner, B.M. (1987). Assessment of major and daily stressful events during adolescence: The Adolescent Perceived Events Scale. *Journal of Consulting and Clinical Psychology, 55,* 534–541.
Compas, B.E., Howell, D.C., Phares, V., Williams, R.A., & Giunta, C.T. (1990). Risk factors for emotional/behavioral problems in young adolescents: A prospective analysis of adolescent and parental stress and symptoms. *Journal of Consulting and Clinical Psychology, 57,* 732–740.

Compas, B.E., Howell, D.C., Phares, V., Williams, R.A., & Ledoux, N. (1989). Parent and child stress and symptoms: An integrative analysis. *Developmental Psychology, 25,* 550–559.

Compas, B.E., & Phares, V. (1991). Stress during childhood and adolescence: Sources of risk and vulnerability. In E.M. Cummings, A.L., Greene, & K.H. Karraker (Eds.), *Life-span developmental psychology: Perspectives on stress and coping.* Hillsdale, NJ: Erlbaum. In press.

Compas, B.E., Slavin, L.A., Wagner, B.M., & Vannatta, K. (1986). Relationship of life events and social support with psychological dysfunction among adolescents. *Journal of Youth and Adolescence, 15,* 205–211.

Deci, E.L., & Ryan, R.M. (1985). *Intrinsic motivation and self-determination in human behavior.* New York: Plenum.

Deci, E.L., & Ryan, R.M. (1987). The support of autonomy and the control of behavior. *Journal of Personality and Social Psychology, 53,* 1024–1037.

Derogatis, L.R. (1983). *SCL-90R Administration, scoring and procedures manual* (2nd ed.). Towson, MD: Clinical Psychometrics Research.

Dweck, C.S., & Elliott, E.S. (1983). Achievement motivation. In E.M. Hetherington (Ed.), *Socialization, personality, and social development* (pp. 643–691). New York: John Wiley.

Elliott, E.S., & Dweck, C.S. (1988). Goals: An approach to motivation and achievement. *Journal of Personality and Social Psychology, 54,* 5–12.

Fergusson, D.M., Horwood, L.J., Gretton, M.E., & Shannon, F.T. (1985). Family life events, maternal depression, and maternal and teacher descriptions of child behavior. *Pediatrics, 75,* 30–35.

Gilligan, C. (1982). *In a different voice.* Cambridge, MA: Harvard University Press.

Grotevant, H.D., & Cooper, C.R. (1985). Patterns of interaction in family relationships and the development of identity exploration in adolescence. *Child Development, 56,* 415–428.

Hammen, C., Adrian, C., Gordon, D., Burge, D., Jaenicke, C., & Hiroto, D. (1987). Children of depressed mothers: Maternal strain and symptom predictors of dysfunction. *Journal of Abnormal Psychology, 96,* 190–198.

Holohan, C.J., & Moos, R.H. (1987). Risk, resistance, and psychological distress: A longitudinal analysis with adults and children. *Journal of Abnormal Psychology, 96,* 3–13.

Hauser, S.T., Powers, S., Noam, G., Jacobson, A.M., Weiss, B., & Follansbee, D.J. (1984). Familial contexts of adolescent ego development. *Child Development, 55,* 195–213.

Johnson, J.E. (1986). *Stressful life events in children and adolescents.* Beverly Hills, CA: Sage.

Joreskog, K.G., & Sorbom, D. (1986). *LISREL VI: Analysis of linear structural relationships by maximum likelihood, instrumental variables, and least squared methods* (4th ed.). Mooresville, IN: Scientific Software.

Kessler, R.C., & McLeod, J.D. (1984). Sex differences in vulnerability to undesirable life events. *American Sociological Review, 49,* 620–631.

Lazarus, R.S., & Folkman, S. (1984). *Stress, appraisal and coping.* New York: Springer.

Montemayor, R. (1983). Parents and adolescents in conflict: All families some of the time and some families most of the time. *Journal of Early Adolescence, 3,* 83–103.

Nisbett, R., & Ross, L. (1980). *Human inference: Strategies and shortcomings of social judgment.* Englewood Cliffs, NJ: Prentice-Hall.

Offer, D., Ostrov, E., & Howard, K. (1981). *The adolescent: A psychological self-portrait.* New York: Basic Books.

Phares, V., Compas, B.E., & Howell, D.C. (1989). Perspectives on child behavior problems: Comparisons of children's self-reports with parent and teacher reports. *Psychological Assessment: A Journal of Consulting and Clinical Psychology, 1,* 68–71.

Rutter, M. (1983). Stress, coping, and development: Some issues and some questions. In N. Garmezy & M. Rutter (Eds.), *Stress, coping, and development in children.* New York: McGraw-Hill.

Selman, R.L. (1980). *The growth of interpersonal understanding.* New York: Academic Press.

Siddique, C.M., & D'Arcy, C. (1984). Adolescence, stress, and psychological well-being. *Journal of Youth and Adolescence, 13,* 459–473.

Silverberg, S.B., & Steinberg, L. (1987). Adolescent autonomy, parent-adolescent conflict, and parental well being. *Journal of Youth and Adolescence, 16,* 293–312.

Taylor, S.E. (1983). Adjustment to threatening events: A theory of cognitive adaptation. *American Psychologist, 38,* 161–1173.

Thomson, B., & Vaux, A. (1986). The importation, transmission, and moderation of stress in the family system. *American Journal of Community Psychology, 14,* 39–57.

Thorbecke, W., & Grotevant, H.D. (1982). Gender differences in adolescent interpersonal identity formation. *Journal of Youth and Adolescence, 11,* 479–492.

Wagner, B.M., & Compas, B.E. (1990). Gender, instrumentality, and expressivity: Moderators of the relation between stress and psychological symptoms during adolescence. *American Journal of Community Psychology, 18,* 383–406.

White, K.M., Speisman, J.C., & Costos, D. (1983). Young adults and their parents: Individuation to mutuality. In H.D. Grotevant & C.R. Cooper (Eds.), *Adolescent development in the family: New directions for child development.* (pp. 61–76). San Francisco: Jossey-Bass.

Youniss, J. (1980). *Parents and peers in social development: A Sullivan-Piaget perspective.* Chicago: University of Chicago Press.

II

Editors' Overview

Sources of Variation in Stress and Stress Responses

These next three papers also advance models for understanding adaptation, distress, and disorder, but as a distinct grouping are nicely illustrative of the theme of variation. How much do the stresses of development and other life problems affect adolescent mental health? Students of this literature know that the answer to this question requires attention to interactive models, such as those we present in Chapter 1, that consider the cumulative effects of a number of relevant variables. Because the effects of particular stresses or clusters of stresses are usually contingent on other situational or personal characteristics, including distal and recent developmental experiences, a focus on configurations of variables that produce excess harm versus configurations that are beneficial, allows us to identify groups of adolescents who are at-risk. In this section, we examine in greater depth the individual and social characteristics as well as developmental trajectories that must be considered to generate a more fine-tuned understanding of youth at-risk in normal populations.

Research on adolescent stress, development and mental health has been strongly guided by an emphasis on the person-situation interaction as the key determinant of variation in behavioral and health outcomes. This person–situation dynamic has long been the basis for behavioral science attention to problems of adaptation (Lewin, 1951; Bronfenbrenner, 1979) and the most recent application of this perspective is in etiologic models of risk and resilience. On the surface, at least, risk and protective factors are easily differentiated: the former are seen as capable of bringing about health changes in and of themselves, while the latter are seen to act in conjunction with risk factors, exacerbating the health effects of stress for some individuals and protecting the health of others. In addition, as Petersen, Kennedy and Sullivan note in their paper, risk factors are usually understood to be social contextual variables, such as socioeconomic status. In contrast, protective factors are often considered to be intrapsychic qualities, such as self esteem and coping styles. While this is a well recognized model, due in large part to research on the resilience of "competent" youth who successfully avoid the ill effects of environmental disadvantage (Garmezy, 1974; Rutter, 1981; Werner & Smith, 1972), we must keep in mind that there is more than one way to model these complex processes of risk and resilience. For example, in some research studies, risk factors are biological processes—like pubertal change—which operate at the individual level rather than as social structural or contextual characteristics. In addition, some contextual risk factors, such as having a mentally ill parent, may operate as a risk through genetic means, so that the mechanism of transmission is in fact at the intra-individual level. Finally, some personality variables have been studied as risk factors, such as locus of control and Type A personality.

Protective factors, similarly, may include both contextual and intra-individual characteristics. In the paper by Dornbusch, Mont-Reynaud, Ritter, Chen and Steinberg in this section, differential sensitivity to stressful life events is examined for sex, ethnicity, family structure and age groups. This type of approach reflects a sociological perspective on the stress-mental health relationship in which even gender and age are regarded as social structural variables, rather than biological statuses. Their focus on family type, socioeconomic status, and ethnicity as vulnerability factors (also known as protective/moderating or stress-buffering factors) is of particular interest, since in some studies these statuses are modeled as risk factors.

Thus, while the currently popular research focus on the stress-moderating role of coping styles or predispositions would suggest that protective processes be seen as intra-individual resources, it is also significant to envision the protective functions and resources available through certain life contexts. In addition, understanding coping resources more broadly as including both intra-individual variables and interpersonal transactions in institutional context fosters consideration of issues such as how social support and self esteem are dynamically interrelated in development, as coping variables in the face of stress, and as foci for intervention and social change.

With this introduction to the complexities of studying variation in health responses to developmental transitions and other life stresses, we now turn to some of the issues addressed in these papers.

There is no doubt that the major focus in research on vulnerability and resistance to the effects of stress has been on gender differences. Here is an example of a significant body of empirical research that has been carefully guided by strong theoretical work. This literature is much too extensive to review, but we can note three major questions that have been important issues in research on adolescent stress and mental health. First, can we locate the point in time during adolescence at which the preponderance of psychological distress among females first occurs? This is an important question in research on the social causation of distress, as research on both adult and adolescent populations points to significant gender-linked socialization processes at this time in life that shape self esteem, coping responses to stress, and mental health related attributional processes, all of which are carried into adult life and influence adult mental health.

The second and third problems are interrelated and often difficult to disentangle. The second concerns whether there are sex differences in exposure to stress. In the literature on adolescent development, this is often asked with regard to the stress of pubertal change and development. We know that both boys and girls are exposed to pubertal development, but are the stressors associated with these biological changes identical? In life events research on adolescents, the problem appears simplified through use of the events inventories, such as the one Dornbusch and associates use in their analysis. Are the same kinds of problems reported by boys and girls to the same degree? The third issue is the question of differential vulnerability to the mental health and behavioral effects of stress. Specifically, this means that when exposed to identical stresses, the impact on boys' and girls' mental health may be similar, or one sex may be more reactive, that is, responding more negatively to stresses.

* * * *

The three papers in this section show distinct but compatible approaches to these general issues. The paper by Petersen and associates uses a longitudinal data set that they have meticulously built over the years. Even among longitudinal data it is striking for its inclusion of both early and later adolescent years, which is an essential feature for consideration of trajectories of mental health and behavior, and for examining the issue of sex differences noted above. Petersen and associates report several key findings on the issue of gender differences. First, by the twelfth grade follow-up, the gender difference in negative affect is the greatest. Although they are not as yet able to pinpoint the reasons for this increasing negative affect among girls, three other findings are especially relevant. First, while for boys childhood and early adolescent depression is a significant predictor of twelfth grade symptoms, this is not true for girls. This gives support to the notion that critical mental health related processes are set in motion for girls during the post-pubertal adolescent years, while for boys behavior is more appropriately seen as a continuation of patterns established in childhood. Second, Petersen and associates also document greater fluctuations in the coping repertoires of girls than boys, suggesting greater difficulty for girls in finding a successful problem solving style, which might be implicated in the increases in negative affect observed in girls. Finally, Petersen and associates report that girls whose puberty preceded the move to secondary school are more distressed than later-developing girls by the time they reach the twelfth grade. These data show the long term impact of pubertal timing, and suggest the need for better understanding of the social and psychological processes that link pubertal timing and school change with girls' higher risk for poor self image and more depressed affect later in their developmental trajectory. Here we should point out that pubertal and school changes are major developmental stressors, and what we are observing is either a sex difference in the secondary stressors associated with these events (the problem of exposure) or differences in vulnerability to these stresses, an issue which Petersen and associates should be able to address in future analyses.

The approach taken by Dornbusch and colleagues presents an interesting contrast in that similar conceptual issues are examined in a large scale cross-sectional data set. Here it is difficult to detect changes in psychological status associated with changing developmental status, as the influence of age is estimated through across-individual analyses. However, the heterogeneous sample and large number of health outcomes are an asset for both internal validity and generalizability, and these are the trade-offs that are usual in research on adolescent stress and mental health. These authors pursue three important questions in the study of adolescent stress: first, whether recent personal, familial and school-related stressors affect several indicators of mental health and functioning; second, whether these stress effects, which are highly significant, should be understood as mediating the impact of macrosocial influences; and third, whether certain subgroups are more vulnerable to the effects of stress than others. As in other studies, these authors also find that the girls are more psychologically distressed in the face of high levels of stress than the boys. However, this pattern does not hold across the other dependent variables, suggesting the vulnerability is limited to the psychological distress arena. In other words, the girls are not more vulnerable to more deviant behaviors and poorer grades in the face of stress. Finally, it is interesting that in the Dornbusch et al. data the girls report experiencing more stressful life events than the boys, and for both boys and girls personal stressors were more significant health influences than family stressors, with school stressors being the least influential. In other data sets as well, family stressors are not found to be as virulent as one would think, and this must be interpreted in developmental context. As Larson and Asmussen discussed in their chapter in Part I, peer and cross-sex relationships come to dominate the everyday thinking of these youth and are a major influence of mood.

In the final paper in this section Brooks-Gunn reviews the research on the stressfulness of adolescence for girls, focusing on the independent and joint effects of pubertal and social changes on mood and affect. This is a fitting conclusion to the discussion of inter-individual differences in stress responses because it so well illustrates our earlier point that the study of girls at puberty is a conceptually and empirically rich field. We see the wealth of existing data demonstrating the interaction of physical, social and psychological events and processes, and Brooks-Gunn brings up to date this research agenda. Here, it is important to note that Brooks-Gunn regards pubertal change as more than physical change. Rather, "puberty acts as a social stimulus for others [and for the girl herself], altering how adults and peers respond to the girl as her body develops" (p. 137). Thus, Brooks-Gunn does not conceptualize pubertal change as a discrete physical event that interacts with other social events, which is one understanding of an interactive model. Rather, in most of the research reviewed here she seeks to address how the timing and effects of these changes are mediated through social contexts. (In this regard, we refer the reader back to our Figures 1 and 2 in Chapter 1 in which we illustrate mediating and moderating processes.) This point is best exemplified in her research on the social factors that condition pubertal timing effects. Brooks-Gunn's work shows quite strikingly that early, and even on-time pubertal development, is especially stressful for girls who are training to be elite dancers as these changes mark the loss of the lean body required for success in this career. She also hypothesizes that one source of parent-child conflict (especially mother-daughter conflict) during the adolescent transition may be the pubertal changes that underlie self-definitional changes. For example, she reports on research showing girls' sense that their mothers and fathers are insensitive to their feelings about their body changes. Thus, there are many possible linkages between pubertal change, mood, and characteristic interpersonal problems during the adolescent transition.

A final issue that is brought into focus in contrasting the findings of Brooks-Gunn with those of Petersen and associates, concerns whether depressive symptoms are greater during the early or later adolescent years. Interestingly, Brooks-Gunn reports higher rates of stressful events and depressed mood during early adolescence, age 13–14, while Petersen and associates, in contrasting eighth and twelfth grade assessments of the same children, find more depressive affect for both boys and girls in the twelfth grade and a larger sex difference at that time. Even longitudinal data sets such as these differ greatly in instrumentation, and the ages of children assessed. Thus, it is impossible to definitively characterize the developmental trajectory of depressive affect through the adolescent years. Differences such as these should encourage collection of new and still better data to answer important questions about the mental health of boys and girls from childhood through adolescence and to early adulthood.

References

Bronfenbrenner, U. (1979). *The ecology of human development: Historical and contemporary variation*. Cambridge, MA: Harvard University Press.

Garmezy, N. (1974). The study of competence in children at risk for severe psychopathology. In E. Anthony and C. Koupernick (Eds.), *The child in his family. Vol 3: Children at psychiatric risk*. New York: Wiley.

Lewin, K. (1951). *Field theory in social science*. New York: Harper.

Rutter, M. (1981). Stress, coping and development: Some issues and some questions. *Journal of Child Psychology and Psychiatry, 22*, 323–356.

Werner, E.E., & Smith, R.S. (1982). *Vulnerable but invincible: A study of resilient children*. New York: McGraw-Hill.

5

Coping with Adolescence

Anne C. Petersen, Robert E. Kennedy, and Patricia Sullivan

Adolescence is a period of the life course involving extensive change. For some young people these changes stimulate further growth. For others, the changes may be overwhelming and lead to developmental decline or problems. This period of life, then, is an excellent one for studying stress and its consequences.

In this chapter, we present a model for understanding stress and its effects on adolescence. Normative developmental stresses and responses to them play a major role in adolescence (Petersen, 1987), and constitute the primary focus of this chapter. Stressful life events (Thoits, 1986) as well as daily strains and hassles (e.g., Compas, 1987a; Folkman & Lazarus, 1986) may also have particular impact in adolescence, but will receive less attention in this chapter.

Our theoretical perspective assumes that it is important to consider biopsychosocial development occurring in major social contexts over the life span (Petersen, 1980). Biological, psychological, and social development interact in significant ways over the course of life. In addition, the nature of key contexts such as the family has been shown to influence development, with different salience at various life stages. Finally, development at any single phase is affected by what has come before and what will be required in the next phase of life.

Emerging ideas about developmental psychopathology are essential to conceptualizations of stress and coping in adolescence (e.g., Garmezy & Rutter, 1983). Garmezy's (1984) concepts of risk and protective factors

integrate consideration of contextual influences with individual characteristics and behavior patterns. Ebata, Petersen, and Conger (1990) have
noted that most of the risk factors that have been identified are contextual
whereas protective factors are more likely to be individual. We could
argue that the risks of adolescence—the stresses—emerge primarily from
key contexts and situations of the developing individual. Successfully
traversing the risks, or stresses, of the adolescent decade could be attributed largely to the effectiveness of the individual's capacity to cope
with these risks or stresses—his or her protective factors. We return to
these concepts toward the end of this chapter.

It is interesting to observe that at least some of the changes of
adolescence have always existed. Why then do these changes seem to be
especially problematic today? There can be no doubt that the complexity
and even risk associated with the opportunities available to and choices
required of youth represents a marked change from the past. Both drugs
and sex, for example, are readily available to most young people in the
present times. With regard to these challenges, we think it important to
emphasize that there is little societal understanding and support for
adolescents during this time in life. The popular stereotypes of adolescents in the United States are quite negative, as a recent study found
(Signorielli, 1987). Examples can be found in the print media, especially
cartoons, in which adolescents are depicted as messy, rude, and moody.
These negative views not only reflect current beliefs but also may affect
adolescents' self-perceptions and behavior in negative ways. Whether
the stereotypes have such effects remains an empirical question that
could be addressed through cross-national comparison or historical
analysis.

At the same time, there has been a dramatic decrease in social cere-
monies noting change in status. There is some evidence that the celebration of transitions can ease adaptation to newly acquired status (Richards
& Petersen, 1987). In the United States, most of the transitions during
childhood and adolescence are seldom celebrated. The major exception is
probably the celebration linked with religious maturity, especially within
the Jewish faith. Rites of passage linked with puberty are virtually
nonexistent in modern society and even former adolescent transitions
such as "sweet sixteen" parties are less frequent. Simply acknowledging
that a transition has taken or will take place would seem to alleviate a
significant part of the confusion and uncertainty experienced by the
young person. In addition, these celebrations are often accompanied by
advice and occasionally real education or training. Given that adolescence
is hard work, we might do well to consider at least acknowledging, if not
celebrating, the growth required of our young people. Further research
on the effects of such celebrations would also be useful.

Stress in Adolescence

A decade ago, when we began our research to test the hypothesis that the emergence of sex differences in mental health was related to puberty, there had been little work in this area. For example, Lipsitz's review of research and programs for young adolescents was titled *Growing Up Forgotten* (Lipsitz, 1977), to dramatize the neglect of research and programs for this age group. Lipsitz also noted that there had been almost no research on girls. Our hypotheses, therefore, were necessarily quite speculative.

The explosion of research on adolescence over the past decade together with increased theorizing and model development have greatly enhanced the entire field, including our own perspectives on the topic (e.g., Petersen, 1988). What we have learned over the past decade is that our initial hypotheses were overly simplistic and occasionally wrong. As we will elaborate, puberty does not appear to operate in a simple, direct way but rather is only one of a large number of changes that affect adolescent development and mental health (e.g., Crockett & Petersen, 1987; Petersen, 1987; Petersen & Crockett, 1985). The pattern of our results has led us to consider the broader issue of developmental transition (e.g., Petersen, 1987; Petersen & Ebata, 1987).

Before turning to a discussion of developmental transitions, we would like to briefly introduce the long-term study that has stimulated and tested much of our thinking over the past decade. This study involves a cohort sequential longitudinal design in which 335 youngsters were sampled randomly from two middle to upper-middle class suburban Midwest school districts (Petersen, 1984). Adolescents were interviewed and tested twice annually from grades 6–8, with interview and test follow-up in grade 12 and 4 years later. Parents were also interviewed and tested when the adolescents were in grades 6, 8, and 12.

Developmental Transitions

Developmental transitions have been conceptualized as those times in life involving significant change, often in both biological and social spheres (e.g., Emde & Harmon, 1984). Examples of developmental transitions include the entry into school in childhood, the transition from childhood to adolescence, and the transition from middle to older adulthood, typically linked with retirement. Each of these sample transitions can be linked to biological changes, with puberty the most dramatic. In addition, developmental transitions are often linked to social role transitions such as the transition to parenthood. The identification of factors that facilitate "more or less successful negotiation of such transitions, that maintain vulnerabilities or protect against them at such periods" (Maughan & Champion, 1988) represents a major focus of research on these important life periods.

A developmental transition, then, involves changes in roles and expectations that are likely to affect self-perceptions. Expectations are, of course, linked to the particular sociocultural context. Therefore, the flavor of a developmental transition for a particular individual may vary significantly from one culture or one cohort to the next. Becoming pubertal, or becoming a parent, may have entirely different meaning from one society to the next, or even from subgroup to subgroup within a society. Such variation will dramatically affect the nature of expectations and the effect of the transition on the individual.

The concept of developmental transition seems particularly well suited to the period of life called adolescence. Adolescence may be thought of as involving two key developmental transitions: from childhood to adolescence and from adolescence to adulthood. If we think of adolescence as involving the second decade of life, the transition into adolescence takes place around age 10 years, with individual variation linked to the timing of puberty. The transition to adulthood occurs about a decade later, around age 20 years, with the greater individual variation in the timing of this transition linked to entry into adult work and family roles.

Childhood to Adolescence: A Developmental Model
of Early Adolescence

The developmental transition from childhood to adolescence, often called early adolescence, may be characterized by tremendous change. Indeed, Hamburg, who first called our attention to this transition as a critical life period (1974), compared the early adolescent transition to entering a lottery, especially from the perspective of youngsters experiencing this transition. Young adolescents know that most everything will be changing and yet they have no idea how it will all turn out. The sense of chance and risk pervades the period and may create anxiety.

All this change is typically stressful, yet not all young adolescents respond to the changes in negative ways (Petersen, Susman, & Beard, 1988). Indeed, because of the variation in responses to changes in adolescence, we have come to refer to them as "challenges" rather than "stresses" to avoid the negative connotation often inferred from the term "stress." To some young adolescents, the changes of this period represent opportunities that they find stimulating and to which they respond with further positive growth. Other adolescents may find all this change overwhelming and be unable to cope. To provide some idea

Table 1. Developmental Changes of Early Adolescence

Puberty	Adult appearance and size
	Reproductive capacity
	Timing (especially if offtime)
	Internal endocrine changes
	Asynchrony (among body parts, among adolescents)
Cognition	Capacity for abstract thought
Peer Groups	Conformity
	Pressure to try new experiences
School	Changing school structure and format
Parents	Parental responses to adult size of adolescent
	Sexual stimulation of newly pubertal child
	Implications for parent's aging
	Impending separation
Society	Hopes and expectations for youth
	Occupational choices and opportunities

of the extent of changes that occur during early adolescence, Table 1 lists some individual changes in biology, cognition, and psychology as well as social changes within the peer group, family, and broader society (Petersen & Spiga, 1982). We could add even more changes to this list. Indeed, there is change in every aspect of individual development and in every important social context in early adolescence (Petersen, 1987).

A model for investigating the effects of the developmental transition in early adolescence is shown in Figure 1. This model is based on our results, and those of others (Petersen & Ebata, 1987). The model considers the timing, nature, and number of changes. It also proposes that parent or peer support might buffer any negative effects of challenge. In addition, we hypothesize that the adolescent's particular coping responses may serve as a buffer, or perhaps as an enhancer of negative effects of challenge during early adolescence. Finally, prior development is important as well; those who come into the transition already vulnerable are likely to have more difficulty with this period.

Following the theoretical model proposed by John Coleman (1978), we considered the effects of *simultaneous change* compared to *sequential change* in early adolescence. Coleman's model for ideal development involves mastering one developmental task or challenge at a time. Our results support Coleman's inference that simultaneous changes are related to more negative outcomes than changes that are sequential. Two changes that may be simultaneous or sequential in early adolescence are puberty and the movement from an elementary to secondary school format. We find, for example, that those who are pubertal prior to or at about the same time as they move from elementary to secondary school have more negative outcomes in early adolescence than those whose

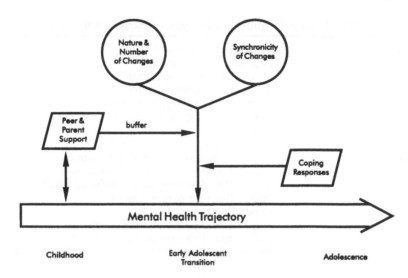

Figure 1. Model of developmental transition in early adolescence. (Reproduced from Petersen and Ebata, 1987, with permission.)

pubertal change occurs after the transition into junior high school (Petersen & Ebata, 1986).

We also hypothesized that particular kinds of changes, typically called stressful life events (Pearlin, Lieberman, Menaghan, & Mullan, 1981), are especially problematic for young adolescents. For example, the loss of a parent, either through death or divorce, is likely to be related to negative outcomes for most youngsters. The loss of a parent not only represents the loss of a loved one but also removes from the life of the young adolescent a potential source of support during this challenging time. To our knowledge, these hypotheses about stronger effects of stressful life events in early adolescence (or transitional periods more generally) and about the reasons for effects have not yet been tested but would be quite interesting to examine. The existing research suggests that the processes related to stressful life events are similar for children and adults but that the effects are weaker for children (Compas, 1987b; Haggerty, 1980; Rutter, 1983). Thus, it is possible that in childhood, any transition effects are dampened relative to possible effects at older ages.

The sheer number of developmental changes is also important to consider. Simmons and colleagues (1987) found, for example, that those youngsters who experienced several changes in early adolescence did more poorly in terms of school achievement and self-esteem. In their study, the absolute number of changes was directly related to negative outcomes.

Two resources were hypothesized to moderate or buffer change: social support and internal coping resources. Social support is a concept that has received a great deal of attention in the research on stressful life events and their effects on mental health among adults (e.g., Kessler, Price, & Wortman, 1985; Thoits, 1986). Although there is accumulating evidence that parent support is important for adolescent mental health (e.g., Sarigiani & Petersen, 1989), less is known about the role of peers at this age. Therefore, we thought it would be important to examine both parent and peer support.

A second kind of resource that could moderate effects of stressful changes or challenges is that of internal coping resources. These internal resources, usually described as coping style (e.g., Lazarus & Folkman, 1984; Nolen-Hoeksema, 1987), have been linked to both the onset and amelioration of depression in adults. Nolen-Hoeksema's theory is particularly relevant for the study of adolescence because it links coping style to sex role socialization, a process thought to change during adolescence with "gender intensification" of appropriate behavior (e.g., Crockett, Camarena, Petersen, & Graber, 1990; Hill & Lynch, 1983). Nolen-Hoeksema argues that "men are more likely to engage in distracting behaviors that dampen their mood when depressed, but women are more likely to amplify their moods by ruminating about their depressed states and the possible causes of these states" (p. 259). The existing literature on adolescent coping styles suggests that the sex-typed adult coping patterns may begin in adolescence (e.g., Cramer, 1979; Newcomb, Huba, & Bentler, 1986; Siddique & D'Arcy, 1984).

Adolescence to Adulthood: Late Adolescence and Young Adulthood

Although we are just now in the process of studying the transition from adolescence to adulthood, we believe that this developmental transition is also full of challenge (e.g., Maughan & Champion, 1988). This period of life is often termed late adolescence or sometimes young adulthood, depending on the particular constructs of interest to the investigator. From our perspective, this developmental transition takes place with the transition into adult family and work roles. This usually occurs at the completion of schooling, although there are instances where the transition into family roles is simultaneous with continued schooling, as is the case with some adolescent pregnancies. Similarly, some young people continue schooling while beginning the work role.

We may hypothesize that the nature of the developmental transition from adolescence to adulthood is conditioned both by the opportunities available to the adolescent as well as by the skills that he or she has accumulated. The availability of few opportunities, regardless of the adolescent's skill, can be quite discouraging. Similarly, adolescents who lack the necessary skills to take advantage of existing opportunities are also likely to feel discouraged about their futures. We are currently examining hypotheses related to these ideas for the transition to adulthood in a rural Pennsylvania sample (e.g., Petersen, Crouter, & Wilson, 1988; Sarigiani, Wilson, Petersen, & Vicary, 1989).

Adolescent Developmental Changes and Trajectories

Given the argument that adolescence may be a difficult period, at least one full of challenge, one way to examine the validity of this argument is to look at the kind of change experienced over the adolescent period. What we see in such an examination are both positive and negative trends. The areas in which these different trends occur suggest something about the developmental phase itself.

Positive Trends

Three examples of positive trends are with biological growth, self-concept, and cognition. As is well documented, pubertal change causes a growth spurt in height and the maturation of reproductive organs and secondary sexual characteristics (e.g., Tanner, 1962). Almost all studies of overall self-concept find that this capacity increases over the adolescent decade. But when specific aspects of the self-concept are examined, not all aspects show this increasing trend. Body image and superior adjustment (a scale that measures self-perceptions related to achievements and competence) decline significantly during early adolescence, especially for girls (Abramowitz et al., 1984). The decline in superior adjustment appears to be an artifact of the move to junior high school, which increases the competition and therefore limits the number of areas in which the youngsters might excel. Body image declines dramatically for girls, and for them, this decline continues to twelfth grade. However, it is important to note that boys recover positive body image after the seventh grade (Petersen, unpublished data).

All aspects of cognition that we have examined increase over the adolescent period. For example, the capacity for abstract thinking or formal operational thought increases during this period, with similarly increasing capacity in spatial visualization ability and verbal fluency (Petersen & Crockett, 1986).

In sum, several aspects of individual growth appear to increase over adolescence. The biggest change in adolescence is with biological growth. In general, however, adolescents also have increasingly positive self-views and increasing cognitive capacity. An exception to this positive trend in individual perceptions or skills is seen with body image in girls.

Negative Trends

There also are areas in which adolescents generally seem to have increasing difficulty. Three of these will be mentioned here: school achievement, problem behavior, and depression.

School Achievement. Most studies report decline in school achievement over the course of adolescence. We find, for example, that school achievement declines for the group as a whole over early adolescence and continues to decline to twelfth grade (Graber, 1988). Simmons and colleagues (e.g., Simmons & Blyth, 1987) also found continued decline. At least part of this decline may be attributable to increasingly difficult grading practices as youngsters move from an elementary school to secondary school format. In addition, there is evidence that some of the decline is due to change in youngsters themselves. For example, boys who are depressed and mildly delinquent (i.e., getting into trouble at school) in the early grades have much sharper grade declines than boys who are neither depressed nor delinquent. The latter group shows almost no decline in achievement (Ebata & Petersen, 1990). Interestingly, we find no relationship between school achievement and depression in girls.

Problem Behavior. All examinations of various kinds of "problem behavior"-cigarette smoking, substance use, alcohol use, sexual behavior, and delinquency—show increasing involvement of adolescents in these behaviors. To some extent this increasing involvement is simply due to the fact that many of these behaviors are considered to be adult, a state toward which these youngsters wish to move. Therefore, young people experiment with behavior that connotes the life stage toward which they are headed. For example, virtually all youngsters have tried drinking by the time they finish high school. Some degree of experimentation with alcohol use can hardly be considered a problem behavior; however, both early use and excessive use are problematic (Jessor & Jessor, 1977; Jessor, 1984).

Depression. The incidence of depressed affect and depressive episodes also increases over adolescence. Reports of emotional tone—a measure of depressed affect that includes both positive and negative items (Petersen et al., 1984)—show significant sex differences favoring boys by 12th grade (Petersen, Sarigiani, & Kennedy, 1990). Similarly, using a clinical epidemiological measure of depressive episodes (Gittleman et al., 1985), the incidence of these episodes increases from early to middle adolescence in both boys and girls, with much greater increase in girls (Petersen et al., 1990). Other analyses reveal that girls are more likely to experience depression for the first time during middle adolescence (Petersen et al., 1990). The depressed boys are more likely to have had previous difficulty in childhood (Ebata, 1987). In other words, when high school depressed affect is considered as a function of junior high depressed affect, analyses reveal that having no early adolescent depression appears to be protective for boys but not girls.

We might ask ourselves, then, whether adolescents are more likely than adults to experience depressed affect. A comparison of adolescents in our sample with their parents suggests that adolescent girls are significantly more likely to experience this state when compared to their mothers. Indeed, adolescent girls reported significantly more depressed affect than all other groups in this comparison.

What is most striking in all of these data on depression is the large gender difference. We found little evidence for gender divergence in the early adolescent years, with the exception of body image. With our twelfth grade follow-up, however, we found dramatically increased sex differences on all measures of self and negative affect (Petersen, Ebata, & Sarigiani, 1987). We also found a stable relationship from sixth to twelfth grade for boys in emotional tone, whereas for girls there was almost no correlation between sixth and twelfth grade emotional tone scores (Petersen et al., 1987).

Why do girls become more depressed in adolescence? One answer lies with the nature of the challenge experienced in early adolescence by girls as compared to boys. Girls are more likely to experience puberty prior to or during the school transition, a factor related to more negative outcomes, as noted earlier.

Effects of Changes on Developmental Patterns

The effects of simultaneous school transition and pubertal change are seen not only in early adolescence; they become even stronger by twelfth grade. For both boys and girls, it is always better to go through peak puberty after (by at least 6 months) moving to secondary school (Petersen et al., 1990). For girls in early adolescence, the effects of early puberty or simultaneous puberty are fairly similar in seventh and eighth grades, producing reports of emotional tone that are on average one-third to two-thirds of a standard deviation lower than that of girls with puberty after school transition. By twelfth grade, those girls whose puberty preceded school change and those girls experiencing simultaneous change still reported poorer emotional tone than those girls whose puberty followed school change.

There are so few boys whose puberty preceded school change by 6 months or more that the comparisons must focus on those boys experiencing simultaneous changes compared to those whose puberty followed school change. At both eighth and twelfth grades, the emotional tone of those whose puberty followed school change was about two-thirds of a standard deviation higher than those whose pubertal and school change was roughly simultaneous.

Pubertal timing effects alone also have long-term impact, especially on girls (Petersen, unpublished data). Early developing girls decline in body image and remain the lowest group by twelfth grade. Similar effects are seen on overall self-image (the average of the nine self-image scales). So both pubertal timing and the relative timing of pubertal change and school change place girls at higher risk for poor self-image and depressed affect.

In addition, girls are three times more likely than boys in our sample to experience a parental divorce in early adolescence. Although this particular result seemed puzzling at first, it is one found in several other adolescent studies, as well as a major national study of divorce (Morgan, Lye, & Condran, 1988). It may be that parents feel more comfortable divorcing when they have a young adolescent girl than when they have a young adolescent boy, because of the typical maternal custody arrangement. In addition to these higher divorce rates for families with young adolescent girls, we also find that girls not living with both biological parents are the only group, in a sex by family type analysis, whose emotional tone fails to increase significantly over adolescence.

Characterization of Adolescent Development

What do these trends tell us about the nature of adolescence, particularly as it pertains to concepts of stress? One way to view the results is that adolescents do increase in capacity over this period, but at least some adolescents experience increasing challenge that they find overwhelming and that leads them to manifest negative outcomes. These results have led us to conclude that the nature of the early adolescent transition influences the subsequent developmental trajectory and that subgoups of youngsters tend to diverge over adolescence.

At first glance, it seems contradictory that some positive characteristics, such as self-esteem, increase during adolescence while negative characteristics, such as depression, also increase. These two apparently contradictory trends can be reconciled by understanding that data on self-esteem are calculated as averages across the entire sample, whereas the changes in negative characteristics like depression often refer to small numbers of youth in the extreme of a distribution. This means that increasing numbers of youth manifest these more negative states. Therefore, we have argued that adolescence is a time of increasing divergence between those who are on positive trajectories as compared to those on negative trajectories. Whether difficulties stem from childhood, which may be more the case for boys, or from the early adolescent transition, there is evidence of increased sorting among youngsters during the adolescent decade. In addition, significant subgroup differences emerge or are maintained through this period.

The nature of change and challenge, however, cannot be the entire story. There is also evidence that individuals vary in their responses to the same change. Some adolescents appear to cope more effectively with change than do others. This has led us to pursue the nature of coping responses to challenges during adolescence.

Coping

In the past few years, there has been increased research on coping responses of adolescents (e.g., Compas, 1987a,b). We have just begun using the Ways of Coping measure (Folkman & Lazarus, 1986) to get at specific coping styles but in our longitudinal data thus far we do have a general coping measure—the Mastery and Coping scale of the Self-Image Questionnaire for Young Adolescents (SIQYA; Petersen et al., 1984). Although there are no sex differences on this measure, it does show strikingly different stability coefficients over time for boys compared to girls. The stability patterns are similar to those for emotional tone, with boys stable over time but with girls' sixth to twelfth grade correlation only .10. These results suggest that girls' perceptions of their coping capacity change dramatically over this period, perhaps in response to actual coping style changes. Other research (e.g., Buescher et al., 1987; Suffi-Krenke, 1988) provides similar data that boys' coping patterns remain stable over adolescence while girls' patterns change over this period.

We also have very striking results suggesting that girls respond differently to interpersonal challenge than do boys. The increased rates of depressed affect that we see among girls may be one result of these different responses. For example, in the face of family stress—such as divorce, death, illness, or exit of a sibling from the home—girls show more depression, whereas boys show no effect (Kennedy & Petersen, 1990). More detail about sex differences in coping was obtained in the doctoral dissertation of Mikesell (1988). Mikesell identified four family types based on patterns among various measures of adolescent–parent relationships. Girls in the most dysfunctional families—those low in cohesion, communication, and organization—reported depressed affect and poor functioning. In contrast, boys reported even better mood and functioning in this family context compared to those in other types of families. On close examination of the interview data, however, Mikesell discovered substantial information from parents and the interviewer suggesting that these boys may have been exaggerating their social skill and popularity. These results, like the earlier ones, are consistent with Nolen-Hoeksema's (1987) hypothesis that girls "amplify" negative moods, in contrast with boys who are more likely to distract themselves from a depressed mood. However, these data also raise the question of whether the responses of the boys are adaptive over the longer term. They may be adaptive and protective for their functioning in instrumental, achievement spheres of life and in the distressed family context, but may be quite maladaptive for future interpersonal relationships. We are interested to learn how these young men are faring now when we follow them up in young adulthood (at about 22 years of age).

The Dilemma: Fix the Kids or Fix the System

The research just described focuses at the individual level of analysis—the protective or coping aspects of individual adolescents. It would be a mistake, however, to focus solely at this level. We also ought to attend to the contextual side of the equation—the primary source of risks and stresses. In the United States today, adolescents face a great many challenges—perhaps more, and of a more difficult nature than they can reasonably handle, however effective their coping responses. The historical trends in various problems (e.g., suicide) in U.S. data (e.g., Frederick, 1985) suggest that our young people are faring increasingly worse throughout adolescence. In addition to finding ways to enhance the effectiveness of coping, we must also ask what we can do to reduce the extent of challenge—and stress—confronting so many young people.

The school system is one obvious focus (e.g., Jackson & Hornbeck, 1988). We currently have a secondary school system developed almost a century ago for the few elite planning to go on to college. But as the recent Grant Foundation report (1988) noted, at least half our young people do not go on to college. Many do not get through high school. This is a serious problem in a country—indeed world—where sophisticated technological and interpersonal skills are increasingly required for productive employment. Our secondary schools in the United States are inhumanely large and anonymous, with order kept by external control. Research of Eccles (Eccles & Midgley, 1990) and Safer (1986) demonstrate a decrease from elementary to secondary school in attributes of the environment and teaching style that enhance learning. Such studies provide growing evidence that we are preparing adolescents in a negative rather than positive direction.

With the several demographic changes in family structure, it is even more imperative that schools be contexts for positive socialization and preparation for adult roles. Although many single mothers are tremendously successful as parents, others simply cannot handle everything alone. Communities, especially through schools, must share responsibility for the future of our young people. Adolescents represent our future—economically and socially. By the year 2030, for example, two workers will be supporting each retiree over age 65; one of these two workers will be from a minority group (Reich, 1988). Minority children are especially poorly served by our current society and schools (Levin, 1986; McDill et al., 1985). Change is essential because we cannot afford to make casualties of our adolescents. And we can do better!

Acknowledgments

This research was supported in part by grants from the National Institute of Mental Health, MH3052/38142, and from the W. T. Grant Foundation, #89127289.

We gratefully acknowledge the contributions of study participants and staff. We also wish to thank Linda Stahl for her assistance in manuscript preparation.

References

Abramowitz, R. H., Petersen, A. C., & Schulenberg, J. E. (1984). Changes in self-image during early adolescence. In D. Offer, E. Ostrov, & K. Howard (Eds.), *Patterns of adolescent self-image* (pp. 19–28). San Francisco: Jossey-Bass.

Buescher, T. M., Olszewski, P., & Higham, S. J. (1987). *Influences on strategies adolescents use to cope with their own recognized talents*. Paper presented at the Biennial Meetings of the Society for Research in Child Development, Baltimore, MD, April 24.

Coleman, J. C. (1978). Current contradictions in adolescent theory. *Journal of Youth and Adolescence, 7*, 1–11.

Compas, B. E. (1987a). Coping with stress during childhood and adolescence. *Psychological Bulletin, 101*(3), 393–403.

Compas, B. E. (1987b). Stress and life events during childhood and adolescence. *Clinical Psychology Review, 7*, 275–302.

Cramer, P. (1979). Defense mechanisms in adolescence. *Developmental Psychology, 15*, 476–477.

Crockett, L. J., Camarena, P. M., Petersen, A. C., & Graber, J. A. (1990). *Masculinity and femininity during early adolescence: Developmental change in self-perception*. Submitted for publication.

Crockett, L. J., & Petersen, A. C. (1987). Pubertal status and psychosocial development: Findings from the early adolescence study. In R. M. Lerner & T. T. Foch (Eds.), *Biological-psychosocial interactions in early adolescence: A life-span perspective* (pp. 173–188). Hillsdale, NJ: Erlbaum.

Ebata, A. T. (1987). *A longitudinal study of gender differences in risk and resilience during adolescence.* Unpublished doctoral dissertation, The Pennsylvania State University, University Park, PA.

Ebata, A. T., & Petersen, A. C. (1990). *Patterns of adjustment during early adolescence: Gender differences in depression and achievement.* Submitted for publication.

Ebata, A. T., Petersen, A. C., & Conger, J. (1990). The development of psychopathology in adolescence. In J. E. Rolf, A. Masten, D. Cicchetti, K. H. Nuechterlein, & S. Weintraub (Eds.), *Risk and protective factors in the development of psychopathology.* Cambridge, NY: Cambridge University Press.

Eccles, J. S., & Midgley, C. (in press). Stage/environment fit: Developmentally appropriate classrooms for early adolescents. In R. E. Ames & C. Ames (Eds.), *Research in motivation in education* (Vol. 3). New York: Academic Press.

Emde, R. N., & Harmon, R. J. (Eds.). (1984). *Continuities and discontinuities in development.* New York: Plenum Press.

Folkman, S., & Lazarus, R. (1986). Stress processes and depressive symptomatology. *Journal of Abnormal Psychology, 95,* 107–113.

Frederick, C. J. (1985). An introduction and overview of youth suicide. In M. L. Peck, N. L. Farberow, & R. E. Litman (Eds.), *Youth Suicide* (pp. 1–16). New York: Springer Publishing Company.

Garmezy, N. (1985). Stress-resistant children: The search for protective factors. In J. E. Stevenson (Ed.), *Recent research in developmental psychopathology* (pp. 213–233). Oxford: Pergamon Press, Ltd.

Garmezy, N., & Rutter, M. (Eds.). (1983). *Stress, coping, and development in children.* New York: McGraw-Hill.

Gittleman, R., Mannuzza, S., Shenker, R., & Bonagura, N. (1985). Hyperactive boys almost grown up. *Archives of General Psychiatry, 42,* 937–966.

Graber, J. A. (1988). *Early-adolescence achievement patterns as trajectories into late adolescence: Effects on self-image and course enrollment.* Unpublished master's thesis, The Pennsylvania State University, University Park, PA.

Grant Foundation Commission on Work, Family, and Citizenship, William T. Grant Foundation. (1988). *The forgotten half: Pathways to success for America's youth and young families.* Washington, DC: Commission Office.

Haggerty, R. J. (1980). Life stress, illness and social supports. *Developmental Medical Child Neurology, 22,* 391–400.

Hamburg, B. (1974). Early adolescence: A specific and stressful stage of the life cycle. In G. V. Coelho, D. A. Hamburg, & J. E. Adams (Eds.), *Coping and adaptation* (pp. 101–124). New York: Basic Books.

Hill, J. P., & Lynch, M. E. (1983). The intensification of gender-related role expectations during early adolescence. In J. Brooks-Gunn & A. C. Petersen (Eds.), *Girls at puberty: Biological and psychosocial perspectives.* New York: Plenum.

Jackson, A. W., & Hornbeck, D. W. (1989). Educating young adolescents: Why we must restructure middle grade schools. *American Psychologist, 44*(5), 831–836.

Jessor, R. (1984). Adolescent development and behavioral health. In J. D. Matarazzo, S. M. Weiss, J. A. Herd, N. E. Miller, & S. M. Weiss (Eds.),

Behavioral health: A handbook of health enhancement and disease prevention (pp. 69–90). New York: John Wiley.

Jessor, R., & Jessor, S. L. (1977). *Problem behavior and psychosocial development: A longitudinal study of youth.* New York: Academic Press.

Kandel, D. B., & Davies, M. (1982). Epidemiology of depressive mood in adolescents. *Archives of General Psychiatry, 39,* 1205–1212.

Kennedy, R. E., & Petersen, A. C. (1990). Stressful family events and adjustment among young adolescents. Submitted for publication.

Kessler, R. C., Price, R. H., & Wortman, C. B. (1985). Social factors in psychopathology: Stress, social support, and coping processes. *Annual Review of Psychology, 36,* 351–372.

Lazarus, R. S., & Folkman, S. (1984). *Stress, appraisal, and coping.* New York: Springer.

Levin, H. M. (1986). *Educational reform for disadvantaged students: An emerging crisis* (National Education Association, Search). Washington, DC: National Education Association.

Lipsitz, J. (1977). *Growing up forgotten: A review of research and programs concerning early adolescence.* Lexington, MA: D.C. Heath.

Maughan, B., & Champion, L. (1988). *Risk and protective factors in the transition to young adulthood.* Paper presented at European Science Foundation Workshop. Longitudinal Research and the Study of Successful Aging, Castle Ringber, Federal Republic of Germany.

McDill, E. L., Natriello, G., & Pallas, A. M. (1985). Raising standards and retraining students: The impact of the reform recommendations on potential dropouts. *Review of Educational Research, 55,* 415–433.

Mikesell, J. (1988). *The relationship between patterns of family functioning and adolescent self-image: A multivariate, multi-process approach.* Unpublished doctoral dissertation, The Pennsylvania State University, University Park, PA.

Morgan, S. P., Lye, D. N., & Condran, G. A. (1988). Sons, daughters, and the risk of marital disruption. *American Journal of Sociology, 94,* 110–129.

Newcomb, M. D., Huba, G. J., & Bentler, P. M. (1986). Desirability of various life change events among adolescents: Effects of exposure, sex, age, and ethnicity. *Journal of Research on Personality, 20,* 207–227.

Nolen-Hoeksema, S. (1987). Sex differences in unipolar depression: Evidence and theory. *Psychological Bulletin, 101,* 259–282.

Pearlin, L. I., Lieberman, M. A., Menaghan, E. G., & Mullan, J. T. (1981). The stress process. *Journal of Health and Social Behavior, 22,* 337–356.

Petersen, A. C. (1980). Biopsychosocial processes in the development of sex-related differences. In J. Parsons (Ed.), *The psychobiology of sex-differences and sex roles* (pp. 31–35). New York: Hemisphere Publishing Corporation.

Petersen, A. C. (1984). The early adolescence study: An overview. *Journal of Early Adolescence, 4,* 103–106.

Petersen, A. C. (1987). The nature of biological-psychosocial interactions: The sample case of early adolescence. In R. M. Lerner & T. T. Foch (Eds.), *Biological-psychosocial interactions in early adolescence: A life-span perspective* (pp. 35–61). Hillsdale, NJ: Erlbaum.

Petersen, A. C. (1988). Adolescent development. In M. R. Rosenzweig (Ed.), *Annual review of psychology* (pp. 583–607). Palo Alto, CA: Annual Reviews, Inc.

Petersen, A. C., & Crockett, L. J. (1985). Pubertal timing and grade effects on adjustment. *Journal of Youth and Adolescence, 14,* 191–206.

Petersen, A. C., & Crockett, L. J. (1986). Pubertal development and its relation to cognitive and pyschosocial development in adolescent girls: Implications for parenting. In J. B. Lancaster & B. A. Hamburg (Eds.), *School-age pregnancy and parenthood* (pp. 147–175). Hawthorne, NY: Aldine Press.

Petersen, A. C., Crouter, A. C., & Wilson J. (1988). Heterosocial behavior and sexuality among normal young adolescents. In M. Levine & E. McAnarney (Eds.), *Early adolescent transitions* (pp. 123–137). Lexington, MA: D.C. Heath.

Petersen, A. C., & Ebata, A. T. (1986). Effects of normative and non-normative changes on early adolescent development. In R. G. Simmons & A. C. Petersen (Chairs), *Adolescent adjustment to the cumulation and synchronization of life transitions.* Symposium conducted at the biennial meeting of the Society for Research on Adolescence, Madison, WI.

Petersen, A. C., & Ebata, A. T. (1987). Developmental transitions and adolescent problem behavior: Implications for prevention and intervention. In K. Hurrelmann, F. X. Kaufmann, & F. Losel (Eds.), *Social intervention: Potential and constraints* (pp. 167–184). New York: Walter de Gruyter.

Petersen, A. C., Ebata, A. T., & Sarigiani, P. A. (1987). Who expresses depressive affect in adolescence? Paper presented in a symposium, *The Development of depressive affect in adolescence: Biological, affective, and social factors,* at the biennial meeting of the Society for Research in Child Development, Baltimore, MD.

Petersen, A. C., Sarigiani, P. A., & Kennedy, R. E. (in press). Adolescent depression: Why more girls? *Journal of Youth and Adolescence.*

Petersen, A. C., Schulenberg, J. E., Abramowitz, R. H., Offer, D., & Jarcho, H. D. (1984). A self-image questionnaire for young adolescents (SIQYA): Reliability and validity studies. *Journal of Youth and Adolescence, 13,* 93–111.

Petersen, A. C., & Spiga, R. (1982). Adolescence and Stress. In L. Goldberger & S. Breznitz (Eds.), *Handbook of stress: Theoretical and clinical aspects.* New York: Free Press.

Petersen, A. C., Susman, E., & Beard, J. (1988). The development of coping responses during adolescence: Endocrine and behavioral aspects (pp. 151–172). In D. Palermo, J. Kagan, & A. C. Petersen (Eds.), *Coping with uncertainty: Biological behavioral and developmental perspectives.* Hillsdale, NJ: Erlbaum.

Reich, R. B. (1988). *Education and the Next Economy.* Washington, DC: National Education Association, Professional and Organizational Development/ Research Division.

Richards, M., & Petersen, A. C. (1987). Biological theoretical models of adolescent development. In V. B. Van Hasselt & M. Hersen (Eds.), *Handbook of adolescent psychology* (pp. 34–52). Elmsford, NY: Pergamon Press.

Rutter, M. (1983). Stress, coping, and development: Some issues and some questions. In N. Garmezy & M. Rutter (Eds.), *Stress, coping, and development in children.* New York: McGraw-Hill.

Safer, D. J. (1986). The stress of secondary school for vulnerable students. *Journal of Youth and Adolescence, 15,* 405–417.

Sarigiani, P. A., & Petersen, A. C. (1990). Perceived closeness with parents and adjustment in adolescence. Submitted for publication.

Sarigiani, P. A., Wilson, J., Petersen, A. C., & Vicary, J. (1990). Self-image and educational plans of adolescents from two contrasting communities. *Journal of Early Adolescence, 30*(1), 37–55.

Siddique, C. M., & D'Arcy, C. (1984). Adolescence, stress, and psychological well-being. *Journal of Youth and Adolescence, 13,* 459–473.

Signorielli, N. (1987). Children and adolescents on television: A consistent pattern of devaluation. *The Journal of Early Adolescence, 7*(3), 255–268.

Simmons, R. G., & Blyth, D. A. (1987). *Moving into adolescence: The impact of pubertal change and school context.* New York: Aldine de Gruyter.

Simmons, R. G., Burgeson, R., Carlton-Ford, S., & Blyth, D. A. (1987). The impact of cumulative change in early adolescence. *Child Development, 58,* 1220–1234.

Suffi-Krenke, I. (1988). *Developmental aspects of health-related behavior in adolescence.* Paper presented at the International Conference on Health Psychology, Trier, West Germany, and at the Center for the Study of Child and Adolescent Development, The Pennsylvania State University.

Tanner, J. M. (1962). *Growth at adolescence.* Springfield, IL: Charles C Thomas.

Thoits, P. A. (1986). Social support as coping assistance. *Journal of Consulting and Clinical Psychology, 54,* 416–426.

6

Stressful Events and Their Correlates among Adolescents of Diverse Backgrounds

**Sanford M. Dornbusch, Randy Mont-Reynaud,
Philip L. Ritter, Zeng-yin Chen, and Laurence Steinberg**

This paper examines the association of stressful events with various measures of well-being among a sample of high school youth from diverse social groups. First, groups of adolescents are compared with respect to their reported exposure to stressful events. Second, although traditional studies of the role of life change events and outcomes have focused on mental and physical symptoms as dependent measures, we have added measures of school performance (self-reported grades) and deviance, thereby tapping more of the life space of our high school sample. Third, across a variety of social groups (parental education groups, ethnicities, and family structures), we test the idea that an increase in perceived stressful events always tends to be associated with negative outcomes.

Stress has been defined in terms of the impact of significant life events that are experienced by individuals and the family as a whole (Holmes & Rahe, 1967). Since the 1950s, the etiological role of stressful life events has been widely accepted (Rabkin & Streuning, 1976). Selye's concept of stress as a "general adaptation syndrome," a set of general psychological reactions to adverse environmental stimuli (1956), has established the study of the correspondence between life changes, stress, and illness as an independent field. Decades of research on the role of socially induced stress in precipitating chronic diseases or illness generally support the idea of a relation between an increase in life change events and an increase in health problems or complaints. Additional research has questioned the simplistic idea that stressful events have a direct etiological connection to health problems; the effects are confounded by the many stressful ongoing social statuses individuals occupy. Thus Gersten and colleagues suggest an indirect, interactive relationship that takes into account the frequency and duration of exposure to stressful events, as well as social status (Gersten, Langner, Eisenberg, & Simcha-Fagan, 1977). Susceptibility to a variety of infections is considered a function of an individual's personal physiological and psychological response to life change events, and not merely a result from mere exposure to microbes or events of stress alone (Rabkin & Streuning, 1976). Some researchers note the limitations of an "events leads to pathology" model.

In stress research, life change events are termed "precipitating factors." Moderating factors are those characteristics of the individual and social support structures that affect sensitivity to life change events. In addition, long-term behavior patterns, the experiences of childhood, and personality characteristics are considered to be "predisposing factors" that affect susceptibility to disease (Rabkin & Streuning, 1976). The concept of stress thus offers possible explanations for individual differences in susceptibility to illness. It also suggests that an understanding of disease states is not possible without consideration of the social environment (Rabkin & Streuning, 1976).

Research among adults supports the link between stressful life events and a variety of psychological and physical health problems, ranging from heart disease to diabetes, from anxiety to depression and social maladjustment (Dohrenwend & Dohrenwend, 1974; Rabkin & Streuning, 1976; Thoits, 1983). There are, however, fewer reports of such relations between stress and health among children and adolescents. The available research on youth does suggest significant associations, similar to those found among adults, between stressful events and various health problems (cf. Boyce, Jensen, Cassell, Collier, Smith, & Raimey, 1977; Pryor Brown, 1985; Sterling, Cowen, Weissberg, Lotyczewski, & Boike, 1985; Vaux & Ruggiero, 1983; Wallerstein & Kelly, 1980). Studies of stress-related correlates among adolescents describe acting-out behavior and depression (Felner, Stolberg, & Cowen, 1975; Johnson & McCutcheon, 1980), delinquency (Vaux & Ruggiero, 1983), impaired school performance (Harris, 1972), depression among adolescents (Hudgens, 1974), accidents and injuries (Padilla, Rohsenow, & Bergman, 1976), and school maladjustment (Pryor Brown, 1985).

Pryor Brown and associates (1989) have shown that urban adolescents experienced a greater number of events and more highly stressful ones than suburban youth. Other reports show that youth from some ethnic groups encounter certain types of life events more often than do others (Newcomb et. al., 1981), supporting the view that there are ethnic-specific sources of stress (Lewis, Siegel & Lewis, 1984), and that culture can both cause and moderate stress effects (Mirowsky & Ross, 1980). Some adult studies conclude that membership in an ethnic group per se does not play a role in the relation of psychological distress to life events (Boyd & Weissman, 1982; Dohrenwend & Dohrenwend, 1974; Hirschfeld & Cross, 1982), and much research has focused on the differential effects of life stressors across social classes. Although some findings indicate that social class, and not ethnicity, is implicated in vulnerability to life stressors (Warheit, Holzer, & Arey, 1975; Dohrenwend & Dohrenwend 1974), other research argues that race is of continuing significance for psychological well-being and quality of life among Black Americans (Thomas & Hughes, 1986).

The operationalization of stress and its correlates has varied considerably as different groups have been studied. This chapter focuses on these important subgroups of adolescents and uses a single set of measures to explore the relation between stressful life events and such correlates as mental and physical health, school performance as measured by grades, and deviance. The diversity and substantial size of the subgroups in our sample permit simultaneous analyses of the correlates of stressful events for male and female adolescents of different social classes, ethnic groups, and family structures.

Sample and Measures

The sample for this study consists of all the high school students in six San Francisco Bay Area schools and three schools in Wisconsin. Approximately 88% of all students registered in these schools participated in our study; there were only a few refusals, but many students were not in class at the time of questionnaire administration. The number of students filling out questionnaires was 10,041. The California schools are all urban and suburban, with considerable diversity in socioeconomic and ethnic composition, while the Wisconsin schools are in a farm area, a suburb of a middle-size city, and inner-city Milwaukee. The variety of these environments is conducive to our central goal: to examine the relation of stressful events to several outcomes across diverse social groupings.

We used a major life events scale, derived from the Cornell Medical Index (Buros, 1965), that asked: "Have any of the following things happened to you in the past 12 months?"

I broke up with my boyfriend or girlfriend.
I began dating or going steady with someone.

A brother or sister left home.
I did not get into a club or sport I really wanted to be involved in.
There was a change in the amount of money my family has.
One of my close friends died or became seriously ill.
One of my grandparents died.
My mother began working.
I was suspended from school.
I became involved in some new religious activities.
One of my parents became seriously ill or was hospitalized.
I moved to a new school district.
One of my parents changed jobs.
I thought that I or my girlfriend was pregnant.
One of my parents lost his or her job.
A new baby was born in our family.
My parents were divorced or separated.
One of my parents remarried.
My mother or father died.
I became seriously ill or was hospitalized.

The number of major events reported by each student was used to form a stressful-events score. Each event was thus given an equal weight in our analyses.

The dependent variables were also derived from the literature on stress and adolescence. The major correlates examined were mental health, physical health, high school grades, and deviance. In analyses relating stressful events to school outcomes, we removed "I was suspended from school" from the events scale. Similarly, in relating stressful events to physical health outcomes, we removed "I became seriously ill or was hospitalized" from the events scale.

Although there is a traditional emphasis in stress research on mental and physical health symptoms as indicators of well-being and adequacy of functioning, we consider it appropriate to include academic performance and deviance for our research on adolescents. For most adolescents, school is a major arena in which they demonstrate their competence. Adolescent deviance, on the other hand, is a negatively evaluated set of behaviors in the eyes of society. Using these four diverse domains and relating them to stressors, we believe we tap a larger proportion of the life-space of most American adolescents. These dependent variables were measured by asking adolescents to report physical and mental health symptoms, grades, and frequency of deviant acts. For reporting mental symptoms, each adolescent was asked, "In the past month, how often have you: Felt over-tired, felt nervous or worried, felt 'low' or depressed, felt tense or irritable, had trouble sleeping, lost your appetite, felt apart or alone, felt as if you were eating too much?"

For physical symptoms, we asked "In the past month, how often have you: Had a headache, had a stomach ache, had a cold or other illness, had a physical injury, had skin problems?"

Some or all the physical complaints could have a psychosomatic component, and some of the emotionally based problems could have physical roots. A strong relation of $r = .54$ obtains between reports of mental and physical health symptoms.

The measure of student performance used throughout this chapter is students' reports of their grades so far in school. The categories were mostly As, about half As and half Bs, mostly Bs, about half Bs and half Cs, mostly Cs, about half Cs and half Ds, mostly Ds, and mostly below D. A numerical scale of self-reported grades was then related to these responses, with 4.0 representing the top category.

The correlation between school-reported grade-point averages and self-reported grades was .79 for a subsample of approximately 5000 students for whom we examined records. We were concerned that there might be a systematic inflation of self-reported grades for students whose academic performance was low. Accordingly, we examined the responses of students at each grade level. There was only a slight tendency to overstate grades when one reached grades near the bottom of the distribution—mean grades of C and below. Because self-reported grades give a close approximation to the distribution of grades on the transcript, the self-reports will be used as the measure of school performance in all analyses.

We measured adolescent deviance by the total score computed from responses to the question "Since the beginning of the school year in September, how often have you done each of these things?" Each student answered whether he or she had "never," "once or twice," "several times," or "often" engaged in the following behaviors:

Copied homework or a class assignment from somebody else.
Smoked cigarettes (other than marijuana) or used chewing tobacco.
Bought beer or liquor yourself or given someone money to buy it for you.
Used a phony I.D.
Cheated on a class test.
Taken something of value from another person.
Run away from home.
Used alcohol excessively or been drunk.
Come to class late.
Smoked marijuana.
Used a drug other than marijuana (for example, "uppers," cocaine).
Got in trouble with the police.
Carried a weapon to school.

Got into a physical fight at school.
Purposely damaged school property.

We used mean level of parents' education as our indicator of socioeconomic status. Every adolescent was assigned to a low, middle, or high
education category. Low level of education refers to an average education
level of parents up to high school graduation, middle refers to some college or technical training, and high indicates college graduation and above.

With respect to household status, we divided our sample into those
youth from two-natural-parent households and youth from all other
types of households (including single mother, single father, mother and
stepfather, father and stepmother, and other possibilities).

Ethnicity was determined by each youth's self-identification in terms of
major ethnic groups. Those groups were Hispanic or Latino, non-Hispanic White, African-American, and Asian-American (including Chinese,
Korean, Japanese, Filipino, Vietnamese, and other South-East Asian
groups, and South Asians). Native Americans, Pacific Islanders, and
Middle-Easterns were excluded from these analyses for insufficient cases.

Findings

Within the category of stressful events, we distinguished three types of
stressors: personal, familial, and school related. Among both males and
females, adolescents showed a greater sensitivity (measured by correlations between types of events and the dependent variables, not detailed
here) to personal events (such as "I broke up with my girlfriend or
boyfriend") than to those that occurred within the family ("My parents
divorced or separated"; "One of my parents remarried") or the school ("I
didn't get into a club"; "I was suspended from school"). Second, family-
related events were more strongly associated with outcomes than were
school-related events. It is striking that this order of strength of association was invariant for each type of outcome: mental symptoms, physical
symptoms, grades, and deviant behaviors. There were no statistically
significant gender differences in sensitivity to stressors of each type.
Regardless of category of event, the health, school performance, and
deviance of adolescent males and females were similarly affected. In sum,
personal events have the most impact in all outcome behavior measures,
among both male and female adolescents, followed in turn by family-
related events and school-related events.

Frequencies of Occurrence of Stressful Events and Adolescent Outcomes

In accord with previous studies of stress among adults (Cleary &
Mechanic, 1983), Table 1 shows adolescent females in our sample re-

Table 1. Means of Stressful Events, Physical and Psychological Symptoms, Grades, and Deviance by Sex, Parental Education, Ethnicity, and Family Structure

	Events	Psych	Physical	Grades	Deviance
Gender					
Males	3.28****	2.24****	2.01****	2.17***	1.61****
	(4325)	(4206)	(4228)	(3644)	(3261)
Females	3.63	2.77	2.29	2.89	1.51
	(4649)	(4528)	(4546)	(3597)	(3499)
Parent-educ					
Males					
Low	3.58***	2.23**	2.02	2.42****	1.63
	(1006)	(925)	(930)	(1152)	(774)
Mid	3.34****	2.28	2.05	2.66****	1.63
	(1256)	(1191)	(1200)	(1370)	(939)
High	3.01	2.32	2.05	2.97	1.61
	(1646)	(1577)	(1583)	(1730)	(1270)
Females					
Low	3.82****	2.76	2.29	2.62****	1.50
	(1243)	(1182)	(1192)	(1311)	(917)
Mid	3.81****	2.83	2.31	2.88****	1.53
	(1340)	(1287)	(1289)	(1389)	(1025)
High	3.39	2.78	2.29	3.15	1.52
	(1702)	(1652)	(1659)	(1740)	(1316)
Ethnicity					
Males					
Black	4.12****	2.17***	2.03	2.37****	1.52****
	(360)	(312)	(314)	(393)	(214)
White	3.14	2.31	2.06	2.78	1.67
	(2381)	(2290)	(2300)	(2526)	(1832)
Asian	2.78****	2.27	1.97***	3.05****	1.44****
	(709)	(673)	(677)	(743)	(572)
Hispanic	3.66****	2.16****	1.98***	2.38****	1.63
	(692)	(628)	(634)	(789)	(500)
Females					
Black	4.46****	2.62****	2.29	2.59****	1.44****
	(492)	(473)	(475)	(495)	(316)
White	3.60	2.85	2.32	2.99	1.58
	(2558)	(2491)	(2496)	(2615)	(1963)
Asian	3.03****	2.69****	2.21****	3.18****	1.34****
	(675)	(634)	(641)	(700)	(543)
Hispanic	3.80**	2.71****	2.27**	2.54****	1.51****
	(764)	(708)	(710)	(796)	(540)
Family structure					
Males					
2 parent	2.87	2.23	2.01	2.79	1.59
	(2646)	(2590)	(2604)	(2878)	(2083)
All others	3.92****	2.26	2.01	2.55****	1.66***
	(1672)	(1604)	(1612)	(1860)	(1178)

Table 1. Continued

	Events	Psych	Physical	Grades	Deviance
Females					
2 parent	3.23	2.76	2.29	3.01	1.49
	(2773)	(2694)	(2708)	(2863)	(2187)
All others	4.26****	2.77	2.29	2.71****	1.54****
	(1856)	(1813)	(1817)	(1938)	(1312)

Numbers in parentheses are number of cases.
**$p < .05$, two-tailed.
***$p < .01$, two-tailed.
****$p < .001$, two-tailed.

ported more stressful events and more mental and physical symptoms compared to males. In addition, female adolescents reported higher grades and lower rates of deviance. Thus we have powerful gender differences in reports of stressful events and outcomes believed to be associated with stressful events. These data do not, however, test the extent to which there are gender differences in susceptibility or vulnerability to stressful events. The relation of stressful events to adolescent outcomes is examined in Tables 2 through 4.

With respect to level of parent education, we see in Table 1 that the mean number of reported stressful events declines with the increase in parental education for both genders. Looking at the four outcome measures, both mental and physical symptoms show little variation by level of parent education; the sole exception is the low incidence of psychological symptoms among low-status males. For grades, there are sharp differences by level of parent education in the expected direction, with high status associated with higher grades. The results for deviance are particularly interesting. There are no differences in deviance rates by parent education levels. There are two explanations for this lack of relation between deviance and social class. First, our choice of indicators includes diverse forms of deviance, in school and outside of school, that extend beyond the usual indicators of delinquency for which class differences are usually observed. Second, with respect to some of the indicators of activities deemed critical, such as carrying weapons or use of hard drugs, many students may choose to under-report.

A comparison of ethnic groups to non-Hispanic Whites showed clear patterns. Asian-Americans of both sexes reported fewer stressful events, fewer physical symptoms, higher grades, and lower deviance compared to non-Hispanic Whites. For psychological symptoms, only female Asian-Americans showed a significantly lower incidence.

Among Black adolescents, both males and females reported more stressful events, fewer psychological symptoms, lower grades, and lower deviance than did non-Hispanic Whites. Hispanics reported more stressful events, fewer psychological and physical symptoms, lower grades, and, in the case of females only, a lower rate of deviance.

Comparing adolescents from two-natural-parent families with those from all other types of family structures (single-parent families and stepfamilies), we noted in Table 1 that youth from intact families report fewer stressful events, higher grades, and lower deviance. The difference in stressful events persists even when we exclude events related to separation, divorce and remarriage.

Outcome Measures among High-Stress and Low-Stress Groups

We now examine the relation of stressful events to each adolescent outcome. In Table 2, each group to be analyzed is divided at the mean of reported stressful events for the total sample. Thus, for example, within a single gender-ethnic group, we compare means on each of the four outcome measures for those youths reporting fewer stressful events and those reporting more stressful events. Comparison of the means is similar to doing a series of zero-order correlations. Subsequent tables will report the results of multiple regressions that simultaneously take into account the contributions of several predictors, as well as interactions between various statuses and the level of stress. Here we limit ourselves to one group at a time.

The pattern of results in Table 2 is clear and can be briefly summarized. Among both males and females, within each ethnic group, parental-education group, family-structure group, and age group, those adolescents reporting more stressful events have more negative outcomes. Psychological symptoms and physical symptoms are more frequent, grades are lower, and reported deviance is greater for those who report experiencing more stressful events. There are no exceptions to this regular pattern, although for Black males and females (the smallest samples), the differences are sometimes not statistically significant.

Examination of Table 2 indicates only slight differences between male and female adolescents in their sensitivity to stressful events. In other words, gender differences in outcomes when high and low stress groups are compared are minor. These gender comparisons are made for each dependent variable within each of the subgroups defined by ethnicity, parental education, family structure, and age. Females show greater differences in response to stress only for psychological symptoms, while the differences for males are greater for reported deviance. For physical symptoms and grades, there is only a slight tendency for female differences to be higher than male differences. Overall, it appears

Table 2. Means of Events, Physical and Psychological Symptoms, Grades, and Deviance of Adolescents Reporting High or Low Incidence of Stressful Events

	Hi/low events	Psych	Physical	Grades	Deviance
Males					
Ethnicity					
Black	Low	2.00	1.90	2.45	1.50
		(147)	(148)	(157)	(98)
	High	2.16*	2.03*	2.34	1.53
		(187)	(188)	(185)	(97)
White	Low	2.20	1.99	2.90	1.60
		(1405)	(1407)	(1421)	(1090)
	High	2.54****	2.23****	2.64****	1.78****
		(884)	(890)	(890)	(617)
Asian	Low	2.19	1.90	3.14	1.40
		(474)	(476)	(470)	(370)
	High	2.44****	2.10****	2.91***	1.56****
		(199)	(201)	(194)	(145)
Hispanic	Low	2.00	1.87	2.51	1.55
		(345)	(347)	(359)	(251)
	High	2.33****	2.09****	2.30***	1.76****
		(283)	(286)	(287)	(179)
Parent-educ					
Low	Low	2.07	1.90	2.54	1.54
		(515)	(517)	(541)	(380)
	High	2.38****	2.13****	2.34****	1.74****
		(466)	(468)	(461)	(297)
Mid	Low	2.15	1.97	2.77	1.57
		(714)	(716)	(722)	(535)
	High	2.50****	2.10****	2.60****	1.72****
		(473)	(479)	(486)	(326)
High	Low	2.23	1.97	3.12	1.54
		(1006)	(1008)	(1009)	(782)
	High	2.46****	2.17****	2.79****	1.73****
		(570)	(571)	(566)	(405)
Family structure					
2-parent	Low	2.16	1.96	2.92	1.53
		(1703)	(1707)	(1709)	(1330)
	High	2.43****	2.18****	2.66****	1.70****
		(831)	(839)	(836)	(578)
All others	Low	2.13	1.92	2.68	1.57
		(741)	(744)	(765)	(524)
	High	2.44****	2.14****	2.47****	1.76****
		(814)	(818)	(811)	(519)
Age group					
13–15 years	Low	2.06	1.93	2.88	1.51
		(1341)	(1345)	(1369)	(1073)
	High	2.34****	2.14****	2.60****	1.67****
		(823)	(833)	(832)	(621)
16–18 years	Low	2.29	1.98	2.82	1.61
		(964)	(967)	(970)	(690)
	High	2.56****	2.18****	2.56****	1.82****
		(688)	(689)	(680)	(416)

	Hi/low events	Psych	Physical	Grades	Deviance
Females					
Ethnicity					
Black	Low	2.45	2.21	2.71	1.41
		(179)	(180)	(173)	(124)
	High	2.72****	2.35**	2.53***	1.47
		(296)	(298)	(289)	(183)
White	Low	2.70	2.23	3.10	1.51
		(1305)	(1307)	(1303)	(1026)
	High	3.06****	2.46****	2.89****	1.66****
		(1178)	(1180)	(1168)	(844)
Asian	Low	2.58	2.14	3.31	1.30
		(381)	(385)	(394)	(332)
	High	2.90****	2.36****	3.01****	1.43****
		(247)	(250)	(244)	(171)
Hispanic	Low	2.46	2.12	2.69	1.42
		(333)	(336)	(346)	(258)
	High	2.91****	2.39****	2.44****	1.58****
		(379)	(378)	(374)	(242)
Parent-educ					
Low	Low	2.55	2.18	2.76	1.42
		(590)	(595)	(600)	(446)
	High	2.95****	2.40****	2.50****	1.59****
		(638)	(643)	(626)	(398)
Mid	Low	2.65	2.19	3.02	1.46
		(634)	(634)	(642)	(505)
	High	3.01****	2.44****	2.77****	1.60****
		(652)	(653)	(649)	(459)
High	Low	2.65	2.22	3.29	1.47
		(884)	(889)	(887)	(710)
	High	2.98****	2.43****	3.03****	1.60****
		(749)	(750)	(745)	(552)
Family structure					
2-parent	Low	2.63	2.20	3.12	1.44
		(1566)	(1576)	(1587)	(1257)
	High	2.98****	2.43****	2.87****	1.59****
		(1100)	(1104)	(1095)	(806)
All others	Low	2.57	2.17	2.86	1.47
		(717)	(717)	(715)	(538)
	High	2.95***	2.41****	2.65****	1.59****
		(1067)	(1071)	(1049)	(683)
Age group					
13–15 years	Low	2.54	2.19	3.07	1.41
		(1344)	(1350)	(1350)	(1129)
	High	2.93****	2.44****	2.77****	1.57****
		(1239)	(1242)	(1224)	(902)
16–18 years	Low	2.74	2.19	3.02	1.51
		(943)	(847)	(855)	(603)
	High	3.03****	2.39****	2.76****	1.64****
		(832)	(835)	(826)	(531)

Numbers in parentheses are number of cases.
 *$p < .10$, two-tailed.
 **$p < .05$, two-tailed.
 ***$p < .01$, two-tailed.
 ****$p < .001$, two-tailed.

that stressful events have about the same association with negative outcomes for both sexes. There is little evidence that female adolescents are, in general, more vulnerable to high stress, although they do evidence more psychological symptoms as a response to an increased level of stressors. Most discussions of vulnerability have focused on psychological symptoms, and it appears that analyses in terms of a larger range of variables yield disparate findings on the vulnerability of females.

We then divided our adolescent sample into a group of younger (13 to 15 years old) and older (16 to 18 years) adolescents. When we then examined differences between youth with high and low stress, we found that, regardless of age, youth with high stress reported moresymptoms, more deviance, and lower grades than did youth with low stress (Table 2). The association of stressful events with adolescent outcomes does not vary with age.

Multiple Regressions to Predict the Four Outcome Measures

Our analyses to this point have used one predictor variable at a time, examining the association of stressful events to each outcome within each subgroup on a specific status variable. Now we report multiple regressions in which all the status variables were simultaneously used as predictors and the stressful events score was entered as the final predictor. This technique enables us to assess the relative strength of stressful events and the status variables in predicting our four adolescent outcomes. We are also able to discern the extent to which a particular relation to a status variable is purely a product of differences in the frequency of stressful events.

In Table 3, which focuses on psychological symptoms, stressful events has the second highest relation to reports of psychological symptoms. Female is the only variable that has a higher β value. The hypothesis that the relation of stressful events to mental health is merely a product of chronic stressors, such as ethnicity or social class, is not supported by these data.

The status variables typically preserve their association with psychological symptoms, shown in Table 3, when the stressful events score is introduced. Females, youth with better educated parents, and older adolescents evidence more psychological symptoms, and Black and Hispanic youth show fewer psychological symptomss when compared with non-Hispanic Whites. With respect to forms of households, there is a major change. Without stressful events in the equation, adolescents in two-natural-parent households are significantly less likely to report psychological symptoms than are adolescents in other types of families (predominantly single-parent or stepparent families). That relation

Table 3. Predictors of Psychological Symptoms, Using Structural Variables and either "With Events" or "Without Events"

Psychological symptoms	Psychological symptoms					
	"Without events"			"With events"		
	b	β	F	b	β	F
Female	.544****	.335	977.1****	.502****	.314	907.2****
	(.017)[a]			(.016)		
Parent-educ level	.025****	.051	20.2****	.021****	.044	16.1****
	(.005)			(.005)		
Black	−.229****	−.081	52.6****	−.281****	−.101	85.9****
	(.031)			(.030)		
Hispanic	−.098****	−.042	13.6****	−.147****	−.065	34.0****
	(.026)			(.025)		
Asian	−.033	−.014	1.7	−.023	−.010	0.9
	(.025)			(.024)		
Age	.088****	.138	167.6****	.080****	.129	153.1****
	(.007)			(.006)		
2 natural parents	−.064****	−.038	12.00****	.015	.009	0.7
	(.018)			(.017)		
Stressful events				.086****	.258	575.0****
				(.004)		
Constant	.3239			.2067		
R^2		.134			.1969	
N		7609			7488	

[a]Numbers in parentheses are standard errors.
****$p < .001$, two-tailed.

seems to be a product of the low frequency of stressful events in two-natural-parent families (see Table 1). When the stressful events score is introduced as a predictor, the relation of family structure to psychological symptoms is not significant.

In Table 4, displaying the results of the multiple regression analysis for physical symptoms, we observe once again that the stressful events score has predictive power. The β for stressful events is higher than that of any status variable in predicting physical symptoms. Being female, having better educated parents, and coming from a two-natural-parent household is associated with more physical symptoms, and being from any minority group is associated with fewer physical symptoms.

As was the case for psychological symptoms, family structure is the only predictor variable sharply affected by the introduction of stressful events as a predictor. But here the finding differs: Children in two-natural-parent households are more likely to exhibit physical symptoms than those in other households once we control for the frequency of stressful events.

Table 4. Predictors of Physical Symptoms, Using Structural Variables and either "with Events" or "without Events"

	Physical symptoms					
	"Without events"			"With events"		
	b	β	F	b	β	F
Female	.276**** (.014)[a]	.217	374.9****	.242**** (.014)	.194	308.3****
Parent-educ level	.012*** (.004)	.031	6.8***	.008* (.004)	.021	3.5*
Black	−.061** (.026)	−.027	5.5**	−.096**** (.025)	−.044	14.6****
Hispanic	−.053** (.022)	−.029	5.9**	−.090**** (.020)	−.051	18.5****
Asian	−.076**** (.021)	−.042	13.5****	−.070*** (.02)	−.040	12.5***
Age	.008 (.006)	.016	2.2	.001 (.005)	.003	.01
2 Natural parents	−.013 (.015)	−.010	0.8	.042*** (.014)	.032	8.0***
Stressful events				.063**** (.003)	.231	416.7****
Constant	1.592			1.544		
R^2		.049			.098	
N		7642			7518	

[a]Numbers in parentheses are standard errors.
*$p < .10$, two-tailed.
**$p < .05$, two-tailed.
***$p < .01$, two-tailed.
****$p < .001$, two-tailed.

We conducted parallel multiple regression analyses (not shown) for self-reported grades and deviance. For grades, the stressful events score is the third best indicator. Having parents with a high education and being female were better predictors of grades, with both associated with higher grades. Being Black, Hispanic, or an older student was associated with lower grades, while being Asian was associated with higher grades.

Finally, in predicting reported deviance, stressful events is the most powerful predictor. With deviance as with grades, family structure shows somewhat reduced predictive power when the stressful events score is introduced. Being female, a member of any minority group, and coming from a two-natural-parent household were all associated with lower deviance, while older adolescents were more likely to be deviant.

In summary, stressful events do affect each outcome, even when we control for a battery of status variables. Family structure is the only status variable whose relation to these outcomes is markedly affected by controlling for stressful events, and this occurs only for the psychological distress and physical symptoms variables.

A further series of regressions was performed in order to determine whether interaction terms combining stressful events with each of the status variables would change the pattern of results. The results are briefly summarized below.

For psychological symptoms, there are significant interaction terms for the combination of stressful events with age, female, Black, and Asian. Only the interaction of events with being female was a positive predictor of psychological symptoms, indicating that females were more vulnerable to high levels of stress for this type of outcome. Older adolescents were less affected, in terms of psychological symptoms, by having many stressful events than were younger adolescents. Compared to non-Hispanic Whites, Black and Asian youth showed fewer psychological symptoms in responses to stressors. Similarly, for physical symptoms, the interaction of being Black and stressful events emerged as a negative predictor, indicating that Black youth, compared to non-Hispanic Whites, were less vulnerable to stressors in terms of this outcome. For grades, there was a positive effect of the interaction of stressful events and age, and a negative effect of the interaction of events and being in a two-parent household. This means that younger adolescents are more sensitive to stressors in terms of their grades, and that adolescents are coming from two-natural-parent households are more affected in their grades by stressful events than are youth from other types of households. Finally, for deviance, there was a negative interaction term of stressful events and being Black, indicating that Black rates of deviance were not affected by stressors as much as were non-Hispanic White rates.

Discussion

Our study of stressful events and their correlates within a large heterogeneous sample of adolescents indicates that stressful events are indeed associated with negative outcomes for youth of all social classes, all ethnic groups and in all types of families. It is impressive that a set of diverse events captures enough of what happens within specific subgroups of the adolescent population so that an overall measure of the number of stressful events predicts symptoms of mental and physical distress, grades, and deviant behavior. Comparing the results for our adolescent population with those found for children and adults, the data provide general support for the role of stressful events, while providing somewhat divergent findings as we examine the impact of stressors in specific social classes, family structures, and ethnic groups.

It has been suggested that women are more burdened with respect to both acute and chronic interpersonal stressors, perhaps because they are more likely to be emotionally distressed by the problems of others (Wethington, McLeod, & Kessler, 1987). Other researchers focusing on adolescence have proposed that this period of life is when intense gender socialization first occurs and that girls are especially vulnerable to stress at this time (Hill & Lynch, 1983).

Women may indeed report more stress and more symptoms, but that does not necessarily imply a greater sensitivity to stress. As other studies have found for adults, our data show that adolescent females do indeed report both more stressful events and more health symptoms than do male adolescents. Yet, only for psychological symptoms do we find that females, compared to males, are more vulnerable to stressful events. Our study, which uses four different measures as outcomes, suggests that preceding studies of female vulnerability may have unwittingly emphasized the one domain where females show increased vulnerability. In contrast to suggestions in the literature (Bush & Simmons, 1987) that male and female adolescents differentially experience and respond to stressors, both male and female adolescents in our sample appear to be equally vulnerable to stressful events in three out of four domains.

A common theme in the research literature on stressors and their correlates is that persons of lower socioeconomic status are exposed to more stressors and consequently manifest more symptoms of distress (Liem & Liem, 1978; McAdoo, 1986; Neff & Husaini, 1980). On the other hand, it has been suggested that "chronic" stress, such as poverty, is more likely than stressful events to engender psychological impairment (Gersten et al., 1977; Kagan, 1982). Research has found that poverty is tied to depression, impaired school functioning, and conduct disorders (Gibbs, 1986; Myers & King, 1983).

Similar to the findings of other researchers, our data also indicate that stressful events were more common among youths from lower parental education groups. We found no tendency for stressful events to have a greater impact among adolescents in the lower parental education groups. Thus, although studies of adults indicate that the relation between stressful events and health impairment is strongest in the lower class (Dohrenwend & Dohrenwend, 1974; Kessler & Cleary, 1980; Liem & Liem, 1978; McAdoo, 1986; Neff & Husaini, 1980), this did not appear to be the case in our adolescent sample.

Previous studies have indicated that children in single-parent households experience more stressful events and show greater sensitivity to them (Belle, 1984; McAdoo, 1986; Pearlin & Johnson, 1977; Weinraub & Wolf, 1983). With respect to major events, for both sexes, all alternative forms of family structure showed a higher frequency of stressful events than was found in two-natural-parent households. (For these analyses we excluded events involving parental separation, divorce, remarriage, and death of a parent. Thus, our findings by household types are not an artifact of these types of stressful events.) When we looked at the associations between stressful events and health symptoms, grades, and deviance for adolescents in different types of families, we noted that the relations are always in the same direction, with stressful events associated with negative behavioral outcomes. There is no evidence of greater vulnerability in the alternative forms of households. Indeed, stress appears to have a greater impact on youth in two-natural-parent households than on youth in other types of households. We thus have an interesting set of findings: youth from two-natural-parent households report fewer stressful events, but there is a tendency for stress experienced by these youth to have a greater negative impact than for youth in other types of households. Alternatively, youth from other types of households report more stressful events but appear less vulnerable to them.

Much previous research indicates that disadvantaged minorities experience more stress and evidence more symptoms of stress (Dohrenwend & Dohrenwend, 1974; Kessler & Neighbors, 1986; Neff, 1984, 1985). When we looked at our heterogeneous sample, there is some support for these perspectives. Non-Hispanic White youths reported fewer stressful events and more health symptoms than do most minorities. Yet Asian-Americans, in contrast to African-Americans and Hispanics, reported fewer major events and fewer health symptoms than all other groups, including the non-Hispanic Whites. Asian Americans also show high grades and low deviance. When we examine the correlates of stressful events within the different ethnic groups, we find a parallel pattern in each. The general relation between stressful events and negative outcomes is found in each ethnic group. Only for African-Americans is there an apparent attenuation of the magnitude of the association between stressful events and outcomes. We do not understand why the relation is weaker among African-Americans. Although we have examined four outcome variables, perhaps we still have not tapped the aspects of health and functioning most salient for this group.

Recent research (Veroff, Douvan, & Kulka, 1981, p. 437) comparing African-American and White adults on social support, coping, and psychological distress found few race differences on psychological symptoms, and concluded that "Blacks live with greater stress, but they have the personal and social resources to maintain a perspective which keeps the stress external."

A recent study of African-Americans concluded that the effects of race and social class on stress responses interact, and models must take the interaction of these variables into account (Kessler & Neighbors, 1986). We do not yet understand the inconsistencies in our data as we look at each gender-ethnic-parental education group.

Finally, this discussion of sensitivity to stress should be linked to the first findings reported on the domains of stress—personal, familial, and school. The impact of stressors in the personal domain was particularly strong in contrast with family and school events. We interpret this differential to reflect the salience of these more personal experiences during this phase of development. This finding may explain the lack of differentiation among status groups in the association between stress and the four outcomes. Many of these personal events cut across groups and may be highly significant to all youth.

Acknowledgments

This research was supported by the Joseph Drown Foundation and the Stanford Center for the Study of Families, Children and Youth. We express here our thanks to Mi-Jeong Ryu for her assistance in the various stages of data analysis, and to Johanna Zeman and Betsy Scroggs for their help in preparing this manuscript.

References

Belle, D. (1984). Inequality and mental health health: Low income and minority women. In L. Walker (Ed.), *Women and mental health policy* (pp. 135–150). Beverly Hills: Sage Publications.

Boyce, T.W., Jensen, E.W., Cassell, J.C., Collier, A.M., Smith, A.H., & Raimey, C.T. (1977). Influence of life events and family routines on childhood respiratory tract illness. *Pediatrics, 60,* 609–615.

Boyd, J.H., & Weissman, M.M. (1982). Epidemiology. In E.S. Paykel (Ed.), *Handbook of affective disorders* (pp. 109–125). New York: Guilford Press.

Buros, O.K. (Ed.), (1965). *Mental measurements yearbook* (6th ed), Highland Park, NJ: Gryphon Press.

Bush, D.M., & Simmons, R. (1987). Gender and coping with the entry into early adolescence. In R. Barnett, L. Biener, & G. Baruch (Eds.), *Gender and stress* (pp. 185–218). New York: The Free Press.

Cleary, P.D., & Mechanic, D. (1983). Sex differences in psychological distress among married people. *Journal of Health and Social Behavior, 24,* 111–121.

Dohrenwend, B.P., & Dohrenwend, B.S. (1974). Overview and prospects for research on stressful life events. In B.S. Dohrenwend & B. P. Dohrenwend (Eds.), *Stressful life events: Their nature and effects* (pp. 313–331). New York: John Wiley.

Felner, R. D., Stolberg, A.L., & Cowen, E.L. (1975). Crisis events and school mental health referral patterns of young children. *Journal of Consulting and Clinical Psychology, 43,* 305–310.

Gersten, J.C., Langner, T.S., Eisenberg, J.G., & Fagan, O.S. (1977). An evaluation of the etiologic role of stressful life-change events in psychological disorders. *Journal of Health and Social Behavior, 18,* 228–244.

Gibbs, J. (1986). Assessment of depression in urban adolescent females: Implications for early intervention strategies: *American Journal of Social Psychiatry, 6,* 50–56.

Harris, P.W. (1972). *The relationship of life change to academic performance among selected college freshmen at varying levels of college readiness.* Unpublished dissertation, East Texas State University, Commerce, TX.

Hill, J.P., & Lynch, M.E. (1983). The intensification of gender-related role expectations during early adolescence. In J. Brooks-Gunn & A.C. Petersen (Eds.), *Girls at puberty: Biological and psychosocial perspectives.* New York: Plenum.

Hirschfeld, R.M.A., & Cross, C. (1982). Epidemiology of affective disorders. *Archives of General Psychiatry, 39,* 35–46.

Holmes, T.H., & Rahe, R.H. (1967). The social readjustment rating scale. *Journal of Psychosomatic Research, 11,* 213–218.

Hudgens, R.W. (1974). Personal catastrophe and depression: A consideration of the subject with respect to medically ill adolescents, and a requiem for retrospective life event studies. In B.S. Dohrenwend & B.P. Dohrenwend (Eds), *Stressful life events: Their nature and effect* (pp. 119–134), New York: John Wiley.

Johnson, J., & McCutcheon, S. (1980). Assessing life stress in older children and adolescents: Preliminary fundings with the life events checklist. In I. Sarason & C. Spielberger (Eds.), *Stress and Anxiety* (Vol. 6, pp. 111–125). New York: John Wiley.

Kagan, J. (1982). *The nature of the child.* New York: Basic Books.

Kessler, R.C., & Cleary, P.D. (1980). Social class and psychological distress. *American Sociological Review, 45,* 463–478.

Kessler, R.C., & Neighbors, H.W. (1986). A new perspective on the relationships among race, social class, and psychological distress. *Journal of Health and Social Behavior, 27,* 107–115.

Lewis, C.E., Siegel, J.M., & Lewis, M.A. (1984). Feeling bad: Exploring sources of distress among pre-adolescent children. *American Journal of Public Health, 74,*(2), 117–122.

Liem, R., & Liem, J.K. (1978). Social class and mental illness reconsidered: The role of economic stress and social support. *Journal of Health and Social Behavior, 19,* 139–156.

McAdoo, H. (1986). Strategies used by black single mothers against stress. In M. Simms & J. Malveaux (Eds.), *Slipping through the cracks: The status of black women* (pp. 153–166). New Brunswick, NJ: Transaction Books.

Mirowsky, John II, & Ross, C.E. (1980). Minority status, ethnic culture, and distress: A comparison of Blacks, Whites, Mexicans, and Mexican Americans. *American Journal of Sociology, 86,* 479–495.

Myers, H.F., & King, L. (1983). Mental health issues in the development of the black American children. In G. Powell, J. Yamamoto, A. Romero, & A. Morales (Eds.), *The psychosocial development of minority group children* (pp. 275–306). New York: Brunner/Mazel.

Neff, J. (1984). Race differences in psychological distress: The effects of SES, urbanicity, and measurement strategy. *American Journal of Community Psychology, 12,* 337–351.

Neff, J. (1985). Race and vulnerability to stress: An examination of differential vulnerability. *Journal of Personality and Social Psychology, 49,* 481–491.

Neff, J., & Husaini, B. (1980). Race, socioeconomic status, and psychiatric impairment: A research note. *Journal of Community Psychology, 8,* 16–19.

Newcomb, M., Huba, G., & Butler, P. (1981). A multidimensional assessment of stressful life events among adolescents: Derivation and correlates. *Journal of Health and Social Behavior, 22,* 400–414.

Padilla, E.R., Rohsenow, D.J., & Bergman, A.B. (1976). Predicting accident frequency in children. *Pediatrics, 58,* 223–226.

Pearlin, L., & Johnson, J. (1977). Marital status, life-strains and depression. *American Sociological Review, 42,* 704–715.

Pryor Brown, L.J. (1985). *Stressful events as perceived by children.* Unpublished doctoral dissertation. Rochester, New York: University of Rochester.

Pryor Brown, L., Powell, J., & Earls, F. (1989). Stressful life events in Black adolescent females. *Journal of Adolescent Research, 4(2),* 140–151.

Rabkin, J., & Struening, E. (1976). Life events, stress, and illness. *Science, 194,* 1013–1020.

Selye, H. (1956). *The stress of life.* New York: McGraw-Hill.

Sterling, S., Cowen, E.L., Weissberg, R.P., Lotyczewski, B.S., & Boike, M. (1985). Recent stressful life events and young children's school adjustment. *American Journal of Community Psychology, 31,* 87–98.

Thoits, P.A. (1983). Dimensions of life events that influence psychological distress: An evaluation and synthesis of the literature. In H.B. Kaplan (Ed.), *Psychological stress* (pp. 33–103). New York: Academic Press.

Thomas, M.E., & Hughes M. (1986). The continuing significance of race: A study of race, class, and quality of life in America, 1972–1985. *American Sociological Review, 51,* 830–841.

Vaux, A., & Ruggiero, M. (1983). Stressful life change and delinquet behavior. *American Journal of Community Psychology, 11(2),* 169–183.

Veroff, J., Douvan, E., & Kulka, R.A. (1981). *The inner American: A self-portrait from 1957 to 1976.* New York: Basic Books.

Wallerstein, J.S., & Kelly, J. (1980). *Surviving the breakup: How children and parents cope with divorce.* New York: Basic Books.

Warheit, G.J., Holzer, C.E. III, & Arey, S.A. (1975). Race and mental illness: An epidemiologic update. *Journal of Health and Social Behavior, 16,* 243–256.

Weinraub, M., & Wolf, B. (1983). Effects of stress and social supports on mother-child interactions in single- and two-parent families. *Child Development, 54,* 1297–1311.

Wethington, E., McLeod, J., & Kessler, R. (1987). The importance of life events for explaining sex differences in psychological distress. In R. Barnett, L. Biener & G. Baruch, (Eds.), *Gender and stress* (pp. 144–156), New York: The Free Press.

7

How Stressful Is the Transition to Adolescence for Girls?

Jeanne Brooks-Gunn

In asking the question, "how stressful is the transition to adolescence for girls?," I feel as though I am decanting old wine into new bottles or at the very least putting new labels on old bottles. The question is as old as the study of adolescence, and probably even predates it. The transition to adolescence has been characterized as stormy and stressful at least since the time of G. Stanley Hall, the father of adolescent psychology (1904). Much of the early research on adolescence conducted in the 1960s and 1970s focused on testing this commonly accepted premise.

Two of the most popular topics of study were whether storm and stress really were characteristic of almost all young teenagers and whether one's self-image changed dramatically during the transition to adolescence (Nesselroade & Baltes, 1974; Offer, 1987). Somewhat surprisingly, most of this research did not focus on either the biological or social changes that accompany the adolescent transition as possible mediators of tumultuous behavior or alterations in self-images (Brooks-Gunn & Reiter, 1990). Generally, these seminal, early studies did not find much evidence for universal storm or for dramatic, discontinuous changes in self-image (Hamburg, 1974).

These findings altered the landscape of adolescent research in the 1980s considerably. Older, more crisis-oriented models were not employed. Instead, the more normative aspects of the transition became the center-piece. After all, every child experiences puberty, has stirrings of sexual arousal, and, in Western countries, moves from elementary school to middle or high school, which places new social and cognitive demands on the individual. Many researchers, including myself, often focused on the fact that many aspects of the adolescent transition were not particularly stressful, at least for the majority of girls. As an example, in the 1970s, Diane Ruble and I began a series of studies on girls' reactions to menarcheal experiences and the factors that influenced their constructions of menarche and menstruation. Perhaps the most widely cited finding has been the lack of an intense, negative response to menarche, as it contradicted prevailing notions about pubertal experiences (Brooks-Gunn & Ruble, 1982; Grief & Ulman, 1982; Ruble & Brooks-Gunn, 1982).

After our excitement about these stereotype-breaking findings died down, we became intrigued with the sometimes large interindividual variations in young adolescents' experiences and outcomes. As the need to defend the view that many aspects of the adolescent transition were not experienced as a crisis for most girls, it became possible to study those subgroups for whom certain events were problematic and the factors that predicted difficulties. In our menarche research, for example, we found that girls who were early maturers, who did not discuss pubertal events with their mothers, and whose fathers were not told about their daughter's menarche immediately were more likely to have negative reactions to menarche (Brooks-Gunn, 1987; Brooks-Gunn & Ruble, 1982). Today, the question is not whether the transition is stressful, but for which girls, in which circumstances, and at what ages is it stressful. This realignment in the types of questions being posed is true of most of the research on young adolescents (Brooks-Gunn, 1989).

The initial characterization of storm and stress really encompasses two overlapping but not exactly identical dimensions. The stress experienced by the young adolescent is defined here in terms of the potentially stressful life events that characterize the transition from childhood to adolescence. A surge of research on this topic has led to the development of a variety of models linking stressful events to adolescent behavior. Thus, more simplistic tests of whether the occurrence of events is associated with behavior have given way to explorations of how, in what circumstances, and at what ages the occurrence of specific events predict adolescent well-being.

In common parlance, storminess refers to moodiness, rapid shifts in moods, and outbursts of often short-lived negative behavior. In this chapter, I will focus on how much of this type of behavior can be attributed to pubertal changes. Hormones are the prime pubertal change candidate for most individuals, given the deference paid to "raging hormones" explanations for young adolescents' behavior. Other pubertal events that are observable to the adolescent herself as well as to others also should be given their due, and I shall do so here. At the same time, since rapid rises in hormones occur at precisely the time that multiple social changes are encountered, comparisons of relative effects of biological and social changes on moodiness and affective behaviors will be considered.

I would be remiss if the colloquial use of storm and stress were not addressed here. The term itself probably arose from adult experiences in the rearing and teaching of young adolescents (Blos, 1979; Hall, 1904). Parental interchanges with young adolescents are almost always portrayed as conflictual. Personal experiences lend face validity to the characterization of conflict and strife. Indeed, confirmatory evidence of this sort has probably impeded the study of parent–child relationships at this age. At the very least, it has hindered the search for mechanisms underlying conflict when it occurs. Conflict has become reified vis-à-vis interactions between parents and young adolescents. In this chapter, our research team's work on parent–child relationships will be touched upon.

Briefly, then, I address the question "how stressful is the transition to adolescence for girls?" by touring some of the current research on the storminess exhibited by the young adolescence, the potentially stressful events experienced by the young girl, and the conflictual aspects of her relationship with her parents. Rather than focusing on the less interesting question of whether storm and stress exist during this life phase, I consider questions of interindividual variability and the mechanisms underlying such variability. Whenever possible, cognitive, biological, and social mechanisms are posed. Although this approach is preferable in the abstract, in reality, more work has been done on possible biological mechanisms than cognitive mechanisms for most adolescent behavior (Keating, 1990). Exceptions do exist. Research on teenage sexual behavior and contraceptive use is concerned with cognitive correlates (Brooks-Gunn & Furstenberg, 1989; Brooks-Gunn & Paikoff, in press; Paikoff & Brooks-Gunn, in press, a). Social cognitive explanations for increased parent–child conflict during the early adolescent years is another (Smetana, 1988, 1989). And the interesting work on the cognitive underpinnings of depressive affect is yet a third example (Nolen-Hoeksema, Seligman, & Girgus, 1990).

Questions about the long-term implications of the biological and social events occurring during adolescence, while of critical importance, cannot be answered satisfactorally, given the paucity of long-term studies with rich information on the young adolescent (see the chapter by Petersen and associates, this volume, for a more in-depth discussion of longitudinal findings; see Brooks-Gunn, Phelps, & Elder, in press for a discussion of opportunities for secondary data analyses with lengthy longitudinal studies).

Stressful Life Events

Most definitions of stress highlight individuals' responses to events. It is said to occur when an individual is confronted with an event that is perceived as threatening, requires a novel response, is seen as important (i.e., needs to be responded to), and for which an individual does not have an appropriate coping response available (Cohen & Wills, 1985; Lazarus, 1966; Lazarus & Launier, 1978). In a vast literature on adults, the occurrence of stressful life events has been associated with physical illness as well as negative emotional states (Broadhead et al., 1983; Kessler, Price, & Wortman, 1985; Thoits, 1983). Most scholars have assumed that events provoking stressful reactions also influence the well-being of adolescents. The measures of well-being in this literature extend past emotional and physical well-being to include school achievement and behavior problems. Like most of the adult literature, little attention is placed on the four criteria just mentioned; it is assumed that particular events are threatening, novel, and important as well as imbued with uncertainty, vis-à-vis the availability of appropriate responses (see Compas & Wagner, this volume, for a discussion of conceptions of stressful events as well as attempts to categorize events along dimensions such as these four).

Is the transition from childhood to adolescence a particularly stressful time in an individual's life? After all, many of the events occurring for most young adolescents are novel, perhaps threatening, and important. Indeed, the concentration of events occurring at this time might be one of two aspects of this transition that marks it as distinct from other life transitions, the other aspect beginning puberty itself (Brooks-Gunn, 1988). Almost no research has addressed the issue of distinctiveness in number or type of social events that the young adolescent faces. Also, whether a limited number of coping responses is available is not known. It seems plausible that few coping responses would be found in a prepubertal child's quiver that would be appropriate for events such as dating; moving to a large, less personal school; and making decisions about behaviors such as smoking, drinking, and sexual intercourse. However, several investigative groups are developing models for studying the timing, sequencing, type, and number of events that young teenagers face.

Three of the more promising approaches are presented here (see Compas & Wagner, this volume and Petersen et al., this volume, for other examples). All three make a distinction between biological and social events taking place at this time, since one of the striking features of this transition is puberty and all that it entails. One model focuses on the interaction of different life events, a second looks at the effects of number of life events occurring in any one year, and the third tests the effects of different features of life events (timing, novelty, number of events, number of events relative to one's peers, and type of event).

Interaction of Pubertal and Social Events

Much of my work delves into the interaction of pubertal and social events. The premise is that certain social events are experienced differently as a function of pubertal development. Puberty acts as a social stimulus for others, altering how adults and peers respond to the girl as her body develops. Given the wide variability in physical development in young adolescents of any given age, studies have been able to tease apart effects of age and pubertal development. Examples include the increased independence given to girls by their parents, interest by boys, and in some cases enhanced same-sex peer relationships, as a function of increases in maturity and controlling for age (Brooks-Gunn, Samelson, Warren, & Fox, 1986; Brooks-Gunn & Warren, 1988; Magnusson, Strattin, & Allen, 1985; Simmons & Blyth, 1987). In other cultures, heightened parental vigilance accompanies pubertal growth as a protection against male interest (Hill & Lynch, 1983).

At the same time, girls' own experiences and interpretations of pubertal events influence how they respond to or interpret social events. As girls mature, they demand more independence from their parents (Simmons & Blyth, 1987). In some cases, they seek out girlfriends who are similar in pubertal maturation (Brooks-Gunn et al., 1986).

More substantive evidence of interactions is found in studies looking at the context in which girls develop physically. David Magnusson and his colleagues (1985) attempted to understand why early maturing girls are likely to engage in smoking and drinking sooner than later maturing girls. They found that the effect was due to many early maturers having older friends who presumably were engaging in such behaviors, which were normative for their age cohort. Roberta Simmons, Dale Blyth, and their colleagues report that early maturing girls have more difficulty moving to middle school in sixth grade than do their peers who are on-time or late maturers and who therefore are not in the midst of puberty during this school transition (Blyth, Simmons, & Zakin, 1985; Simmons, Blyth, & McKinney, 1983).

Our research team has reported that timing of maturation is associated with dating behavior in dancers but not in nondancers (Gargiulo, Attie, Brooks-Gunn, & Warren, 1987). We posited that early and on-time maturing dancers, because their bodies do not fit the prevailing standards for elite dancers (and we were working with national ballet school companies, which are the training ground for elite dancers), begin to turn away from dance. They do not have the long linear bodies that are valued in the dance world (Hamilton, Brooks-Gunn, Warren, & Hamilton, 1988). Such a mismatch becomes evident at puberty, and the late maturing dancers continue their focus on dance, while their earlier maturing peers move toward the nondance peer culture. Additional support for these speculations come from another study in which on-time dancers had poorer emotional well-being, more negative body images, and higher eating problem scores than did late maturing dancers; such differences were not found for nondancers (Brooks-Gunn & Warren, 1985b). Comparisons with other athletic groups also reinforce our beliefs that effects such as those discussed here are due to an emphasis on thinness, not on athletics per se (Brooks-Gunn, Attie, Burrow, Rosso, & Warren, 1989; Brooks-Gunn, Burrow, & Warren, 1988).

Another window on possible interactions between pubertal and biological events is provided by a study of fifth to seventh graders where depressive symptomatology was the outcome. Main effects of pubertal events (menarche, breast growth, and timing of maturation) and negative and positive social events (family, peer, school) were examined simultaneously. Negative social events occurring in the past 6 months were associated with more depressive affect, while positive events were not (as expected from the adult literature). Somewhat surprisingly, pubertal events were not associated either. However, interactions between pubertal and negative social events were found: For example, premenarcheal girls who experienced negative family events were more depressed than postmenarcheal girls who experienced the same events (Brooks-Gunn, Warren, & Rosso, 1990). We suggested that the postmenarcheal girls had more opportunity to receive social support from peers than premenarcheal girls, a premise that was partially supported.

Cumulative Effects of Events

Simmons and her colleagues (1988) have conducted an elegant study demonstrating the effects of sheer number of events on middle school children's well-being. In these analyses, the addition of life events increased the report of school problems, both academic and behavioral, and decreased self-esteem scores. The associations were primarily linear and were found for both boys and girls. In these analyses, social events as well as one biological event were entered into the equations; separate effects of each were not explored, except to say that all events contributed to the decrements in well-being via a cumulative pathway.

Type, Novelty, and Relativity of Events

In a recent analyses, Nazli Baydar and I attempted to build on the two approaches just mentioned to extend them in several ways. Our earlier work and that of Simmons and her colleagues demonstrated that the number of life events, particularly negative social ones, is linked to decrements in well-being. However, we still did not know what it was about the events that contribute to decrements. Accordingly, we specified five hypotheses to test in our 4-year longitudinal study using depressive symptomatology as our measure of decrement in well-being: (1) The multitude of life experiences during a given time period will increase depressive symptoms due to their cumulative load on resources for coping. (2) The number of experiences in excess of that experienced by an adolescent's peers will increase depressive symptoms. This premise has not been tested in previous studies. (3) The novelty of a particular kind of experience will increase depressive symptoms more than subsequent experiences. This premise is particularly important to test in that it is believed that young adolescents experience more novel events than other age groups. (4) The occurrence of a novel experience will have an increased impact for young adolescents, due to an increase in emotional vulnerability prior to age 14. (5) Particular types of events will lead to an increase in depressive symptoms. Family and peer events were the most likely candidates (Baydar & Brooks-Gunn, 1990, p. 2).

We also tested three hypotheses with respect to pubertal events: (1) Pubertal growth will affect depressive symptoms due to the meaning of these changes to the self and to others, as previously discussed. (2) The timing of maturation will be associated with depressive symptoms, although most research has looked at body image and self-esteem decrements rather than depressive symptoms (Blyth et al., 1985; Brooks-Gunn & Warren, 1985b; Magnusson et al., 1985; Petersen & Crockett, 1985). Generally, pubertal timing efforts are stronger than pubertal status effects (Brooks-Gunn & Reiter, 1990). (3) Tempo of pubertal development may influence depressive symptoms, although this has been rarely studied (Brooks-Gunn & Warren, 1985a; Eichorn, 1975).

Depressive symptoms increased most between the ages of 13 and 14, although increases occurred through age 15. This confirms beliefs that depressive symptoms are quite high for the young adolescent (although we have no measure of depressive symptoms in late childhood in this study for true across life phase comparisons). The peak of increase in depressive symptoms at ages 13 to 14 was due primarily to the large number of life events experienced at this age, not to pubertal changes directly.

Number of life events are associated with an increase in depressive symptoms over the 4 years; these effects were due to the number of events in any year, rather than to an increase in the number of events experienced over time. Importantly, the number of events experienced relative to one's peers was more important than the sheer number of events, although both made significant contributions. Novelty of events was not important, nor was the type of events.

Pubertal changes played a much less significant role than did life events in the developmental course of depressive affect in this sample of girls. Pubertal changes or rate of changes did not contribute to depressive symptoms. However, late maturation acted as a protective factor against depressive symptoms. These findings parallel previous findings for body image (Brooks-Gunn, 1988; Petersen, Sarigiani & Kennedy, 1990).

Storminess in the Young Adolescent Girl

Storminess, as evidenced by intense, negative, and labile moods, is believed to characterize the young adolescent's emotional landscape. Results are mixed on whether, or in what circumstances, this is true. Research on girls has focused on depressive symptoms more than on lability or other emotional states. Studies of clinical depression report a dramatic rise in the pubertal and postpubertal period (Rutter, Graham, Chadwick, & Yule, 1976). Depressive symptoms have been reported to be higher at ages 13 and 14 in our research as just mentioned as well as by others (Brooks-Gunn & Petersen, 1991). However, not all studies report such rises. These across study differences in part are due to the different measures used, the different ages tested, and the different composition of the samples (see special issue of *Journal of Youth and Adolescence*; Brooks-Gunn & Petersen, 1991).

Hormonal factors have been suggested as a contributor to the expected increases in depressive symptoms. Hormonal levels rise rapidly during the pubertal years. Since no one-to-one correspondence exists between secondary sexual characteristics and hormonal levels, it is possible to examine the contribution of internal and external pubertal changes on the young adolescent's emotions (Brooks-Gunn & Reiter, 1990; Petersen & Taylor, 1980). Such a separation is critical since we know that the changes in secondary sexual characteristics influence how others treat the developing child and how the child perceives herself, as discussed earlier.

Several investigative groups are examining hormone-behavior links during the pubertal period (see Paikoff & Brooks-Gunn (1990) for a review of pubertal hormone-behavior links across a variety of domains of well-being). All studies are focusing on what is called activational effects of hormonal functioning at puberty; these are possible direct effects of hormonal rises on emotional states or on arousal levels, which in turn might influence emotional states. In contrast, organizational effects involve the effects of prenatal levels of circulating hormones on brain organization that might influence subsequent pubertal rises or hormones or more likely, the brain's responses to the increased levels at puberty. Currently, no study has gathered data on hormonal environment both prenatally and pubertally (Paikoff & Brooks-Gunn, 1990).

Depressive Symptomatology

Two research groups have examined the links of hormonal levels during puberty and depressive symptoms, lability, and hormonal environment. In our Adolescent Study Program, 100 girls in fifth to seventh grade had hormonal data available. We have found links between reported emotions and hormones. Michelle Warren has classified hormonal functioning into four categories based on the effects of estradiol on internal reproductive functioning. There are four groupings: (1) Levels of less than 25 pg/ml of estradiol have little effect. (2) Levels of 25–50 pg/ml have early visible physiological effects such as secondary sexual development, and effects on the vagina estrogens at this level are generally not significant enough to cause proliferation of the endometrium and withdrawal bleeding with a progesterone challenge. (3) Levels of 50–75 pg/ml typically are commensurate with middle or late puberty and early follicular levels in menstruating girls. These levels have significant effects on endometrial growth and other organs such as the breast. (4) Levels greater than 75 pg/ml are associated with cyclicity in women (Gold & Iosimovich, 1980; Grumbach & Sizonenko, 1986; Warren & Brooks-Gunn, 1989). Although these groupings were based on estradiol levels, they also take into account levels of luteinizing hormone (LH) and follicle-stimulating hormone (FSH). Looking at these levels, we found that depressive symptomatology increases from level 1 to level 3 but not from level 3 to level 4 (Warren & Brooks-Gunn, 1989). Pubertal stage of development did not influence these findings (Brooks-Gunn & Warren, 1989).

Another research group looking at hormonal links with depressive symptoms reports no associations for girls (Susman et al., 1987). When our data are analyzed in a similar fashion, no effects are found, either. A difference between studies is that our research group used self-reports and maternal reports of depressive symptoms while the other group used maternal reports of depressive symptoms only. Our depressive symptom–hormone link findings exist for self-reports but not for maternal reports (Warren & Brooks-Gunn, 1989).

Our group has also looked at short-term longitudinal effects of hormonal levels on girls' reports of depressive symptoms. Higher levels of estradiol at the initial testing are associated with higher levels of depressive symptoms 1 year later, even controlling for initial depressive symptoms (Paikoff, Brooks-Gunn, & Warren, 1991). Pubertal status and age did not influence these results.

What is the relative influence of hormonal levels? We know from the previous discussion that social events are more predictive of depressive symptoms than are pubertal events other than hormonal levels. In an analysis entering social events and hormonal events, hormonal levels as characterized by estradiol levels accounted for about 1% of the variance in depressive symptoms while negative life events accounted for 8% of the variance (Brooks-Gunn & Warren, 1989). Such findings suggest that hormonal functioning plays a role, albeit a small one, in the young adolescent's report of depressive symptoms.

Mood Lability

Only one research group has looked at mood swings with respect to hormonal functioning (see Csikszentmihalyi & Larson, 1984, for an excellent study of mood lability in and of itself, rather than on the biological mechanisms underlying mood lability). An unpublished doctoral thesis in which hormonal concentrations and variability and mood intensity and variability were studied over a day and a month in 24 girls suggested that high follicle-stimulating hormone (FSH) variability, but not variability in progesterone or testosterone, was associated with moodiness within a day. High FSH concentration was associated with moodiness over a month (Buchanan & Eccles, 1989). Pubertal status was associated with mood intensity and variability over the 1-month period as well. Since estradiol could not be measured, as this study used saliva samples to estimate hormonal levels and measures of estradiol from saliva in pre- and early-pubertal girls are unreliable, it is difficult to compare these results to those found by our research group for depressive symptoms.

Aggressive Symptomatology

Links between hormonal levels and aggressive behaviors or emotions have been found for boys and girls (Olweus, Mattsson, Schalling, & Low, 1980, 1988). Higher levels of testosterone were associated with increases in impatience and irritability, which in turn increased the tendency toward aggressive-destructive behavior in the study by Dan Olweus and colleagues. Estradiol levels were negatively and androstenedione levels were positively associated with parental reports of aggression and delinquency in boys in another study (Inoff-Germain, 1986; Susman et al., 1987).

In girls, adrenal androgens, specifically dehydroepiandrosterone (DHEA) and dehydroepiandrosterone sulfate (DHEAS), were negatively associated with reports of aggressive behavior in the two studies of girls already discussed (Brooks-Gunn & Warren, 1989; Susman et al., 1987).

Also, in our study, estradiol category was associated with aggressive symptoms in a similar fashion to the depressive symptom findings (Warren & Brooks-Gunn, 1989). Progesterone and aggression also were associated in the two studies that measured progesterone rather than estradiol (Udry & Talbert, 1988; Eccles et al., 1988).

Putting these findings into a richer context, our research group compared the relative effects of hormonal functioning and social events. We found that DHEAS accounted for 4% of the variance in aggressive symptoms while negative events accounted for 18% of the variance and an interaction of negative events and DHEAS for an additional 15% of the variance (Brooks-Gunn & Warren, 1989). These findings suggest that hormones play a larger role in aggressive than in depressive symptomatology.

Storm and Stress in Parental Relationships

The cornerstone of the storm and stress characterization has to do not with how social and biological events influence the young adolescent's well-being, but how the young adolescent interacts with others. And perhaps the greatest concern, at least from an adult perspective, is how parent–child interchanges are affected during the adolescent transition. Not only are such interactions believed to be transformed but they are thought to be rife with conflict. The transformations are portrayed as a change from unilateral authority to mutuality, from a more vertical to a somewhat more horizontal relationship (Hartup, 1989; Youniss, 1985). However, conceptual models stressing renegotiation models have not been applied to the young adolescent or to the pubertal years directly, instead being used for older adolescents (Grotevant & Cooper, 1985).

Instead, the measures that have been used to study parent–child interactions at this time include time spent with parents, perceptions of relationships as less positive, emotional distance, and yielding to parents in decision making. All four decrease from early to middle adolescence (Csikszentmihalyi & Larson, 1984; Hill, 1988; Montemayor & Hanson, 1985; Steinberg, 1987; Youniss, 1985).

Much of the research focuses on conflict. Conflict seems to be higher in early adolescence, although the frequency of conflict is similar in early and middle adolescence (Montemayor & Hanson, 1985). The conflict is not intense and does not necessarily presage a diminution of a strong bond between parents and children. Although mild, both parents and children agree that these conflicts are significant (Smetana, 1988, 1989). Adolescents tend to see conflicts occurring more frequently than do parents.

These increases have been postulated to be due to self-definitional change, social cognitive alterations, direct biological changes,
and psychodynamic processes (see Brooks-Gunn, Zahaykevich, 1989
and Paikoff & Brooks-Gunn, in press b, for a discussion of each of
these perspectives). We have argued that self-definitional changes
are in part due to the meaning of pubertal changes. The underlying
mechanism could be based on conflicting feelings being elicited by
pubertal change or a reorganization of self-definitions based on bodily
changes and the social role alterations that accompany such bodily
changes. For example, although almost all girls learn about pubertal
changes, in particular menarche, from their mothers, they tend not to
discuss their feelings with her, instead turning to girlfriends (Brooks-
Gunn & Ruble, 1983). In some cases, girls perceive their mothers and
fathers as insensitive to the concerns about body changes. An example is
the fact that fifth and sixth graders perceive their parents' comments
about their breast development as teasing (Brooks-Gunn, 1984). In one
study where sixth to eighth graders were shown a picture of an adult
woman showing a girl and an adult male a bra that she has just taken out
of a shopping bag, the most common responses are embarrassment
about the father's presence and anger at the mother for showing the
bra to the father (Brooks-Gunn, Newman, & Warren, 1990; Brooks-Gunn
& Zahaykevich, 1989). I suspect that these research findings are in-
dicative of girls' reluctance to discuss pubertal events in any detail at
home and, even more strongly, in front of their fathers. Such situations
may elicit conflict.

Biological changes also may contribute to conflict. The mechanism here
would be increased moodiness or lability, which plays itself out as
storminess in parental interactions. Hormonal changes do influence
moods, making this pathway plausible. At the same time, social events
have an even greater role in emotional well-being. Given that the young
adolescent is experiencing a number of events, the cumulative load of
events (or events relative to her peers) may be triggering conflictual
interactions via low impulse control and depressive and aggressive
symptomatology.

Social cognitive perspectives on conflict have been elegantly studied by
Smetana (1988). She finds that teenagers and parents disagree as to the
legitimacy of parental authority in many situations. Teenagers tend to
classify more situations as involving personal choice, and parents categorize more situations as involving social conventions. The greatest shift
toward personal choice categorizations by children occurs between fifth
and sixth and to seventh and eighth grade for teenagers. Parent–child
disagreements are largest in the middle school years. It is important that
many of the seventh and eighth graders understand but reject their

parents' perspective for issues in which they believe personal jurisdiction is legitimate.

Psychodynamic perspectives are the least studied of the possible mechanisms listed here. Generally, this perspective predicts that young adolescent girls will go through an initial aggressive and oppositional phase of interaction with their parents, before reverting to more passive modes of resistance to parental authority, such as indifference and denial. A few studies find support for this thesis (Brooks-Gunn & Zahaykevich, 1989; Hill, 1988). The psychodynamic perspective is especially valuable for highlighting parents' needs to recognize the separateness of their daughters, not just daughters' needs to be more autonomous (Blos, 1979).

Thus far, I have considered conflicts between parents and daughters with no consideration of possible differences in conflicts for mothers and fathers. Generally, mother–daughter conflicts are more pronounced than conflicts in other parent–child combinations (Montemayor, 1982; Smetana, 1989). Why this is the case has not been studied extensively. Following many theorists, I believe that mothers and daughters may have more extreme conflicts because their relationship may be closer than that of mothers and sons or fathers and daughters or sons. Chodorow (1978) argues that mothers get gratification from parenting because they experience feelings of closeness and that such feelings are stronger with their daughters because of same-sex identification. This premise has not been tested extensively. However, comparisons of observational studies of mothers with sons and daughters do highlight differences in interactions as function of sex of the pubertal child (Steinberg & Hill, 1978; Hill, 1988). However, whether the mother–daughter relationships are more difficult than mother–son ones has not been studied.

Another approach to the issue of conflict involves looking at parent–child agreements as to the climate of the home. Carlton-Ford, Paikoff & Brooks-Gunn (in press) are conducting such analyses, finding that disagreements are associated with decrements in adolescent girls' well-being. In a recent study, Ilana Attie and I (1989) found that maternal perceptions of a difficult home environment were associated with the daughters' eating problems while the daughters' perceptions were not. Such research, while not focusing on conflict *qua* conflict, provides a window on how differing perceptions of the family and parent–child relationships influence young adolescents' well-being.

Conclusion

I hope that this brief tour of some of our recent findings, as well as those of others, sheds some light on more than just whether the transition to adolescence is stressful, but on what aspects are stressful and what mechanisms account for some events being perceived or experienced as stressful. Clearly, the concentrations of events occurring during the transition to adolescence are a major aspect of stress at this time. Experiencing more events than one's peers also is a stressor. Finally, being a late maturer protects some young adolescents from the untoward effects of negative events.

Although storminess also seems to characterize the transition, the results are more mixed. Hormonal influences play a role, albeit a small one. However, social events are more predictive of negative affect than are hormonal changes.

The storm and stress of parental conflict is seen across studies. Recent research is focusing on the mechanisms underlying such conflict. The richness and diversity of perspectives being studied are heartening and appropriate, given how complex the transition towards adolescence actually is.

Acknowledgments

The research presented in this chapter was supported by the National Institute of Child Health and Human Development and the W. T. Grant Foundation; their support is greatly appreciated. Rosemary Deibler and Florence Kelly are to be thanked for their help in manuscript preparation. The research discussed here could not have been done without the collaboration of Roberta Paikoff, Nazli Baydar, Linda Hamilton, Michelle Warren, and our research staff and students; I am pleased to have had the opportunity to work with them.

References

Attie, I., & Brooks-Gunn, J. (1990). The development of eating problems in adolescent girls: A longitudinal study. *Developmental Psychology, 25*(1), 70–79.

Baydar, N., Brooks-Gunn, J. (1990, March). *Determinants of negative emotional expression in adolescent girls: A four year longitudinal study.* Paper presented in a Symposium entitled, "Timing of Maturation and Adolescent Problem Behavior in Differing Cultural Contexts," at the Society for Research on Adolescence, Atlanta, GA.

Blos, P. (1979). *The adolescent passage.* New York: International Universities Press.

Blyth, D. A., Simmons, R. G., & Zakin, D. F. (1985). Satisfaction with body image for early adolescent females: The impact of pubertal timing within different school environments. *Journal of Youth and Adolescence, 14*(3), 207–225.

Broadhead, W. E., Kaplan, B. H., et al. (1983, May). The epidemiologic evidence for a relationship between social support and health. *American Journal of Epidemiology, 117*(5), 521–537.

Brooks-Gunn, J. (1984). The psychological significance of different pubertal events to young girls. *Journal of Early Adolescence, 4*(4), 315–327.

Brooks-Gunn, J. (1987). Pubertal processes and girls' psychological adaptation. In R. Lerner & T. T. Foch (Eds.), *Biological-psychosocial interactions in early adolescence: A life-span perspective* (pp. 123–153). Hillsdale, NJ: Lawrence Erlbaum Associates.

Brooks-Gunn, J. (1988). Antecedents and consequences of variations in girls' maturational timing. *Journal of Adolescent Health Care, 9*(5), 365–373.

Brooks-Gunn, J. (1989). Adolescents as children and as parents: A developmental perspective. In I. E. Sigel and G. H. Brody (Eds.), *Methods of family research: Biographies of research projects, Volume I: Normal families* (pp. 213–248). Hillsdale, NJ: Lawrence Erlbaum Associates.

Brooks-Gunn, J., Attie, I., Burrow, C., Rosso, J. T., Warren, M. P. (1989). The impact of puberty on body and eating concerns in different athletic and nonathletic contexts. *Journal of Early Adolescence, 9*(3), 269–290.

Brooks-Gunn, J., Burrow, C., & Warren, M. P. (1988). Attitudes toward eating and body weight in different groups of female adolescent athletes. *International Journal of Eating Disorders, 7*(6), 749–758.

Brooks-Gunn, J., & Furstenberg, F. F., Jr. (1989). Adolescent sexual behavior. *American Psychologist, 44*(2), 313–320.

Brooks-Gunn, J., Newman, D., and Warren, M. P. (1990). Significance of breast growth. Unpublished manuscript.

Brooks-Gunn, J., & Paikoff, R. L. (in press). "Sex is a gamble, kissing is a game": Adolescent sexuality, contraception, and pregnancy. In S. P. Millstein, A. C. Petersen, & E. Nightingale (Eds.), *Promotion of Health Behavior in Adolescence.* NY: Carnegie Corporation.

Brooks-Gunn, J., & Petersen, A. C. (Eds.). (1991). The emergence of depression in adolescence. *Journal of Youth and Adolescence, 19*(6).

Brooks-Gunn, J., Phelps, E., & Elder, G. H. (in press). Studying lives through time: Secondary data analyses in developmental psychology. *Developmental Psychology.*

Brooks-Gunn, J., & Reiter, E. O. (1990). The role of pubertal processes in the early adolescent transition. In S. Feldman & G. Elliott (Eds.), *At the threshold: The developing adolescent* (pp. 16–53) Cambridge: Harvard University Press.

Brooks-Gunn, J., & Ruble, D. N. (1982). The development of menstrual-related beliefs and behaviors during early adolescence. *Child Development, 53,* 1567–1577.

Brooks-Gunn, J., & Ruble, D. N. (1983). The experience of menarche from a developmental perspective. In J. Brooks-Gunn & A. C. Petersen (Eds.), *Girls at puberty: Biological and psychosocial perspectives* (pp. 155–177). New York: Plenum Press.

Brooks-Gunn, J., Samelson, M., Warren, M. P., & Fox, R. (1986). Physical similarity of and disclosure of menarcheal status to friends: Effects of age and pubertal status. *Journal of Early Adolescence, 6*(1), 3–14.

Brooks-Gunn, J., & Warren, M. P. (1985a). Measuring physical status and timing in early adolescence: A developmental perspective. *Journal of Youth and Adolescence, 14*(3), 163–189.

Brooks-Gunn, J., & Warren, M. P. (1985b). Effects of delayed menarche in different contexts: Dance and nondance students. *Journal of Youth and Adolescence*, 14(4), 285–300.

Brooks-Gunn, J., & Warren, M. P. (1988). The psychological significance of secondary sexual characteristics in 9- to 11-year-old girls. *Child Development, 59*, 161–169.

Brooks-Gunn, J., & Warren, M. P. (1989). Biological contributions to affective expression in young adolescent girls. *Child Development, 60*, 372–385.

Brooks-Gunn, J., Warren, M. P., & Rosso, J. (1990). The impact of pubertal and social events upon girls' problem behavior. Unpublished manuscript.

Brooks-Gunn, J., & Zahaykevich, M. (1989). Parent-child relationships in early adolescence: A developmental perspective. In K. Kreppner & R. M. Lerner (Eds.), *Family systems and life-span development* (pp. 223–246). Hillsdale, NJ: Erlbaum.

Buchanan, C. M., & Eccles, J. (1989). Evidence for activational effects of hormones on moods and behavior at adolescence. Unpublished manuscript.

Carlton-Ford, S., Paikoff, R., Brooks-Gunn, J. (in press). Models for assessing effects of disagreement on adolescents and their parents. In R. L. Paikoff & W. A. Collins (Eds.), *New directions for child development: Implications of disagreements about family functioning for adolescents and their parents.*

Chodorow, N. (1978). *The reproduction of mothering: Psychoanalysis and sociology of gender.* Berkeley: University of California.

Cohen, S., & Wills, T. A. (1985). Stress, social support, and the buffering hypothesis. *Psychological Bulletin, 98*(2), 310–357.

Csikszentmihalyi, M., & Larson, R. (1984). *Being adolescent: Conflict and growth in the teenage years.* New York: Basic Books.

Eccles, J. S., Miller, C., Tucker, M. L., Becker, J., Schramm, W., Midgley, R., Holmes, W., Pasch, L., & Miller, M. (1988). *Hormones and affect at early adolescence.* Paper presented at the Biannual Meeting of the Society for Research on Adolescence, Alexandria, VA.

Eichorn, D. E. (1975). Asynchronizations in adolescent development. In S. E. Dragastin and G. H. Elder, Jr. (Eds.), *Adolescence in the life cycle: Psychosocial change and the social context* (pp. 82–96). Hillsdale, NJ: Halsted Press, (Wiley).

Gargiulo, J., Attie, I., Brooks-Gunn, J., & Warren, M. P. (1987). Girls' dating behavior as a function of social context and maturation. *Developmental Psychology, 23*(5), 730–737.

Gold, J. J., & Iosimovich, J. (1980). *Gynecologic endocrinology.* New York: Harper & Row.

Grief, E. B., & Ulman, K. J. (1982). The psychologic impact of menarche on early adolescent females: A review of the literature. *Child Development, 53*, 1413–1430.

Grotevant, H. D., & Cooper, C. R. (1985). Patterns of interaction in family relationships and the development of identity exploration in adolescence. *Child Development, 56*, 415–428.

Grumbach, M. M., & Sizonenko, P. C. (Eds.). (1986). *Control of the onset of puberty II.* New York: Academic Press.

Hall, G. S. (1904). *Adolescence: Its psychology and its relations to physiology, anthropology, sociology, sex, crime, religion and education.* NY: Appleton & Co.

Hamburg, B. A. (1974). Early adolescence: A specific and stressful stage of the life cycle. In G. V. Coelho, B. A. Hamburg, & J. E. Adams (Eds.), *Coping and adaptation* (pp. 101–124). New York: Basic Books.

Hamilton, L. H., Brooks-Gunn, J., Warren, M. P., & Hamilton, W. G. (1988). The role of selectivity in the pathogenesis of eating disorders. *Medicine and Science in Sports and Exercise, 20*(6), 560–565.

Hartup, W. W. (1989). Social relationships and their developmental significance. *American Psychologist, 44*(2), 120–126.

Hill, J. P. (1988). Adapting to menarche: Familial control and conflict. In M. R. Gunnar & W. A. Collins (Eds.), *Development during the transition to adolescence* (Vol. 21, pp. 43–77). Hillsdale, NJ: Erlbaum.

Hill, J. P., & Lynch, M. E. (1983). The intensification of gender-related role expectations during early adolescence. In J. Brooks-Gunn & A. C. Petersen (Eds.), *Girls at puberty: Biological and psychosocial perspectives* (pp. 201–228). New York: Plenum.

Inoff-Germain, G. (1986). *Hormones and aggression in early adolescence.* Paper presented at the first Biennial meeting of the Society for Research on Adolescence, Madison, WI.

Keating, D. P. (1990). Adolescent thinking. In S. Feldman & G. Elliott (Eds.), *At the threshold: The developing adolescent.* Cambridge: Harvard University Press.

Kessler, R. C., Price, R. H., & Wortman, C. B. (1985). Social factors in psychopathology: Stress, social support, and coping processes. *Annual Review of Psychology, 36*, 531–572.

Lazarus, R. S. (1966). *Psychological stress and the coping process.* New York: McGraw-Hill.

Lazarus, R. S., & Launier, R. (1978). Stress-related transactions between person and environment. In L. A. Pervin, & M. Lewis (Eds.), *Perspectives in interactional psychology.* New York: Plenum Press.

Magnusson, D., Strattin, H., & Allen, V. L. (1985). Biological maturation and social development: A longitudinal study of some adjustment processes from mid-adolescence to adulthood. *Journal of Youth and Adolescence, 14*(4), 267–283.

Montemayor, R. (1982). The relationship between parent-adolescent conflict and the amount of time adolescents spend alone and with parents and peers. *Child Development, 53*, 1512–1519.

Montemayor, R., & Hanson, E. A. (1985). A naturalistic view of conflict between adolescents and their parents and siblings. *Journal of Early Adolescence, 5*, 23–30.

Nesselroade, J. R., & Baltes, P. B. (1974). Adolescent personality development and historical change: 1970–1972. *Monographs of the Society of Research in Child Development, 39*(1) (Serial No. 154).

Nolen-Hoeksema, S., Seligman, M. E. P., & Girgus, J. S. (1991). A longitudinal study of depression in pre-adolescents: Sex differences in depression and related factors. *Journal of Youth and Adolescence, 20*(1).

Offer, D. (1987). In defense of adolescents. *Journal of the American Medical Association, 257*(24), 3407–3408.

Olweus, D., Mattsson, A., Schalling, D., & Low, H. (1980). Testosterone, aggression, physical, and personality dimensions in normal adolescent males. *Psychosomatic Medicine, 42*(2), 253–269.

Olweus, D., Mattsson, A., Schalling, D., & Low, H. (1988). Circulating testosterone levels and aggression in adolescent males: A casual analysis. *Psychosomatic Medicine, 50,* 261–272.

Paikoff, R. L., & Brooks-Gunn, J. (1990). Physiological processes: What role do they play during the transition to adolescence? In: R. Montemayor, G. Adams, & T. Gullotta (Eds.), *Advances in adolescent development: Vol. 2, The transition from childhood to adolescence* (pp. 63–81). Newbury Park, CA: Sage.

Paikoff, R. L., & Brooks-Gunn, J. (in press a). Taking fewer chances: Teenage pregnancy prevention programs. *American Psychologist.*

Paikoff, R., & Brooks-Gunn, J. (in press b). Do parent-child relationships change during puberty? *Psychological Bulletin.*

Paikoff, R. L., Brooks-Gunn, J., & Warren, M. P. (1991). Long-term effects of hormonal change on affective expression in adolescent females. *Journal of Youth and Adolescence, 20*(1).

Petersen, A. C., & Crockett, L. (1985). Pubertal timing and grade effects on adjustment. *Journal of Youth and Adolescence, 14*(3), 191–206.

Petersen, A. C., Sarigiani, P. A., & Kennedy, R. E. (1991). Adolescent depression: Why more girls? *Journal of Youth and Adolescence, 20*(1).

Petersen, A. C., & Taylor, B. (1980). The biological approach to adolescence: Biological change and psychological adaptation. In J. Adelson (Ed.), *Handbook of Adolescent Psychology* (pp. 117–155). New York: John Wiley.

Ruble, D. N., & Brooks-Gunn, J. (1982). The experience of menarche. *Child Development, 53,* 1557–1566.

Rutter, M., Graham, P., Chadwick, O. F., & Yule, W. (1976). Adolescent turmoil: Fact or fiction. *Journal of Child Psychology and Psychiatry, 17,* 35–56.

Simmons, R. G., & Blyth, D. A. (Eds.) (1987). *Moving into adolescence: The impact of pubertal change and school context.* New York: Aldine de Gruyter.

Simmons, R. G., Blyth, D. A., & McKinney, K. L. (1983). The social and psychological effects of puberty on white females. In J. Brooks-Gunn & A. C. Petersen (Eds.), *Girls at puberty: Biological and psychosocial perspectives* (pp. 229–272). New York: Plenum Press.

Simmons, R. G., Burgeson, R., & Reef, M. J. (1988). Cumulative change at entry to adolescence. In M. Gunnar & W. A. Collins (Eds.), *Development during transition to adolescence: Minnesota symposia on child psychology* (Vol. 21, pp. 123–150). Hillsdale, NJ: Erlbaum.

Smetana, J. G. (1988). Concepts of self and social convention: Adolescents' and parents' reasoning about hypothetical and actual family conflicts. In M. Gunnar & W. A. Collins (Eds.), *Development during transition to adolescence: Minnesota symposia on child psychology* (Vol. 21, pp. 79–122). Hillsdale, NJ: Erlbaum.

Smetana, J. G. (1989). Adolescents' and parents' conceptions of parental authority. *Child Development, 59*(2), 321–335.

Steinberg, L. D. (1987). The impact of puberty on family relations: Effects of pubertal status and pubertal timing. *Developmental Psychology, 23,* 451–460.

Steinberg, L. D., & Hill, J. P. (1978). Patterns of family interaction as a function of age, the onset of puberty, and formal thinking. *Developmental Psychology, 14,* 683–684.

Susman, E. J., Inoff-Germain, G., Nottelmann, E. D., Loriaux, D. L., Cutler, G. B., & Chrousos, G. P. (1987). Hormones, emotional dispositions, and aggressive attributes in young adolescents. *Child Development, 58,* 1114–1134.

Thoits, P. A. (1983). Dimensions of life events that influence psychological distress: An evaluation of synthesis of the literature. In H. P. Kaplan (Ed.), *Psychosocial stress: Trends in theory and research* (pp. 33–103). New York: Academic Press.

Udry, J. R., & Talbert, L. M. (1988). Sex hormone effects on personality at puberty. *Journal of Personality and Social Psychology, 54*(2), 291–295.

Warren, M. P., & Brooks-Gunn, J. (1989). Mood and behavior at adolescence: Evidence for hormonal factors. *Journal of Clinical Endocrinology and Metabolism, 69*(1), 77–83.

Youniss, J. (1985). *Adolescent relations with mothers, fathers and friends.* Chicago: University of Chicago Press.

Steinberg, L. D., & Hill, J. P. (1978). Patterns of family interaction as a function of age, the onset of puberty, and formal thinking. *Developmental Psychology, 14,* 683–684.

III

Editors' Overview

Youth at High Risk: The Social Situation and Mental Health of Adolescents Under Adversity

In the previous section we focused on the diversity of models and methodologies for understanding which subgroups of youths are most at risk for mental health problems when exposed to normative developmental stressors or cumulative life stress. We must keep in mind that in these large and small cross-sections of adolescents most youth are within the range of adaptive functioning, and many who are experiencing difficulties will weather the stresses of this period to make a relatively successful transition to adulthood. The authors, however, have identified some problematic patterns for girls and for boys. Recall, Brooks-Gunn has identified early developing girls as at-risk, and Petersen and associates have shown that depressed, mildly delinquent boys at early adolescence are at heightened risk for significant grade declines in later adolescence. Finally, Dornbusch and colleagues have uncovered greater vulnerability to stress among girls, in the area of distress symptoms, and vulnerability to behavioral problems among children living in non-two parent households.

In this section we focus on subgroups of youth whose development has already been at least somewhat compromised, who, by virtue of their capacities, behavior, or environment are at extreme risk for poor mental health, understood in the broadest possible way. Specifically, the papers

consider: mildly mentally retarded adolescents, the developmental trajectories of youth who were abused in early childhood, the social milieu of
female teenage parents, and the social situation and stresses of male gay
and runaway adolescents. We introduce these chapters with our own
paper that focuses on adolescents who have a number of mental health
problems—depressive symptoms, school failure, drinking problems,
delinquent behavior, sexual risk-taking, other affective disturbances, etc.
Although our sample is much like those described in the earlier chapters
of the volume, that is, drawn from regular high school classrooms in three
communities, we show how by focusing on these multi-problem "syndromes" we can provide alternative perspectives on questions about sex
differences, and, importantly, make data from community samples speak
to the problem of severe risk.

As we shift attention to these special populations, we face the task of
deriving new perspectives on risk, and, specifically, on the nature and
meaning of stress and mental health. As we noted in Chapter 1 and in
other section overviews, much of the research on adolescent mental
health has been guided by fairly well articulated ideas about risk and
resilience, formulated from the viewpoint of primary prevention, that is,
early identification of risk factors and intervention prior to the appearance
of any form of disorder. For groups of adolescents who are reasonably
well functioning in appropriate social roles, we also know that it is
incorrect to chart a narrow range of adaptive functioning, as this is a time
of normal developmental experimentation, both with respect to behaviors and the emerging coping repertoire.

But for some groups of adolescents, mental health and the developmental trajectory has already been somewhat compromised, and there is
evidence that they are nearing the periphery of the range of adaptive
functioning. Following the thinking of Jessor (1982) on their at-risk status,
we suggest that the subgroups discussed in the following papers *are in
jeopardy because the effects of risk-taking behaviors and life situations have not
been delayed, insulated or minimized.* They may already evidence distress,
and they are wide open for other problems as well. Here, we are not
focusing solely on psychiatric dysfunction; in fact, the papers in this
section place more emphasis on problematic ingredients of daily life and
the implications for the developmental trajectory. As Petersen and
associates so thoughtfully noted in their paper, adolescence is a pivotal
time from mental health perspectives because this is when youth who are
on positive and negative trajectories become increasingly divergent.
Thus, we might say that youth at serious risk are those whose trajectories
are likely to show continued movement in a negative direction. In sum,
from both the stress and developmental perspectives, the question of risk

must be reformulated to consider starting points in which problems of some kind may already be evidenced at the psychological level and/or in the developmental trajectory. As in all research on adolescent mental health, this trajectory pertains not only to intra-individual characteristics and interpersonal relationships, but also to an orderly progression of life roles.

* * * *

Turning now to the papers in this section, we ask the reader to appreciate both the specifics of the problems discussed and the study methodologies and conceptualizations of risk and disorder. For example, contrast the data in our chapter on the nature of multi-problem profiles with the analyses in earlier papers that have focused on age differences in depressive affect. Although much attention has focused on the period of early adolescence as a time of increased risk, our data show that this conceptualization does not fit the experience of boys—who initiate more problem behaviors as they move from grades 10 through 12. Such increases in the numbers of affective and problem behaviors over time are one indicator of increased risk and this suggests yet another perspective on the stages of development in which youth are considered to be most at risk. Our data on the clustering of affective and problem behaviors also provide support for more comprehensive approaches to the question of sex differences in distress and disorder. All too often we speak of so-called feminine and masculine styles of deviant expression and then give selective attention to single variables that are likely to show such sex differences. It is important to focus on all relevant health outcomes and describe the various forms of stress responses that boys and girls actually evidence. We find that many girls are at high risk for problems other than depressive disorders, and that it is important not to overlook the significant numbers of boys who are at risk for internalizing and not just externalizing symptoms of distress.

Widom's investigation of the causal linkage between childhood victimization and subsequent arrest for delinquency is striking for its methodological precision. It establishes not only the critical etiological link between childhood victimization and later disturbance but, within this strong study design, also shows that sex differences in stress-related outcomes are not always in the direction we expect them to be. Specifically, Widom finds that abused and neglected girls have higher rates of arrest for violence against others than abused and neglected boys. The girls' high rates of arrest for theft and vandalism as well are evidence that there are no clear feminine and masculine domains of distress response.

This reinforces our earlier point about the tendency to stereotype the troubles of boys and girls as fitting a clear masculine and feminine mold. Widom's discussion of the significantly greater impact of early childhood victimization on the later arrest records of black males and females is similarly revealing.

The paper by Rotheram-Borus and associates complements Widom's paper in several ways. First, it also focuses on subgroups of adolescents who have experienced some level of harm in their families of origin. Second, it concerns itself with runaways, one of the "status" offenses for which some of the adolescents in Widom's sample are arrested. Third, as Widom notes, her archival data give an incomplete portrait of these youths' lives, and do not allow for study of processes that mediate victimization and later deviance. We see some of the needed descriptive richness regarding the life situation of runaway youth in the Rotheram-Borus paper. The details are disturbing. From this research and other studies we know that: runaway and male gay youth experience four times the rate of stressful life events than those reported in studies of "normal" populations; 38% of runaway youth meet DSM III criteria for a diagnosis of substance abuse; runaway boys and girls are highly sexually active, boys especially so, and they manifest a high rate of HIV positive; there is considerable history of parental alcoholism and experience with teenage pregnancy for the girls; and, finally, 33% of runaway girls and 15% of runaway boys have attempted suicide, rates much higher than those reported in studies of normal cross-sections of youth. These analyses underscore the risk-taking lifestyles of children not living with their parents, or who are otherwise estranged from primary ties, and provide some insight into the deviant pathways that Widom has documented in her research.

Importantly, both Widom and Rotheram-Borus and associates question what outcomes or behaviors we should consider successful adaptation. Widom points to the large proportion of victimized youth who do not become delinquent, but cautions that there are other negative adaptations to childhood victimization that were not assessed in her research. She further suggests that delinquency as a long term consequence of victimization may be more adaptive than other outcomes. Rotheram-Borus and associates also present data to indicate that there appears to be considerable variation within their sample, that some youth report satisfying relationships with parents and peers, success in school, and adequate levels of support. This suggests a psychosocial resiliency that bears further investigation but, as data of this sort contrast with levels of deviant and risk-taking behavior and reports of stress, we may be seeing a pattern of accomodation that includes a certain acceptance of the life style and social ties available, with few expectations about their quality. This preliminary research into these neglected populations further underscores the need for more grounded research on the meaning and nature of social support, an issue that Gottlieb discusses in the final section of the volume.

The third paper in this section considers the intersection of two problems that have occupied much attention in the field of adolescent health: substance use and teenage pregnancy and parenting. While many theoretical frameworks have been brought to bear on each of these problems, it is significant that co-authors Amaro and Zuckerman are focusing their most recent studies of teenage parents on the norms and behaviors of significant others in their social networks. In line with the "problem-proneness behavior" theory advanced by Jessor and Jessor (1977), their data show high rates of alcohol and drug use among pregnant and parenting teens. Importantly, we see "support" for these behaviors—both normatively and behaviorally—in their immediate social networks, including family, peers and partners. Data of this nature have heretofore been advanced to speak to the issue of "initiation into drug use," but Amaro and Zuckerman also point to the higher rates of violence and life stresses in the lives of drug-using pregnant adolescents, findings suggesting the complexity of the psycho-social environment of parenting teens and the likelihood of drug use as a coping response to stress. Further, the fact that there is considerable alcohol and drug use in the social networks of non-drug using teenage mothers points to the need for timely interventions to help these mothers maintain their more healthful status.

The final paper in this section, by Siperstein and Wenz-Gross, focuses on mildly mentally retarded adolescents. They review existing data on stress, development and mental health, and highlight the limitations of our knowledge and understanding of this significant population. Drawing upon the conceptualization of stigma, Siperstein and Wenz-Gross show how existing literature from stress perspectives takes the adolescent as the stressor and concerns itself with the difficulties of the family. The stresses of the adolescent go unstudied, although a small body of evidence indicates that these youth suffer from social isolation and poor mental health. Not only do Siperstein and Wenz-Gross outline an agenda for stress studies, they also suggest that the timing of normal developmental processes differs for these youth and that the atypical nature of this trajectory needs to be understood from both developmental and stress perspectives. In sum, this is a fitting conclusion to this section as it also brings home the point that much more research is needed in many areas of adolescent stress and development.

References

Jessor, R. (1982). Critical issues in research on adolescent health promotion. In
    T. J. Coates, A. C. Petersen, & C. Perry (Eds.), *Promoting Adolescent Health.*
    NY: Academic Press.
Jessor, S., & Jessor, R. (1977). *Problem behavior and psychological development: A
    longitudinal study of youth.* New York: Academic Press.

8

The Patterning of Distress and Disorder in a Community Sample of High School Aged Youth

Mary Ellen Colten, Susan Gore, and Robert H. Aseltine, Jr.

In 1982, Richard Jessor urged adolescent researchers to pursue the findings from research accumulated over the previous decade indicating that there is "substantial *covariation*" among many adverse mental health and health-related behaviors. He noted that while drug use, drinking, sexual behavior, and deviance have been shown to cluster together, researchers have generally failed to extend research on multiple problems to other concerns such as depression and anxiety (Jessor, 1982, p. 453).

In the years since Jessor's exhortation, there has been only modest progress in moving beyond a behavior–specific orientation to an exploration of the links between the diverse indicators of poor mental health and high risk in adolescents. This paper is designed to advance that process and, we hope, to prompt the inclusion of these concerns in future research.

Most of the work on multiple problems has been limited to one side or the other of the "internalizing–externalizing" dichotomy. This rubric for classifying disorder, reflected in a widely used instrument constructed and refined by Achenbach and colleagues (Achenbach, 1966; Achenbach & Edelbrock, 1987), makes a distinction between the "externalizing" group of problems, those with an overt, active, and outward expression, and the "internalizing" problems whose orientation is cognitive, emotional, or psychosomatic. Among the externalizing problems are drug use, delinquency, drinking, sexuality, and school problems; the internalizing category includes problems such as depression, anxiety, suicidal thoughts and feelings, psychosomatic symptoms, and eating disorders. There is mounting evidence within the externalizing category, for example, of the covariation of drinking and drug use, or of antisocial and delinquent behaviors with poor school performance or dropping out (Jessor, 1982; Newcomb & Bentler, 1989). Similarly, within the internalizing category links have been made between depression and suicidal thoughts and behaviors, and between depression and anxiety, among others (Rubenstein et al., 1988; Kashani, Carlson et al., 1987).

A major impetus for looking at the joint occurrence of internalizing and externalizing problems and for considering alternate expressions of distress, has been interest in adolescent depression. The current research literature on adolescent mental health shows a prominent emphasis on depression in light of epidemiologic evidence showing increases in rates of depression since World War II (Klerman & Weissman, 1989), and data showing that current rates are at least as high as those reported for adults. Evidence is accumulating for the central role of depressed mood as a precursor or risk factor for other forms of emotional and behavioral disorders and as a mediator of environmental/genetic influence (such as stress) on other problem outcomes. Depressed mood in adolescence is associated with suicidal feelings and behaviors (Rubenstein et al., 1988; Robbins & Alessi, 1985) and with poor school performance, dropping out, and other indicators of deviance, including drug and alcohol use (Newcomb & Bentler, 1988; Carlson & Cantwell, 1979). In addition, longitudinal analyses by Kandel and associates (Kandel, Kessler, & Margulies, 1978) have shown that depressed mood is an important determinant of initiation into illicit drug use of drugs other than marijuana, and that many adolescents continue to use drugs as a means of alleviating depression (Kandel & Davies, 1982). Weiner (1980) argues that children and early adolescents are unable to express depression in the usual adult forms and so use acting out behaviors both as attempts to ward off depression and as appeals for help. In later adolescence, sex and drugs may be significant mechanisms for expressing depression.

One concept linking depression to other problems, especially externalizing problems, is "masked depression" (Carlson & Cantwell, 1980; Kovacs & Beck, 1977), which suggests that problems such as antisocial behaviors, conduct disorders, and poor school performance may be forms of behaviors and symptoms that "mask" underlying depressive feelings that are essentially inaccessible to the child or adolescent. For example, Rutter (1986) notes that depression is commonly found among children who have conduct disturbances. Puig-Antich (1982) reports that treatment of prepubescent boys for depression resulted in the virtual disappearance of their conduct disorder.

From middle adolescence on throughout adulthood, females evidence higher rates of depression (Cleary, 1987; Gove & Herb, 1984). Much research and debate has focused on the meaning and etiology of these observed gender differences (Weissman & Klerman, 1977; Kessler & McLeod, 1984). The view that the existence of gender differences in depression does not necessarily imply that females are more distressed, but rather than males and females are predisposed or socialized to different, sex-role congruent *expressions* of distress, has fostered research on multiple problems in youth, with an eye toward linking the internalizing problem of depression to externalizing problems that may share some common etiologic processes (Horowitz & White, 1987). The position that each sex has a distinct style of expressing disturbance is supported by prevalence data showing that conduct disorders are three times more prevalent in adult men than women.

A particular issue of interest is whether for boys, or other subgroups, deviant behavior is an alternative expression of distress, that is, one not necessarily accompanied by depressive symptoms. To explore this issue in their community sample, Kandel and Davies (1982) cut depression scores at the median and coded delinquency as an ever/never occurrence. Their measure of delinquency included minor delinquent acts, drinking, and school problems. Using these gross classifications, and with other cut-offs as well, they found identical proportions (23% for the median split) of the boys and girls in the "neither highly depressed nor delinquent" category, twice the number of boys than girls in the "delinquent only" category, and the reversed pattern for the "depressed only" category. From this perspective, boys are seen as disturbed as girls, but as having an "externalizing," rather than "internalizing" pattern of symptom expression. In the Kandel and Davies data, girls were more likely than boys to be both depressed and delinquent, suggesting that delinquent girls are more likely to be psychologically disturbed than delinquent boys.

In a recent study of 18 year-old boys and girls not in treatment, Gjerde, Block, and Block (1988) report that the correlates of depression differ for boys and girls: the boys with depressive tendencies were seen by observers as "disagreeable, aggressive, and antagonistic to others," while the girls—who similarly saw themselves as aggressive and alienated—were rated as "ego-brittle, unconventional, and ruminating." Therefore, even when boys and girls are identified as depressed, this affective state may have different self- and other- reported behavioral correlates. They observe that boys and girls respond to stressful experiences in ways that are compatible with their socialization history. Other extensive research has pursued this issue in examining differential responses to family divorce, separation, and conflict, noting that girls respond to these stressors along an "overcontrolled" dimension and boys respond along an "undercontrolled" dimension.

Research on gender differences in depression and other indicators of distress clearly shows that there is considerable variability in the experience and expression of distress across a wide range of measures both between and within the sexes. The next steps are to identify syndromes and patterns of symptoms that hang together in meaningful ways. A good example is the work of Earls and colleagues (1988), who report that a *combination* of emotional and conduct problems most distinguish children of alcoholic parents from a group of controls. And, as Magnusson and Bergman (1988) point out in their defense of such a person-oriented pattern approach (as opposed to a variable based approach) to research on risk, a behavioral problem can have quite a different meaning when it appears in a syndrome or cluster with one set of variables than when it appears with another set. Furthermore, Rutter and Sandberg (1988) make the point that "disorders associated with a wide range of emotional or behavioral difficulties tend to have a worse outcome than those associated with a single symptom or a narrow range of problems." A possible explanation for this difference lies in the fact that the contagion of distress through more and more role behaviors and institutional spheres is itself a sign of greater severity of disorder. That is, not only does functioning within each role domain become more inadequate, but any protected arenas of competence are jeopardized as well.

These are strong arguments for the broad assessments of distress and disorder presented in this chapter. In the analyses that follow, we describe the pattern of mental-health relevant distress and deviance in a normal, community sample of youth, giving attention to the number, types and range of dysfunction. As much of the research in the field focuses on the psycho-social correlates of distress and disorder in adolescents (e.g., Felner et al., 1985; Wells, Deykin, & Klerman, 1985; Compas et al., 1986; Garmezy & Rutter, 1983), we also briefly consider the role of life stress and its relationship to patterns of problems in youth.

Methods

Study Population and Design

Data for these analyses were collected in 1989 as part of the second wave of a prospective study of the stress process in the high school years. The first wave sample, interviewed one year earlier, was comprised of a random sample of ninth, tenth, and eleventh graders in three community high schools in the Boston area. The second wave sample consists of 1033 students: 323 high school sophomores, 362 juniors, 323 seniors, and 25 dropouts. This Wave II data set consists of interviews with 86% of those interviewed at Wave I. Eighty percent of the eligible students had agreed to take part in the first wave of the study.

The three communities were selected to represent a range of socioeconomic status and life situations. The median incomes of the three communities according to the 1980 census were: $19,004; $22,097, and $29,055. As a whole the sample does not include many youth from extremely disadvantaged circumstances.

The sample consists of 436 boys and 597 girls, 99% of whom were between 15 and 18 years of age at the time of the interview. Over three-fourths (77%) were living in two parent households, 21% in single parent households, with the remainder in living situations with neither parent.

Structured personal interviews of approximately one hour in length were conducted with the students by professional interviewers from the Center for Survey Research of the University of Massachusetts at Boston. In addition to the data reported here on emotional and behavioral problems and symptoms, the interview covered life stress, social supports, coping behaviors, and a number of other personality, predispositional, and demographic variables.

Measures

Measures of 13 mental health problem areas are used in these analyses. Some of the measures are dichotomies indicating presence or absence of a problem while others, such as the measure of depression, the Center for Epidemiologic Studies-Depression scale (CES-D), have well established criteria for a cut-off level for "risk" or "caseness." In the case of nondichotomous variables with no established cut-off criterion, our goal is to designate those scoring above the eightieth percentile as having a problem, so we have segmented the distribution of scores at the value that most closely approximates this break.

Problem areas are conceptualized along two lines. The first is the distinction discussed earlier between *internalizing* problems—those with an affective, cognitive, or psychosomatic orientation, and *externalizing* problems—those with a behavioral orientation such as substance use problems and those involving role behavior and performance. Included in the internalizing category are measures of depression, anxiety, suicidal thoughts, hostility, eating disorders, and psychosomatic symptoms. Included in the externalizing category are measures of problems related to drinking and drug use, school behavior problems, delinquency, school performance (grade point average and dropping out of school), and sexual risk taking.

In order to provide more detail about functioning, we then split the internalizing problems into affective and body domains and the externalizing problems into role and substance use domains. The four categories are: (1) *affect:* depression, anxiety, hostility, suicidal thoughts; (2) *body:* eating disorder, psychosomatic symptoms; (3) *substance use:* drinking problems, drug use; (4) *role problems:* school behavior problems, delinquency, grades, dropping out, sexual risk-taking.

Depression: The measure of depressive symptoms is the Center for Epidemiologic Studies Depression Scale (CES-D), a 20 item self-report measure of the number of days symptoms of depressive mood and feelings were experienced over the past week (Radloff, 1977). Although the CES-D was not designed as a diagnostic measure of depression, a score of 16 or over has been used as an indicator of clinically significant symptoms and "caseness." We use this criterion of 16 as the cut off point for distinguishing the "depressed" group from the "nondepressed" group.

Eating Disorder: Eating disorder is determined by responses to the question: "Have you ever had an eating disorder like anorexia or bulimia in the past twelve months?"

Anxiety: The measure of tension and anxiety consists of 10 items (e.g., feeling tense or keyed up; nervousness or shakiness inside; feeling easily annoyed or irritated). The respondent rates the extent of being distressed by each in the past month on a 5 point scale from "not at all" to "extremely." The index is adapted from the SCL-90 (Derogatis, 1977) and has previously been used in a large study of high school students (Locksley & Douvan, 1979; Kelly, 1979). We designate those scoring in the top 17% (scores of 19 and above on a 50 point scale) on the index as the high anxiety group, the group with potential problems with symptoms of tension and anxiety.

Hostility: The index of hostile, aggressive, and resentful feelings consists of five items, also from the SCL-90 (e.g., temper outbursts that you could not control; having urges to beat or harm someone, getting into frequent arguments), rated by respondents on the same scale and drawn from the same source as the index of anxiety. Those in top 17% (15 or above on a 30 point scale) are designated as having problems with hostile and aggressive feelings. Both the anxiety and hostility measures have demonstrated acceptable inter-item and test-retest reliability coefficients.

Suicidal Thoughts: Respondents were asked: "In the past year, how often have you thought about killing yourself—often, sometimes, rarely, or never?" The 11% of the sample reporting that they thought about suicide often or sometimes are considered to be high in this problem area.

Psychosomatic Symptoms: Frequency of being distressed by headaches or pains in the head and stomachaches or upset stomach in the past month was rated on the same scale as the Anxiety and Hostility Indices. The cut-off for high psychosomatic symptoms is a score of 5 or more (out of a possible 10); 29% of the respondents have high psychosomatic symptoms.

Drinking: Responses to the following items are combined to establish a drinking index: "During the past 12 months, how often have you had a drink of beer or wine or liquor—every day, 4 or 5 days a week, 2 or 3 days a month, about once a month, once or twice, or never?"; "In the past month, how many times have you had 5 or more drinks in a row—never, once, 2–5 times, or 6 or more times?"; "In the past year have you had any fights or disagreements with your parents about your drinking?"; "In the past year have you gotten into trouble because of drinking, like having an accident or being arrested for drunk driving?"; "In the past year have you had any school or job troubles because of drinking?" Respondents are labeled as having problems with drinking if they meet at least two of three criteria: (1) Answering yes to any of the three questions about problems with drinking; (2) had 5 or more drinks in a row in the past month; (3) reported a drinking frequency of at least once a week.

Drug Use: Drug use is assessed as use in the past year of marijuana or hash, cocaine or crack, barbiturates, tranquilizers, amphetamines, heroin, or hallucinogens.

Delinquent Behaviors: The delinquency index is based on reports of committing in the past year 10 delinquent acts (e.g., stole or tried to steal things, purposely damaged or destroyed property that did not belong to you). Items are drawn from the Monitoring the Future Studies (Bachman, Johnston, & O'Malley, 1986). Those engaging in three or more of these acts in the past year are designated as having problems with delinquency.

School Problems: Students designated as having school problems met at least two of the following criteria regarding "this year in school": (1) expelled or suspended from school; (2) kicked out of class; (3) in the upper 17% of times skipped school (3 or more days); (4) late to school 7 or more days (19%); (5) reported committing at least 4 behaviors out of 8 items on the school behavior problem index (18%): e.g., wise off and disrupt a class; cheat on a test, quiz, or another classwork; refuse to participate or work in a class.

School Performance: Bad grades is a self-reported cumulative grade point average of less than a "C." *Dropout* includes only those students not enrolled in school at the time of the interview.

Sexual Risk Taking: Respondents who reported that they had intercourse in the past year either without a condom or without birth control (including condoms) were designated as engaging in sexual risk-taking.

The analyses that follow describe the patterning of these distress and behavior problems. As much of the research in the field focuses on psychosocial correlates, we briefly consider the role of life stress. The measures of stressful life events draw upon items used in the research of Compas, Davis, and Forsythe (1985), Johnson and McCutcheon (1980) and Newcomb, Huba, and Bentler (1981). Events happening in the past year are divided into four groupings: (1) *Events to self* such as illness, assault, accident, work problems, and financial problems (7 items); (2) *Relationship events* including conflict with family and friends, loss of friendship or romantic relationship (4 items); (3) *Family events*—events happening to parents and siblings (13 items); and (4) *Friend events*— events happening to friends (8 items). Each of the event groupings is dichotomized into high and low stress groups. The proportion in the high stress groups are: events to self 28.2%, relationship events 31.9%, family events 28.1%, and friend events 27.1%.

Results

The Distribution of Problems

Table 1 shows the percentage of students having the various problems. We should point out that for the continuous variables the criteria for presence or absence of problem is relative, as in taking the upper 20% of the distribution. However, the stress analyses presented below indicate that these breaks in the distributions are meaningful. Also, there is considerable variation in the stringency of the criteria across problem areas and the absolute values or rates cannot be seen as comparable—one unit of depression does not equal one unit of delinquency. Thus, except in a few cases where the criterion for presence or absence of a problem is very well established or is a true dichotomy, we will not make comparisons between the rates of problems in this sample and rates reported in other studies. Comparison with other studies of the *relative* rates of incidence of problems for males and females can appropriately be made.

Given the powerful, and not unexpected, sex differences in these problems, all analyses are shown for males and females separately. In addition to comparisons across grade levels, comparisons are shown of those in two parent households as opposed to other family types.

Table 1. Percent of Boys and Girls Having Problems by Grade and Household Type

| | BOYS | | | | | GIRLS | | | | | | |
| | Household | | Grade | | | Household | | Grade | | | All Boys | All Girls |
Problem	non-2-Parent %	Two-Parent %	10 %	11 %	12 %	non-2-Parent %	Two-Parent %	10 %	11 %	12 %	%	%
Depression	21.1	17.1	13.3	20.5	19.1	35.0	27.5	33.2	27.1	27.2	17.9	29.2***
Anxiety	29.2	11.8***	10.9	18.1	16.9	27.7	27.2	24.8	25.6	31.6	15.6	27.3***
Hostility	31.3	13.5***	16.3	19.9	15.4	18.2	16.1	13.9	18.1	17.9	17.4	16.6
Suicidal thoughts	9.4	5.0	0.8	8.8	7.4*	21.9	13.1*	14.9	11.6	19.0	6.0	15.1***
Eating problems	2.1	0.9	0.8	1.8	0.7	6.6	3.9	7.4	3.0	3.2	1.2	4.5**
Psychosomatic	19.8	14.7	14.0	19.9	12.5	46.7	36.5	38.1	47.2	41.3	15.8	38.9***
Delinquent behav.	38.5	19.7***	18.6	24.0	28.7	15.3	9.3	9.9	9.5	12.8	23.9	10.7***
Drug use	38.5	26.5*	19.4	33.9	32.4*	44.5	26.5***	30.2	27.1	34.7	29.1	30.7
Drinking problems	33.3	22.4*	10.1	29.2	33.1***	21.9	15.4	18.3	16.6	15.8	24.8	16.9**
School behavior	41.7	21.2***	20.2	25.7	30.9	22.6	12.4**	16.3	12.6	15.3	25.7	14.7***
Dropout	6.3	0.9**	0.8	1.8	3.7	8.0	1.1***	3.5	2.5	2.0	2.1	2.7
Bad grades	36.5	19.7**	20.2	27.5	21.3	21.9	13.9*	19.8	16.6	10.7*	23.4	15.7**
Sexual risktaking	45.7	24.7*	20.8	28.7	37.5*	43.4	19.9***	20.3	22.4	33.2**	29.2	25.3
(N)	(96)	(340)	(129)	(171)	(136)	(137)	(460)	(202)	(199)	(196)	(436)	(597)

* p < .05
** p < .01
*** p < .001

Comparisons by parent's level of education also were made; they yielded few significant differences so those distributions are not shown in Table 1, but will be referred to in the text.

In Table 1 we see significant sex differences for 9 of the 13 problem areas. These findings are consistent with the hypothesis that distress is largely expressed through different routes for males and females (Achenbach & Edelbrock, 1987). The proportion of girls with affective problems—anxiety, depression, and suicidal feelings—far exceeds that of boys. These findings are consistent with evidence from most other community studies of adolescents over age 14 or 15 (Kandel & Davies, 1982; Kashani, Beck et al., 1987; Horowitz & White, 1987; Lewinsohn et al., 1988; Gove & Herb, 1974; Kashani & Orvashel, 1988; Petersen & Craighead, 1986). The percent of girls reporting body-related problems, both eating disorders and psychosomatic symptoms, is more than double that of boys, a finding also consistent with previous research (Bemis, 1978; Boskind-Lodahl, 1976).

As is the case in most other studies of adolescents, we find that many more boys than girls report high levels of role related problems: delinquent behavior, problem behavior at school, and poor grades (Colten & Marsh, 1984; Canter, 1984; Leland, 1982; Simmons & Blyth, 1987). More boys than girls also have drinking problems. Failure of role performance and alcohol–related problems clearly are more the province of adolescent males than females.

Interestingly, there is no reported difference in use and abuse of most illicit substances other than alcohol and, by any criteria, the boys in this study cannot be considered to have more of a problem with drug use than girls. The lack of sex difference in drug use holds up even when a more stringent criterion of use of two or more drugs is applied to the definition and when frequency of use is the criterion. Boys are slightly more likely than girls to use hallucinogens and much more likely to use steroids, but the use of all other drugs is the same for the two sexes in this sample. Because girls are most often initiated into drug use by boys (Marsh et al., 1982) and there is a tendency for females to associate with older males, it is not surprising that the tenth grade girls far exceed tenth grade boys in the proportion reporting drug use, while the proportions in the later two grades are the same. Block and Gjerde (1990) found that as late as age 18, the illicit drug use of females exceeded that of males, while Horowitz and White (1987), in a longitudinal study of a large community sample, found no sex differences in drinking or drug use until age 18, when male use overcame female use.

While both boys and girls appear to be responsive to family structure, they express their reactivity differently, with family structure affecting a wider range of problems for boys than for girls. Rutter (1970) has made a strong theoretical and empirical case that implicates family discord in externalizing problems for boys (but not for girls) and Emery (1982) suggests that the greater apparent reactivity of males to family discord may be due to the type (and visibility) rather than the intensity of the reaction. Werner and Smith (1982), in their study of resilient children, also report a greater impact of family circumstances on boys, considerably more boys in non-two parent families suffer from heightened anxiety and hostility. Girls in non-two parent families tend more to have suicidal thoughts and psychosomatic symptoms. Notably, family structure per se is not related to heightened depression for either sex. As might be predicted from Rutter's work, every externalizing problem we measured occurs with greater frequency for boys who do not reside in two-parent households. For girls, there is also a pattern of greater problems in non-two parent households. However, although girls in two-parent households report fewer problems with drinking and delinquency than those in non-two parent households, the differences are not statistically significant.

When we shift to consideration of the four domains of affective, body, substance, and role problems, all four domains appear to be affected by family structure for girls. For boys, body-related problems is the one domain unaffected by family structure.

In general, then, for both sexes, problematic responses to family circumstances, even on a structural level without regard to the present emotional context, appear in both externalizing and internalizing forms. In future analyses, we will disaggregate the two-parent households into those with and without stepparents to obtain a more fine-tuned picture. In addition, we caution against placing too much emphasis on family structure as an etiologic influence, as we are not working with a causal model and there are important control and intervening variables in such a model.

Looking at the distribution by grade level, we note that for girls, only bad grades and sexual risk taking change significantly between sophomore and senior year. Fewer girls than boys have problems with grades as they advance through school. This may be an example of girls becoming more attuned to the requirements of the student role and learning how to cater to adult role demands. Locksley and Douvan (1979) have documented the importance for girls of meeting adult expectations and the distress that accrues to adolescent girls who fail to do so and, in this volume, Smetana and colleagues report on the heightened conflict behavior of girls and their mothers in early adolescence regarding conventional expectations. Alternatively (or in addition), by senior year girls may have begun to emerge from the disruption of puberty (Brooks-Gunn & Petersen, 1983), and the intensification of gender role demands (Bush, 1985; Hill & Lynch, 1983) and may be freer to concentrate on performance in the school role without threats to femininity or success in the female role. Clearly, to adequately address this issue we must examine our longitudinal data and identify subgroups with different trajectories, as Petersen and colleagues have done in their paper.

In these communities equal proportions of boys and girls report that they are sexually active. The increase in sexual risk-taking over the high school years appears to be concomitant with the increase in sexual activity and although there may be increased use of birth control, unprotected sex may also increase. The increased risk for those not in two parent households is cause for concern. Further, sexual risk-taking is one of the few problem areas related to parents' educational level, even though the occurrence of most other problems we studied does not vary according to the education of the parents. Children of more highly educated parents report engaging in substantially less risk taking.

The dropout rates reported here are only of those students whom we were able to relocate and reinterview for the second wave of the study. The lack of sex difference may not reflect the actual rates of dropping out in these communities, but rather the relative ease of locating male and female dropouts. Dropping out of school is more often linked to pregnancy or family responsibilities for girls.

It is important to remember that the measure of hostility includes angry and hostile feelings and the sense of loss of control, but does not cover aggressive acts. The strong relationship between family circumstances and those feelings in boys, but not in girls, is an issue that warrants further inquiry.

Relationship among Problems

Table 2 begins our consideration of these problems in conjunction with one another, presenting the intercorrelations of all the problems for boys and girls. In general, difficulties in the various problem areas are strongly associated with one another. For boys, as well as girls, internalizing problems relate strongly to one another, but eating problems affect a minuscule fraction of boys and the disorder is mostly unrelated to other behavioral and emotional problems in boys' lives. Eating problems are also unassociated with other body related problems for boys. For the 27 girls in the sample reporting eating problems, these problems are clearly related to a wide range of both internalizing and externalizing problems.

Both grades and dropping out are associated with most other externalizing problems for boys and girls. These indicators of school performance are also related to internalizing problems for girls, but not for boys. This is consistent with the findings of Locksley and Douvan (1979), but runs counter to Ebata and Petersen's (in press) report of a relationship

Table 2. Intercorrelation of Problems by Sex

Problem	CESD M	CESD F	Anxiety M	Anxiety F	Hostile M	Hostile F	Suicidal Thoughts M	Suicidal Thoughts F	Psycho-somatic M	Psycho-somatic F	Eating Problems M	Eating Problems F	Delin-quency M	Delin-quency F	School Behavior M	School Behavior F	Drug Use M	Drug Use F	Drinking M	Drinking F	Bad Grades M	Bad Grades F	Drop Out M	Drop Out F
Anxiety	.60c	.59c	—	—																				
Hostility	.48c	.57c	.59c	.66c	—	—																		
Suicidal Thoughts	.43c	.53c	.31c	.49c	.29c	.37c	—	—																
Psycho Somatic	.39	.44c	.46c	.54c	.32c	.48c	.12b	.34c	—															
Eating Problems	.07	.19c	.09a	.25c	.01	.12b	-.02	.11a	.02	.22c	—													
Delin- quency	.21c	.23c	.27c	.29c	.40c	.34c	.20c	.23c	.16b	.23c	.02	.12b	—											
School Behavior	.09a	.22c	.20c	.23c	.32c	.31c	.11b	.21c	.07	.18c	.09a	.19c	.63c	.46c	—									
Drug Use	.13b	.21c	.14b	.25c	.35c	.34c	.16c	.23c	.09a	.23c	-.03	.09a	.52c	.46c	.43c	.48c	—							
Drinking	.09a	.19c	.11a	.19c	.24c	.24c	.18c	.16c	.09a	.15c	.01	.13b	.44c	.36c	.40c	.41c	.47c	.45c	—					
Grades	.03	.21c	.03	.06	.10a	.18c	.01	.11b	.02	.09a	.09a	.05	.29c	.18c	.38c	.39c	.32c	.33c	.27c	.20c	—			
Drop Out	.02	.14c	.06	.11b	.12b	.11b	.01	.12b	-.02	.06	-.02	.11b	.15b	.13b	.05	.08a	.17c	.17c	.10b	.10b	.08a	.23c	—	
Sexual Risk	.14b	.16c	.12b	.13b	.20b	.24c	.06	.10a	.09a	.13b	-.02	.12b	.38c	.27c	.29c	.30c	.36c	.39c	.33c	.29c	.27c	.24c	.05	.26c

a = p < .05
b = p < .01
c = p < .001

between depression and poor grades in middle school for boys, but not for girls. Other researchers have noted links between academic performance and depressive symptoms among children (Achenbach & Edelbrock, 1981). As our sample is older, it may be hard to reconcile such differences. Other kinds of school behavior problems are linked to internalizing as well as externalizing problems for both boys and girls.

Depression and Other Problems

Turning now to a focus on depression and its correlates, we can see in Table 3 the relationship between depressed mood and other problem behaviors. The analyses presented here have two aims. One is to illuminate the links between depression and other problems in adolescence, and the second is to address the meaning of sex differences in depression during adolescence with its implications for the more general question of sex differences in the modes of expression of distress.

A first observation from Table 3 is that depression is more consistently related to other problems for girls than for boys. For every one of the 12 other problems we measured, a significantly higher proportion of the highly depressed than less depressed girls evidenced the problem. While the difference between the depressed and less depressed girls is

Table 3. Percent of High vs. Low Depressed Boys and Girls Reporting Other Problems

	Boys		Girls			
Problem	CESD <16	CESD >16	CESD <16	CESD >16	All Boys	All Girls
Anxiety	8.4%	48.7%***	14.9%	56.9%***	15.6%	27.3%***
Suicidal Thoughts	2.2	23.1***	5.9	37.4***	6.0	15.1***
Hostility	12.6	39.7***	8.1	36.8***	17.4	16.6
Eating Problems	1.1	1.3	2.6	9.2***	1.2	4.5**
Psychosomatic	11.5	35.9***	28.7	63.8***	15.8	38.9***
Drug Use	29.4	28.2	26.8	40.2**	29.1	30.7
Drinking Problems	24.1	28.2	14.7	22.4*	24.8	16.9**
School Problem	24.9	29.5	10.7	24.7***	25.7	14.7***
Delinquency	21.0	35.9**	8.8	15.5*	23.9	10.7***
Bad Grades	24.6	17.9	11.1	27.0***	23.4	15.7**
Drop Out	1.7	3.8	0.9	6.9***	2.1	2.7
Sex Risk-Taking	28.5	32.9	22.4	31.8*	29.2	25.3
N	(357)	(78)	(422)	(174)	(435)	(596)

*p < .05
**p < .01
***p < .001

most pronounced among the affective and body problems, the differences between the two groups for all the externalizing problems is also consistent and overwhelming. There is also a significant difference between more and less depressed boys in rates of reported affective and psychosomatic problems. However, in contrast to the girls, depression in boys is not as systematically related to presence or absence of externalizing problems. In the case of delinquency, the rates of depressed and nondepressed boys do significantly differ, but this pattern is not replicated in the other externalizing measures. Kandel and Davies (1982) also report a stronger association between externalizing behaviors and depression for girls compared to boys.

The Four Domains of Problems

A look at the proportions of boys and girls reporting any single problem in isolation from the other problems could lead to the conclusion that (except for psychosomatic difficulties in girls) about a third of the sample is presently manifesting difficulties that indicate present or future risk. When we aggregate problems into the domains of affective problems (depression, anxiety, hostility, suicidal thoughts), body problems (eating disorder, pyschosomatic symptoms), substance problems (drinking, drug use) and role problems (delinquency, school behavior, grades, drop-out, sexual risk-taking), we see a very different picture.

Table 4 summarizes the data, with the entire sample as the base, on the number of youth in various problem configurations. Over 70% of both boys and girls have problems in at least one domain, with only 29% of the girls and 28% of boys having no problems in any domain. About a third of the boys (32%) and a quarter of the girls (24%) have problems in only one domain. *A sizable group of boys and girls have problems in more than one domain—40% of the boys and 47% of the girls have problems in at least two domains.* Among boys, 21% have problems in two domains and 19% have problems in three or four domains. For girls the comparable figures are 23 and 24%. This suggests that problem types are not simply substitutions for one another. These problems co-exist with considerable frequency among youth and the probability of an adolescent having problems in any domain is enhanced if he or she already has a problem in another area.

Substantial sex differences in the nature of problems are evident. Among boys with problems in only one domain, the externalizing problems of substance use (32%) and role problems (38%) are most common. For girls, we see only half the rate of role related problems and five times greater risk for body-related problems. Although girls have higher rates of affective distress and boys higher rates of substance problems, these differences among the "one problem only" youth are not as great as might be expected. When youth having two domains of problems are considered, boys tend to expand further into externalizing problems and girls tend to expand into more internalizing problems. The most frequent combination of two domains for boys is substance problems and role problems. Nearly 45% of those with two problem domains have the substance/role problem combination, while only 16% have the combination of the two internalizing domains of affect and body problems. For girls with problems in two domains, the most frequent configuration of problems is the combination of the two internalizing domains of affective and body problems. While 48% of girls with two problem domains have the internalizing combination, only 17% have the problem configurations of both externalizing domains of substance and role problems that is so common among boys. In these sex differences, we see most clearly evidence of the internalizing/externalizing dichotomy. Boys and girls are equally likely to have a combination of internalizing and externalizing problems, 27.3% of boys and 32% of girls have both, suggesting a considerable degree of cross-domain (internalizing-externalizing) problems for both sexes. We

Table 4. Percent of Sample with Problem Domain Combinations by Sex

Domains	Boys	Girls
No Domains	28.4%	29.0%
One Domain		
Affect	7.8	7.4
Body	1.6	6.0
Substance	10.1	6.5
Role	11.9	4.2
Two Domains		
Affect/Body	3.4	11.2
Affect/Substance	2.1	3.0
Affect/Role	3.9	2.0
Body/Substance	0.7	2.2
Body/Role	1.6	1.0
Substance/Role	9.4	4.0
Three Domains		
Affect/Body/Substance	0.7	5.7
Affect/Substance/Role	9.6	3.7
Affect/Body/Role	2.5	3.0
Body/Substance/Role	3.0	2.2
Four Domains		
Affect/Body/Substance/Role	3.2	8.9
Total	100%	100%
N	(435)	(596)

continued this line of comparison for the three problem clusters, finding that 61% of these boys evidenced the substance/role/affective problem pattern, while the largest group of girls (39%) had the affective/body/substance problem combination.

Of special note is that 9% of the boys have the substance/role problem combination and another 10% have the substance/role/affective problem combination. Nine percent of girls have problems in all four domains. Certainly these additional problems are portents of increased severity of mental health problems.

The Relationship of Mutliple Problems to Stressors

We turn now to the question of the relationship between problems in the various domains and stressful events in the adolescents' lives. Displayed in Table 5 is the percentage of boys and girls with problems in each domain by the various levels and kinds of stressful life events—high or low in stressful events to self, relationship stressors, stresses in the lives of family members and stresses in the lives of friends. In the last row of the table is the mean number of problem domains for each subgroup of youth.

Considering the domains of problems separately, we see that among girls high levels of each of the stressors is associated with a high rate of problems in each of the four domains. These effects are consistently large. In the case of each stressor, one and one half to more than two times as many girls in the high stress group as in the low stress group have problems in each and every domain. Each one of this wide range of stressors is related to high presence of problems in each domain of problem behavior.

The same pattern of relationships generally holds for boys but is, as a whole, somewhat less powerful than for girls. Boys high in stress to self are much more likely than those low in stress to self to have problems in all four domains. Boys high in each kind of stress—self, relationship, family, and friend—are much more likely to have affective problems than their less stressed counterparts. Other combinations of stress and problems follow this pattern, and are statistically significant, but with less strong effects. The association between relationship stress and the proportion of boys experiencing role problems and between family stress and boys experiencing body problems also are in the direction of more boys in the high stress groups having problems, but they are of borderline (p < .10) statistical significance. There are two exceptions to the findings—no significant relationship exists between family stress and rates of substance problems or between the stress of friends and body problems.

Table 5. Percent of Boys and Girls with the Four Problem Domains by Kinds and Level of Stress Experienced

Problem Domain	Self Stress				Relationship Stress				Family Stress				Friend Stress			
	Boys		Girls		Boys		Girls		Boys		Girls		Boys		Girls	
	Low	High	Low	High	Low	High	Low	High	Low	High	Low	High	Low	High	Low	High
Affect	26.6	50.4c	36.2	66.9c	25.9	55.0c	35.4	61.5c	27.8	50.0c	35.7	65.9c	29.4	48.4c	36.1	63.7c
Body	11.5	30.1c	20.6	50.3	14.2	24.3a	33.5	51.8c	15.0	22.2*	35.2	51.6c	15.4	22.0	33.4	54.7c
Substance	32.7	54.5c	35.4	61.5c	35.2	49.5b	31.1	45.0c	37.3	43.5	31.3	47.3c	36.0	49.5a	28.3	53.2c
Role	39.1	60.2c	29.0	54.4c	42.6	52.3*	23.5	38.5c	42.2	53.7a	23.1	42.3c	42.2	56.0a	22.1	43.7c
Mean Number of Domains	1.1	2.0	1.2	2.3	1.2	1.8	1.2	2.0	1.2	1.7	1.3	2.0	1.2	1.8	1.2	2.2
t	-7.40		-9.72		-5.17		-6.96		-3.77		-7.47		-3.99		-8.98	
df	(433)		(595)		(433)		(595)		(433)		(595)		(433)		(595)	
t	<.001		<.001		<.001		<.001		<.001		<.001		<.001		<.001	

* = $p < .10$
a = $p < .05$
b = $p < .01$
c = $p < .001$

Across the board, there are large and significant differences in the mean number of problem domains for boys and girls who are high in stress compared to those who have experienced fewer events in each of the four arenas of stress. In other words, higher stress appears to have effects beyond the intensification of a single problem or even exacerbation of problems within a domain. It appears to increase the likelihood that the adolescent's problem behaviors will expand into new domains of functioning. Of course, we also recognize that youth with multiple problems in turn manage to more often expose themselves to stressful events.

Finally, in addition to the relationship between individual stressors and the rate of reported problems in the various domains, there is a very strong correlation between the number of arenas in which an adolescent experiences stress and the number of domains in which he or she has problems (Boys: $r = .38$, $p < .001$; Girls: $r = .48$, $p < .001$). Table 6 shows the consistency of this relationship between the number of arenas of stress and the number of problem domains. Of those youth who have no arenas of high experienced stress in the past year, 40.7% of the boys and 50% of the girls have problems in no domains. However, among those exposed to high levels of stressors in three or four arenas, only 12% of the boys and 5.8% of the girls have no manifest problems. Similarly, boys and girls with very low exposure to stressful events (low stress in all four arenas) are much less likely to have problems in several domains. Only 8.8% of the boys and 7.7% of the girls who have low stressors in all arenas have problems in three or four domains, while fully half (boys 50%, girls 51.5%) of those who have been exposed to high numbers of stressful events in three or four arenas have problems in three or four domains. In combination, Tables 5 and 6 make clear the

Table 6. Number of Problem Domains by Number of Arenas of Stressors Experienced

Problem Domains	Stressors							
	No Arenas		One Arena		Two Arenas		Three-Four Arenas	
	Boys	Girls	Boys	Girls	Boys	Girls	Boys	Girls
None	40.7%	50.0%	25.0%	27.9%	16.2%	13.8%	12.0%	5.8%
One	33.5	25.7	39.0	28.5	17.6	24.1	20.0	13.6
Two	17.0	16.5	23.5	26.7	29.4	25.9	18.0	29.1
Three-Four	8.8	7.7	12.5	16.9	36.8	36.2	50.0	51.5

Boys: $X^2 = 88.70$ (df $= 16$) $p < .0001$
Girls: $X^2 = 155.07$ (df $= 16$) $p < .0001$

very strong linkages between exposure to stress and multiple problems in adolescence.

These descriptive analyses have not been designed to establish a direction of causality. Although previous research strongly supports the assumption that stressful life events have an impact on distress and problem behavior, there are evident routes by which most of the problems themselves could increase a youth's exposure to further stressors. For example, heavy drinking could lead to relationship problems within the family or an adolescent who is delinquent may be more likely to find or place him or herself in the company of friends who have problems with the law or who are acting out because of their own family problems. The source of the observed relationship between relationship stress and drinking problems would then be the drinking and the source of the link between friends' stress and delinquency would be the delinquency.

Conclusion

The data in this chapter remind us that, just as we must remain attuned to the reciprocal effects between problem behaviors and social (stress) context, reciprocal effects between problems also merit serious attention. It is not hard to discern mechanisms through which many of these problems might be linked to one another, particularly as mediated through the social and interpersonal consequences of the problems. The earlier sections of this volume, which focus on basic social and interpersonal processes, identify critical family and peer processes.

Clearly, greater understanding of *configurations* of difficulties is called for, especially those crossing the boundaries between externalizing and internalizing behaviors. Can we contrast the epidemiology of patterns crossing domains to those that do not? Which patterns of problems place youth at higher risk for expanding problems into new domains of functioning and, which patterns are more easily contained? How will these patterns and their associated risks differ for boys and girls?

While we know that these adolescent problems are risk factors for adult adjustment we know that many youth who have these problems in adolescence do manage to make a satisfactory adaptation in adulthood. More information is needed about the configurations of patterns that are likely to be consolidated by the end of adolescence and to foretell adult functioning, and about configurations that are looser, more transient constellations. Just as we look to social resources and liabilities as exacerbating or reducing risk, coexisting patterns of problems must be considered as having the potential to intensify vulnerability and psychosocial risk.

Acknowledgment

This research was supported by NIMH Grant MH42909.

References

Achenbach, T. M. (1966). The classification of children's psychiatric symptoms: A factor-analytic study. *Psychological Monographs*. (Whole No. 615).

Achenbach, T. M., & Edelbrock, C. S. (1981). Behavioral problems and competencies reported by parents of normal and disturbed children aged 4 through 16. *Monographs of the Society for Research in Child Development*, 46 (Serial No. 188).

Achenbach, T. M., & Edelbrock, C. S. (1987). *Manual for the Youth Self-Report and Profile*. Burlington, VT: University of Vermont Department of Psychiatry.

Bachman, J. G., Johnston, L. D. & O'Malley, P. M. (1986). *Monitoring the Future*. Ann Arbor, MI: Institute for Social Research.

Bemis, K. (1978). Current approaches to the etiology and treatment of anorexia nervosa. *Psychological Bulletin*, 85, 593–617.

Block, J. & Gjerde, P. F. (1990). Depressive symptomatology in late adolescence: A longitudinal perspective on personality antecedents. In J. E. Rolf, A. Masten, D. Cicchetti, K. Neuchterlein, & S. Weintraub (Eds.) *Risk and protective factors in the development of psychopathology* (pp. 334–360). NY: Cambridge University Press.

Boskind-Lodahl, M. (1976). Cinderella's stepsisters: A feminist perspective on anorexia nervosa and bulimia. *Signs*, 2, 341–356.

Brooks-Gunn, J., & Petersen, A. C. (Eds.). (1983). *Girls at puberty: Biological and psychosocial perspectives*. NY: Plenum.

Bush, D. M. (1985). The impact of changing gender role expectations upon socialization in adolescence. In A. C. Kerckhoff (Ed.), *Research in sociology of education and socialization* (Vol. 5, pp. 269–297). Greenwich, CT: JAI Press.

Carlson, G. A., & Cantwell, D. P. (1979). A survey of depressive symptoms in a child and adolescent psychiatric population: Interview data. *Journal of the American Academy of Child Psychiatry*, 18, 587–599.

Carlson, G. A., & Cantwell, D. P. (1980). Unmasking masked depression in children and adolescents. *American Journal of Psychiatry*, 137, 445–449.

Canter, R. J. (1982). Sex differences in self-report delinquency. *Criminology*, 20, 373–393.

Cleary, P. D. (1987). Gender differences in stress-related disorders. In R. C. Barnett, L. Biener & G. K. Baruch (Eds.), *Gender and stress* (pp. 39–72). The Free Press.

Colten, M. E., & Marsh, J. C. (1984). A sex-roles perspective on drug and alcohol use by women. In C. S. Widom (Ed.), *Sex roles and psychopathology* (pp. 219–248). NY: Plenum.

Compas, B. E., Davis, G. E., & C. J. Forsythe. (1985). Characteristics of life events during adolescence. *American Journal of Community Psychology*, 13, 677–691.

Compas, B. E., Slavin, L. A., Wagner, B. M., & Vannatta, K. (1986). Relationship of life events and social support with psychological dysfunction among adolescents. *Journal of Youth and Adolescence, 15*, 203–219.

Derogatis, L. R. (1977). *SCL 90: Administration, scoring, and procedures manual for the revised version.* Baltimore, MD: Johns Hopkins University.

Earls, F., Reich, W., Jung, K., & Cloninger, C. (1988). Psychopathology in children of alcoholic and antisocial parents. *Alcoholism: Clinical and experimental research, 12*, 481–487.

Ebata, A. T., & Petersen, A. C. (in press). *Patterns of adjustment during early adolescence: Gender differences in depression and achievement.* Submitted manuscript.

Emery, R. E. (1982). Interparental conflict and the children of discord and divorce. *Psychological Bulletin, 92*, 310–330.

Felner, R. D., Aber, M. S., Primavera, J., & Cauce, A. M. (1985). Adaptation and vulnerability in high-risk adolescents: An examination of environmental mediators. *American Journal of Community Psychology, 13*, 365–379.

Garmezy, N., & Rutter, M. (1983). *Stress, coping and development in children.* NY: McGraw Hill.

Gjerde, P. F., Block, J., & Block, J. H. (1988). Depressive symptoms and personality during late adolescence: Gender differences in the externalization-internalization of symptom expression. *Journal of Abnormal Psychology, 97*, 475–486.

Gove, W. R., & Herb, T. R. (1974). Stress and mental illness among the young: A comparison of the sexes. *Social Forces, 53*, 256–265.

Hill, J. P., & Lynch, M. E. (1983). The intensification of gender-related role expectations during early adolescence. In J. Brooks-Gunn & A. C. Petersen (Eds.), *Girls at puberty: Biological and psychosocial perspectives* (pp. 201–228). NY: Plenum.

Horwitz, A. V., & White, H. R. (1987). Gender role orientations and styles of pathology among adolescents. *Journal of Health and Social Behavior, 28*, 158–170.

Jessor, R. (1982). Critical issues in research on adolescent health promotion. In T. J. Coates, A. C. Petersen, & C. Perry (Eds.), *Promoting Adolescent Health* (pp. 447–465). NY: Academic Press.

Johnson, J. H., & McCutcheon, S. (1980). Assessing life events in older children and adolescents. In I. G. Sarason & C. D. Spielberger (Eds.), *Stress and anxiety* (Vol. 7), Washington, DC: Hemisphere.

Kandel, D. B., & Davies, M. (1982). Epidemiology of depressive mood in adolescents. *Archives of General Psychiatry, 39*, 1205–1212.

Kandel, D. B., Kessler, R. C., & Margulies, R. Z. (1978). Antecedents of adolescent initiation into stages of drug use: A developmental analysis. *Journal of Youth and Adolescence, 7*, 13–39.

Kashani, J. H., & Orvashel (1988). Anxiety disorders in mid-adolescence. *American Journal of Psychiatry, 145*, 960–964.

Kashani, J. H., Beck, N. C., Hoeper, E. W., Fallahi, C., Corcoran, C. M., McAllister, J. A., Rosenberg, T. K., & Reid, R. C. (1987). Psychiatric disorders in a community sample of adolescents. *American Journal of Psychiatry, 144*, 584–589.

Kashani, J. H., Carlson, G. A., Beck, N. C., Hoeper, E. W., Corcoran, C. M., McAllister, J. A., Fallahi, C., Rosenberg, T. K., & Reid, J. C. (1987). Depression, depressive symptoms and depressed mood among a community sample of adolescents. *American Journal of Psychiatry, 144*, 931–934.

Kelly, J. G. (1979). *Adolescent boys in high school: A psychological study of coping and adaptation.* Somerset, NJ: Erlbaum.

Kessler, R. C., & McLeod, J. D. (1984). Sex differences in vulnerability to undesirable life events. *American Sociological Review, 49*, 620–631.

Klerman, G. L., & Weissman, M. M. (1989). Increasing rates of depression. *JAMA, 261*(15), 2229–2235.

Kovacs, M., & Beck, A. T. (1977). An empirical clinical approach towards a definition of childhood depression. In J. Schulterbrandt & A. Raskin (Eds.), *Depression in childhood.* NY: Raven Press.

Leland, J. (1982). Gender, drinking, and alcohol abuse. In I. Al-Issa (Ed.) *Gender and psychopathology.* New York: Academic Press.

Lewinsohn, P. M., Hops, H., Roberts, R., and Seeley, J. R. (1988). *Adolescent depression: Prevalence and psychosocial aspects.* Paper presented at the Annual meeting of the American Public Health Association, Boston.

Locksley, A., & Douvan, E. (1979). Problem behavior in adolescence. In E. S. Gomberg & V. Franks (Eds.), *Gender and disordered behavior* (pp. 71–100). New York: Brunner/Mazel.

Magnusson, D., & Bergman, L. R. (1988). Individual and variable-based approaches to longitudinal research in early risk factors. In M. Rutter (Ed.), *Studies of psychosocial risk: the power of longitudinal data* (pp. 45–61). NY: Cambridge University Press.

Marsh, J. C., Colten, M. E., & Tucker, M. B. (1982). Women's use of drugs and alcohol: New perspectives. *Journal of Social Issues, 38*, 1–8.

Newcomb, M. D., & Bentler, M. D. (1988). *Consequences of adolescent drug use: Impact on the lives of young adults.* Newbury Park, CA: Sage.

Newcomb, M. D., & Bentler, M. D. (1989). Substance use and abuse among children and teenagers. *American Psychologist, 44*, 242–248.

Newcomb, M. D., Huba, G. J., & Bentler, P. M. (1981). A multi-dimensional assessment of stressful life events among adolescents: Derivations and correlates. *Journal of Health and Social Behavior, 22*, 400–415.

Petersen, A. C., & Craighead, W. E. (1986). Emotional and personality development in normal adolescents and young adults. In G. L. Klerman (Ed.), *Suicide and depression among adolescents and young adults* (pp. 17–52). Washington, DC: American Psychiatric Press.

Puig-Antich, J. (1982). Major depression and conduct disorder in prepuberty. *Journal of the American Academy of Child Psychiatry, 21*, 118–128.

Radloff, L. S. (1977). The CES-D scale: A self-report depression scale for research in the general population. *Applied Psychological Measurement, 1*, 385–401.

Robbins, D. R., & Alessi, N. E. (1985). Depressive symptoms and suicidal behavior in adolescents. *American Psychiatric Association, 142*, 588–592.

Robins, L. N., Helzer, J. E., Weissman, M. M., Orvaschel, H., Gruenberg, E., Burke, J. D., & Regier, D. A. (1984). Lifetime prevalence of specific psychiatric disorder in three sites. *Archives of General Psychiatry, 41*, 929–958.

Rubenstein, J. L., Heeren, T., Housman, D., Rubin, C., & Stechler, G. (1988). *Suicidal behavior in "normal" adolescents: Risk and protective factors*. Paper presented at biennial meeting, The Society for Research in Adolescence. Alexandria, VA.

Rutter, M. (1986). The developmental psychopathology of depression: Issues and perspectives. In M. Rutter, C. E. Izard, & P. B. Read (Eds.), *Depression in young people* (pp. 3–30). NY: Guilford Press.

Rutter, M. (1970). Sex differences in children's responses to family stress. In E. Anthony & C. Koupernki (Eds.), *The Child in his family* (Vol. 2, pp. 165–196). NY: Wiley.

Rutter, M., & Sandberg, S. (1988). Epidemiology of child psychiatric disorder: Methodological issues and some substantive findings. *Child Psychiatry and Human Development, 15*, 209–233.

Simmons, R. G., & Blyth, D. A. (1987). *Moving into adolescence: The impact of pubertal change and school context.* NY: Aldine de Gruyter.

Stroufe, L. A., & Rutter, M. (1984). The domain of developmental psychopathology. *Child Development, 55*, 17–29.

Weiner, I. B. (1980). Psychopathology in adolescence. In J. Adelson (Ed.), *Handbook of adolescent psychology.* New York: Wiley.

Weissman, M. M., & Klerman, G. L. (1977). Sex differences and the epidemiology of depression. *Archives of General Psychology, 34*, 98–111.

Wells, B., Deykin, E., & Klerman, G. (1985). Risk factors for depression in adolescence, *Psychiatric Developments, 3*, 83–108.

Werner, E. E., & Smith, R. S. (1982). *Vulnerable but invincible: A longitudinal study of resilient children and youth.* New York: McGraw Hill.

9

Minority Youths at High Risk: Gay Males and Runaways

Mary Jane Rotheram-Borus, Margaret Rosario, and Cheryl Koopman

The futures of Black and Hispanic youths in the United States are often not as bright as for their White peers (Furstenberg, 1987; Manoff, Gayle, Mays, & Rogers, 1989). Minority youths are less likely to have a job (William T. Grant Foundation, 1988), but more likely to drop out or not to enter college (Bock & Moore, 1986), to become single parents (Zelnik & Kantner, 1980), or to die early by homicide (Alers, 1978). Although these statistics on minority youths are alarming, there are subgroups of minorities with even fewer chances for healthy adjustment.

Runaway and gay male minority adolescents are two groups that have reduced chances for healthy adjustment. As adolescents these youths have experienced even greater stress, have fewer resources, and engage in more risky acts than their same-ethnic peers. This chapter will describe the stresses experienced by runaway and gay youths, their social supports, and the risk behaviors that have been observed.

Runaways

The number of runaways has been increasing over the last 15 years. In 1975 it was estimated that there were between 519,500 and 635,000 runaways and homeless youths (DHHS, 1984). This number rose to approximately 733,000 in 1982 (Chelimsky, 1982) and today it is estimated that there are approximately 1.5 million runaway and homeless youths (Children's Defense Fund, 1988).

One of the problems in understanding risk behaviors among runaways has been confusion and mislabeling of subgroups of runaways. Bucy (1990) has identified five categories of youths:

1. *Runaway children* have left their families overnight without parental or caretaker permission, usually because they are unable to deal with some family or personal problem. Running away often occurs repeatedly (Shaffer & Caton, 1984). Those who runaway repeatedly are more likely to stay away from home longer, are less likely to return home voluntarily, are more likely to come from troubled homes, have more difficulties in school, and have more trouble with the law.

2. *Homeless or throw-away youths* have left with the full knowledge of their parents/guardians, even though they may have no alternative home. Robertson (1989) found that approximately 31% of youths in Los Angeles runaway shelters had been asked to leave home. Rotheram-Borus and colleagues (Rotheram-Borus, Koopman, & Bradley, 1989) found 63% of youths in New York City to be throw-aways.

3. *Street kids* are long-term homeless or runaways who have become adept at fending for themselves "on the street." They are likely to engage in illegal, high-risk activities to survive, such as selling drugs or exchanging sex for money.

4. *System kids* have been removed from their families for their own protection. Often these children are placed in a series of unsuccessful foster care placements. Approximately 50% of runaway youths come from foster care placement, delinquent detention facilities, or group homes (Robertson, 1989).

5. *Victimized children* have been verbally, physically, or sexually abused by their parent, guardian, or other family member. In San Francisco approximately 60% of the runaway girls have reported sexual abuse (Hermann, 1988), while in Los Angeles service providers estimated that about 26% of their clients had been sexually abused (Rothman & David, 1985). In New York, 50% of shelter runaways reported having been sexually and/or physically abused by one or both parents (Shaffer & Caton, 1984).

These categories of youths are not mutually exclusive. For example, "throw-away children" who are currently living on the streets may be turned over to the local Social Services for Children Bureau next week, becoming "system kids." Although recognizing the importance of these distinctions, we focus on problems common among these categories of homeless and runaway youth.

Approximately equal numbers of girls and boys are served in residential shelters, although more boys are typically on the street (Robertson, 1989; Shaffer & Caton, 1984). The ethnic breakdown of runaways typically reflects that of the surrounding geographic area. Nationally, 70% of runaways are white, 19% Black, and 7% Hispanic (Children's Defense Fund, 1988). Ninety percent of the runaways in New York City are minority youths. Furthermore, while shelter staff frequently report a large number of youths migrating from rural to urban areas, the epidemiological studies do not support these assertions. Shaffer and Caton (1984) found more than 90% of runaways in New York City to be from the New York area. However, the West Coast is believed to have a different pattern, as suggested by research by Yates, MacKenzie, Pennbridge, and Cohen (1988).

A number of factors have been associated with running away and/or being homeless. For girls, it may be a consequence of teenage pregnancy. In Illinois in 1985, it was estimated that 35% of the 20,000 homeless youths were teen mothers or pregnant. One-third of displaced and homeless families have children, but adolescents are often not allowed to receive shelter in the same welfare hotel as their parents. For example, in New Jersey 18% of the adolescents are in foster care because their families cannot find shelter (Fagan, 1987). Thus, some adolescents enter the residential shelter system due to their parents' homelessness.

The families of runaways have often been perceived as the source of the youth's problems (Chelimsky, 1982). Many of the youths have been physically and sexually abused within their families, with estimates from 25 to 75% (Chelimsky, 1982; Hermann, 1988; National Network of Runaway and Homeless Youths, 1985; Robertson, 1989). Robertson found that the majority of parents of runaways were alcoholic, 14% of the parents had received treatment for their alcoholism, and 23% of youths reported that parents' alcoholism was the precipitant for leaving home, similar to the findings of Shaffer and Caton (1984). Solarz (1988) found that mothers of runaways were more likely to have psychiatric problems, abuse illicit substances, and to have fewer social supports. Only 37% of runaways come from two-parent families (Shane, 1989).

Among runaways, there are reports of high rates of alcohol and substance abuse, unprotected sexual intercourse, trouble at school and with the law, and emotional distress (Council on Scientific Affairs, 1989). Although alcohol or substance abuse is not typically the cause of leaving a stable living environment, high rates of life-time use are often associated with homelessness. Yates et al. (1988) found that 84% of runaways receiving services at a health clinic used alcohol or drugs, compared to 35% among nonrunaways. Robertson (1989) found 38% of runaway youths met DSM III criteria for a diagnosis of substance abuse, which was five times that of nonrunaway adolescents.

Runaways have been perceived at high risk for HIV infection and as a potential vector for infecting the heterosexual community with HIV (Daley, 1988). In our research on largely minority youth, approximately 65% of the runaway girls and boys engaged in intercourse in the last 3 months (Rotheram-Borus & Koopman, 1990), with sexually active boys and girls having averaged 4.7 to 2.0 sexual partners, respectively, during the last 3 months. There are no adequate normative data for comparing sexual behavior patterns among minority youths in the United States, although we found that approximately 12% of the runaway girls have had more than ten sexual partners during their lifetime (Rotheram-Borus, et al., 1990), compared to 3% reported in a 1970 probability sample of urban girls (Turner, Miller, & Moses, 1989). Runaway boys have been relatively more active, with 42% reporting more than 10 lifetime partners compared to approximately 9% of boys in the same report.

Unlike their peers in stable home environments, runaways—particularly the boys—often resort to trading sex for money or drugs. In one study (Rotheram-Borus, et al., 1990) we found 22% of the boys to have engaged in prostitution at some point, mostly with opposite-sex partners. Only 7% of the girls reported these behaviors. Robertson (1989) reported that 30% of runaways in Los Angeles engaged in prostitution, and Yates et al. (1988), in a medical outpatient clinic, reported 26% had traded sex for money or drugs at some point. It is more likely that the choice of partners, rather than the frequency of the sexual activity of these youths, places them at risk for HIV infection, since they are especially likely to know other HIV-infected persons, and runaways are similar to their nonrunaway peers in their use of condoms. Most disturbing are the results of screening youths at Covenant House, a large runaway shelter in NYC, for HIV infection in a blind seroprevalence study (Stricof, Novick, Kennedy, & Weisfuse, 1988). Among the youths, 6.7% were HIV seropositive; 7.4% of the adolescent boys and 5.4% of the girls were found to be positive.

Children living in homeless shelters have been found to demonstrate serious developmental and emotional problems (Bassuk & Rosenberg, 1988). Approximately half of runaway youths have been suspended or expelled from school (Price, 1987; Shaffer & Caton, 1984). Frequently they are below average in their academic performance: Robertson (1989) found in Los Angeles that 25% had repeated at least one grade and 25% also attended special education classes. Shaffer and Caton (1984) also reported that 25% of girls and 50% of boys had been arrested or jailed at some point.

It is not surprising that in this unstable living context, emotional distress also has been reported to be high. Shaffer and Caton (1984) found 38% of runaway and homeless adolescents believe they needed help for emotional problems; 70% were depressed or having behavior problems; 33% of the girls and 15% of the boys had previously attempted suicide. Similar findings were reported in Los Angeles, with Robertson (1989) finding that 49% had attempted suicide. In addition, meeting basic survival and security needs is a difficult problem. Robertson (1989) found that hunger was a problem for 57% of runaways within the last month, and that 19% had a serious but untreated health problem within the last year.

The high rates across each of these five risk behaviors indicate that a substantial percentage of runaways are likely to exhibit a "multi-problem behavior syndrome" (Jessor & Jessor, 1977). That is, an adolescent who engages in one of these behaviors is more likely to engage in several, since these risk behaviors often cluster together (Biglan et al., 1989)

Gay Youths

Gay youths are a much more difficult group to describe. There are scant data available on which to base conclusions (Remafedi, 1987a). Some argue that adolescents are too young to self-identify gay (Sullivan & Schneider, 1987), while others argue that the development of a gay identity typically begins prior to puberty (Troidan, 1988). Sexual relationships are particularly paramount in adolescence, and youths need opportunities to feel close without fear of ridicule or exploitation (Berlin, 1980). Yet, for gay youth, failure to conform to traditional roles elicits harassment, violence, and rejection from family, peer groups, and religious institutions (D'Augelli, 1989). Many youths, therefore, meet sexual needs by engaging in anonymous sex, resulting in loneliness and isolation for gay males (Martin, 1982). Kellog (1978) describes the loneliness accompanying breaking up, while Harding (1986) discusses suicides that follow break-ups.

Problems in school are a major concern for adolescents, and gay male adolescents are especially likely to experience difficulties. Of the gay male youths interviewed in Minneapolis/St. Paul (Remafedi, 1987a), 80% had deteriorating school performance, and 28% dropped out of high school.

Gay youths also typically do not have ready access to health care that recognizes and addresses their sexual concerns (Paroski, 1987). Remafedi (1987a) found that nearly three-quarters of gay male youths preferred attending a public health or gay venereal disease clinic than visiting a private or family physician.

There has been little research on risk behaviors of gay male adolescents, and even less on those who are Black or Hispanic. A sample of largely white, middle class gay male adolescents from Minneapolis/St. Paul was found to engage in a number of risk behaviors, including substance abuse, running away, having sexually transmitted diseases, and attempting suicide (Remafedi, 1987a). The generalization of these findings to Black and Hispanic gay males is unclear.

A Study of Stressful Life Events and Social Supports in a Sample of Runaway and Gay Youths

We are in the first phase of a 5-year longitudinal study of HIV (the AIDS virus) prevention. We recruited a consecutive series of male and female runaway youths who were provided shelter at two New York City residential runaway programs for at least 48 hours. We also recruited male youths who participated in the activities of a community agency for gay and lesbian adolescents in Manhattan, the Hetrick-Martin Institute. In 15 months, only 2 youths seeking services at these agencies refused to voluntarily participate in the study.

There were 43 female runaways, 47 male runaways, and 36 gay males, aged 12 to 18 years old. The youths were predominantly minority: 55% Black, 36% Hispanic, 5% White, and 4% other. There were more Black male runaways (59%) than Black gay males (31%), but more Hispanic gay males (57%) than Hispanic male runaways (34%). As for sexual orientation, 93% of the male runaways and 95% of the female runaways described themselves as heterosexual, while 93% of the gay males described themselves as homosexual or bisexual. All of the youths described here as "gay males" were recruited from the Hetrick-Martin Institute.

Assessments

In this study, we focused on the youths' stressful life events, social supports, and sexual risk behaviors. Choosing assessment instruments is difficult when conducting research with populations that have rarely been studied. On the one hand, we wanted to use existing measures to compare and to replicate findings across studies. On the other hand, there was a need to be sensitive to the uniqueness of the groups. We attempted to meet both demands.

Johnson and McCutcheon's (1980) adolescent stressful life events instrument appeared to be the most useful measure for high risk youths. This instrument focuses on the occurrence of desirable and undesirable life events and also asks youths to evaluate the impact of each event. It does not, however, assess daily hassles, such as subway delays. Following focus group discussions and piloting, our revised instrument consists of 62 items that monitor events over the last 3 months. Its response scale allows examination of two questions: whether the event occurred or not, and, when it did occur, did it have a positive or negative impact. In this report, we will focus primarily on the undesirable events.

Barrera's (1981) Arizona Social Support Interview Schedule was the major social support measure. Five different types of support were assessed: (1) intimate support, focusing on those persons who provided advice and those with whom the youth discussed "very personal and private" matters; (2) physical support, identifying the persons who instrumentally assisted the youth with such things as "driving you someplace you needed to go, helping you do some work around the house, going to the store for you, and things like that"; (3) socializing support, focusing on those persons with whom the youth interacted "to have fun or to relax"; (4) sexual information, identifying those persons to whom the youth turned for information "about sex, birth control, AIDS, and so on"; and (5) alcohol/drug information, identifying those persons to whom the youth turned for information about "drugs or alcohol." Youths can turn to a drug pusher or to a parent for information about alcohol. Therefore, a support person may be a source who encourages or discourages drug use.

For each type of support over the last 3 months, four different types of information were gathered: the number of available supporters, the number of supporters the youth actually contacted, satisfaction with actual support received using a 7-point Likert response rating (7 = high satisfaction), and need for support using a 5-point Likert response scale (5 = great need). In addition, we asked about the age, ethnicity, and the relationship to the youth of each person giving support. Finally, to focus on sexual risk behavior, youths identified the numbers of people in their support group who used drugs and engaged in unsafe sexual acts.

Given that the ongoing study is concerned with HIV prevention, we closely examined the sexual risk behaviors of these youths. Experienced sex researchers developed our assessment instruments. Again, focus group discussions were held with runaway and gay youths and all measures were extensively piloted. The Sexual Risk Behavior Assessment Schedule—Youth Baseline Interview (Meyer-Bahlburg, Ehrhardt, Exner, & Gruen, 1988) provides indices of the number of sexual occasions, partners, and condom use over the last 3 months.

What Stresses Do These Youths Experience?

We summarized the frequency of stressful life events reported by these youths in Table 1. We have organized the events into subcategories, based on the type of stressful event.[1] The table shows that runaway and gay youths experience a great deal of stress. The stress data indicate that 62% of the events for male runaways, 72% of the events for female

Table 1. Percentage of Youths Experiencing Each Stressor during Past Three Months[a]

	Male runaways (N = 53)	Female runaways (N = 52)	Gay males (N = 22)	Total (N = 127)
Family Stress				
New stepparent	17	27	14	21
Increased arguments between parents	32[c]	65	46	48
Increased parental absence	30[d]	44	9	32
Parents separated	28	37	18	30
Parents divorced	17	23	9	18
Increased arguments with parents	45	60	50	52
Changes in parents' financial status	28[d]	33	9	19
Parent lost job	17[c]	39	5	24
Parent having legal trouble	11	19	9	14
Parent going to jail	17	19	9	17
Increased trouble with sibling	28[b]	44	27	35
Sibling left home	17[c]	40	5	24
Family member having drug problems	40[d]	39	14	35
Family member having illness or injury	25	33	14	26
Family member died	30	44	36	37
Move Stress				
Changing to a new school	32[c]	54	41	43
Moving to a new home	51[c,d]	73	23	55
Changing residences more than twice	40[d]	39	14	35
School Stress				
Failing a grade	40[b]	58	57	45
Failing grades on report card	26[c]	56	27	39
Trouble with classmates	34[b]	50	23	39
Trouble with teacher	40	44	46	43
School suspension	36[d]	33	14	31
School expulsion	23[d]	23	5	20
Not making an athletic team	21	29	14	23
Peer Stress				
Breaking up with girlfriend/ boyfriend	36	31	18	31
Losing a close friend (other than by death)	26	35	27	30
Close friend's drug problem	30[b]	15	23	23
Close friend's serious illness or injury	19[c]	42	18	29
Close friend's death	11[c]	35	27	24
Self Stress				
Losing a job	26	27	27	27
Trouble with police but not arrested	21	23	23	22
Arrested but not convicted of a crime	17	15	9	15

	Male runaways (N = 53)	Female runaways (N = 52)	Gay males (N = 22)	Total (N = 127)
Convicted of a crime	19^d	12	5	13
Jailed	26	17	14	21
Robbed or burglarized	21	19	14	19
Physically assaulted	13	21	27	19
Raped or sexually assaulted	15	27	14	20
Health Stress				
Having a drug or alcohol problem	13	23	14	17
Major personal illness or injury	23	37	14	27
Getting pregnant	NA	25	NA	25
Having an abortion	NA	21	NA	21
Girlfriend getting pregnant (males only)	25^d	NA	0	17
Girlfriend having an abortion (males only)	13	NA	5	11
Gay/Bisexual Stress				
Came out to parents	9	2	31	10
Came out to sibling	4	4	32	9
Came out to friends	8	4	64	16
Parents discovered that you are gay	6	4	23	8
Other family members discovered that you are gay	8	6	27	10
Friends discovered that you are gay	8	0	36	10
Someone ridiculed your sexual identity	9	2	55	14
Positive events				
Parent getting a new job	23^d	31	5	23
Getting a job on your own	43	37	32	39
Special recognition for good grades	42^b	60	40	49
Making the honor roll	25	39	36	32
Making an athletic team	30	21	23	25
Special recognition for athletic performance	17	27	23	22
Joining a club	32	21	27	27
Acquiring a new girlfriend/ boyfriend	34	23	40	31
Making up with a girlfriend/ boyfriend	32	23	27	28
Getting a new sibling	11^c	31	14	20

^{a}Comparisons of percentages were performed via the z test, using the arcsine transformation. Two sets of comparisons were made: between runaway males and females and between runaway and gay males.
^{b}p < .10 between runaway males and females.
^{c}p < .05 between runaway males and females.
^{d}p < .05 between runaway and gay males.

runaways, and 32% of the events for gay males were reported by more than 20% of youths in these groups. These rates are about four times as large as those reported in other populations of adolescents (Newcomb, Huba, & Bentler, 1981; Swearingen & Cohen, 1985).

These youths had experienced an increase in arguments with and between their parents. Among the runaways, parents had been absent from home more often in the last 3 months, lost a job, and the family finances had changed. Even more important, many of the runaways' parents were reported to have problems with drugs (about 40%). As might be expected, the runaways had moved more frequently than the gay youths.

Problems at school were also common. Runaway girls reported more trouble academically and with peers. However, both runaway girls and boys were suspended or expelled more frequently than the gay youths. Friends and romantic relationships appeared to be important stressors for youths, despite their potential to provide support. About one-third of the runaways had ended a romantic relationship in the last 3 months, as did 18% of the gay youths. In addition, large percentages of all youths had lost friendships, had friends who died or were injured, as well as had friends with drug problems.

The most striking reports were those documenting the stressors indicating victimization. In the last 3 months, approximately one in five youths had been physically assaulted, one in five youths had been raped or sexually assaulted, and one in five youths had been robbed or burglarized. However, in addition to being victimized, one in five also had been in trouble with the police, but had not been arrested, one in six had been arrested, one in six had been convicted of a crime, and one in five had been jailed.

Personal stressors also extended into the areas of sex and substance abuse behaviors, those which place youths at higher risk for HIV. Overall, 17% reported having a problem with drug and alcohol use. Disturbingly, 25% of runaways, both males and females, reported being involved in a pregnancy. Many of these pregnancies reportedly resulted in abortions. It is difficult to interpret these data, however, since we have little information on base rates of sexual behaviors among inner-city minority youths.

Do the Stresses Differ by Group?

Overall, runaways reported more stressful life events than the gay males in this sample (with the exception of gay-related stressors). In addition, a rank order of stress appeared: runaway females experienced more stress than runaway males, who in turn experienced significantly more stress than gay males. Of the 12 significant differences between runaway males and females, 11 followed this trend. When runaway males and gay males were compared, all of the 8 significant differences were in this direction. In this sample, the gay male adolescents had more stable home lives, and were less likely to report problems with school, peers, and the law.

Differences between runaway males and females were concentrated in certain areas: family, moving, school, and peers. In each of these domains, a higher percentage of the girls than the boys experienced the stressful life events. Problems with health issues and personal stress due to assaults, work, and legal trouble were similar across runaway males and females. Runaway males, however, did report having more close friends with drug problems than did runaway females.

Is There a Unique Stress in Being Gay?

Gay youths have unique sources of stress, issues of disclosing or being discovered by family or friends, reactions by others to their homosexuality, and chronic stress associated with their homosexuality. One- to two-thirds of gay youths reported experiencing stressors in the gay domain.

Within the previous 3 months more youths disclosed their sexual orientation to friends (64%) than to parents (31%), a pattern also found among middle-class gay adolescents in Minneapolis/St. Paul (Remafedi, 1987b). Interestingly, Strommen (1989) suggested that siblings are told before parents, but our gay youngsters' rates of disclosure to siblings and parents were practically identical.

Hunter (1990) reports that the earlier one self-identifies as gay, the greater the emotional distress and the greater the punishment one receives from adults. However, even among youths who self-identify as gay and attend a gay-identified community agency, one-third have not come out to friends and two-thirds have not disclosed to their parents. These data suggest that many youths may hide their gay sexual orientation until late adolescence or adulthood.

Gay youths may have chosen not to disclose, but others may have discovered their gay sexual orientation. In the previous 3 months, approximately one-quarter of parents and one-third of friends have discovered the youths' homosexuality. Therefore, half of the youths had come out to or had been discovered by at least one parent and all were known to be gay by at least one friend.

Despite the stress necessarily associated with disclosure, discovery by an important other may be even more stressful. Our data offer a preliminary test of this hypothesis. We found that more youths rated disclosing events as positive experiences than they did discovery events: 71% of youths disclosing to friends rated disclosing as positive, while 50% of youths who were discovered by friends rated the discovery as positive. Whether gay youths disclose or others discover their sexual orientation, they have little control over others' reactions, i.e., will they be accepted or rejected? Perhaps it is this inability to predict the outcome that makes gay events stressful in their contemplation and actual occurrence, and explains cover-up of a gay sexual orientation.

In addition, rejection by others can have important repercussions. Remafedi (1987b) found that a sizable proportion (41%) of gay male youths had lost a friend over the youths' homosexuality, making us wonder about the extent to which this issue played a role for the 27% of gay youths who lost a close friend. More importantly, in a study of young gay male suicidal attempters and nonattempters, Schneider, Farberow, and Kruks (1989) found that recent attempters, unlike nonattempters, rated rejecting others as more important to them and were more dependent on those who rejected them.

Gay youths are at risk for abuse by family and others (Martin & Hetrick, 1988) and therefore, must be chronically vigilant. The data (Table 1) indicate that more than half of the gay male youths had been ridiculed during the previous 3 months for their sexual orientation. Remafedi (1987b) found that over half his sample experienced verbal abuse from classmates and about a third were assaulted physically ("gay bashing"). We, therefore, wonder to what extent the physical assaults experienced by our gay youths (27%) were related to their sexual orientation.

The documentation of gay stressful events presents an interesting paradox. Typically, the absence of an event implies a condition of nonstress, but this does not hold for gay stress. For gay youths who hide their sexual orientation, not to disclose to family and friends may be a more significant stressor than coming out. In this case, in the absence of disclosure, the individual may be evading and hiding, a circumstance that may be more stressful than disclosing.

Although our assessment measure was developed after holding several focus groups, consulting clinicians, and reviewing charts, the scale was not constructed with an appreciation for the chronic stress attributable to nondisclosure of one's sexual orientation. More generally, the existence of acute and chronic gay stress underscores the omission in the literature, as no gay stressful life events are included in any adult or adolescent stressful life events instrument with which we are familiar.

Positive Events

Although the runaway and gay youngsters have alarming rates of negative events, they also have high rates of positive events, a welcomed finding since positive events may bring joy into their lives and highlight their social skills. Over a third of the youths in each sample had gotten a job on their own, underscoring the youngsters' social skills and abilities to interact with the larger society. These positive attributes also are implied in their high rates (over 20% of each sample) of athletic and club membership. Moreover, substantial numbers of youth reported receiving special recognition for academic performance. These data are at odds with the stressful event data of the school domain and, therefore, suggest subpopulations of well-functioning youths among these high risk adolescents. There are some who may avoid stress, others who experience it and fail to cope with it in a way that eradicates the stress, and still others who may experience it but may cope with it effectively. For example, the rates for failing a grade and special recognition for good grades are both high for the runaway girls. Runaway and gay adolescents are not a homogeneous group; only a detailed, longitudinal analysis of their stress, coping strategies, social supports, and adaptation will be able to shed light on this issue.

Who Do Youths Go to for Social Support?

Next, we examined the social support systems of the youths. In Table 2, we see that both nuclear and extended family members are sources of support to youths. It was somewhat surprising to find this characterizing runaway adolescents who did not significantly differ from gay youths, as this is contrary to the view in the popular press that runaway youths sever family ties (Hersch, 1988). Perhaps this popular view is inaccurate

Table 2. Youth's Identification of Supporters[a]

	Percent			
	Male runaways (N = 50)	*Female runaways (N = 38)*	*Gay males (N = 30)*	*Total (N = 118)*
Father	20	21	20	21
Mother	43	42	50	44
Sibling	39	32	30	34
Extended family adult	42	29	33	36
Extended family children	14	24	7	15
Peer	98[b]	90	90	93
Informal adult	18[c]	21	3	15

[a]The overall patterns of support identification for males and females were significantly different at $p < .05$.
[b]$p < .10$ between runaway males and females.
[c]$p < .05$ between runaway and gay males.

or it may apply only to street youths, a different population from the runaway youths who attend shelters. However, it is important to note that we do not as yet have comparison data from a normal cross section of youth. We suspect that estimates of parental and familial support for all these groups are quite low.

Mothers were cited as sources of support more so than fathers (42–50% vs. 20–21%) for each of the three groups of youths. Also it is striking that only 3% of gay youths reported having a network of adult informal supports, whereas approximately 20% of runaways have an adult as a resource who is not in a formal role toward the youth. This suggests that many runaways, especially the boys, adapt for forging ties with supportive adults outside the immediate family.

We also found that over 90% of each sample turned to peers for support. Unfortunately, the number of runaway and gay youths who lost a close friend or whose close friend had a drug problem or a serious illness/injury (Table 1) was high; therefore, we wonder just how supportive these friends actually can be. It is particularly questionable whether peers who used drugs could usually provide socially acceptable advice and information.

The three groups also differed significantly on the number of supporters who used drugs, alcohol, and were knowledgeable about AIDS. Runaway males reported that more members of their support network used drugs and alcohol than did runaway females and gay males. This picture is consistent with data from the measure of stressful life events for family members' and close friends' drug problems (Table 1). The runaway males had the highest reports of these problems, followed by the females and the gay males.

What Are the Youths' Social Supports?

We next examined the availability, use, and satisfaction with the support provided in different domains: closeness, instrumental help, socializing, and sexual, drug and alcohol information. For intimacy and help, youths typically identified more than two potential supporters and had utilized these sources of support in the last three months. Although youths reported a relatively high level of need for support in each of these domains, they also reported relatively high satisfaction in these domains. In the area of support for socializing, youths reported more than twice the number of potential supporters than in the other areas. In other words, youths had strong socializing networks, but many fewer supporters available for the other functions: closeness and instrumental help. This would suggest that many of the socializing ties are *not* strong ties capable of offering other important support resources. Similar to their ratings in other domains, youths were relatively satisfied with the support they received.

Youths reported a somewhat different pattern for sexual information and advice regarding the use of illicit substances. First, the number of potential resources appeared lower, as was the utilization of help from members of these networks. Youths appeared to perceive less need for help in these domains, while their satisfaction remained relatively high. There is no doubt that many of these youths have adopted risky sexual and drug-related life-styles but do not see themselves as needing help in these areas. We must consider these critical areas for intervention.

There were significant differences among the groups on support for physical care, socializing, and sexual information. Overall, runaway males reported less satisfaction with their support than runaway females. This may indicate that females are more likely to have their requests for support met either because others are more sympathetic and forthcoming to females or females go about seeking support in a way that ensures a satisfying return. Second, gay males were less satisfied with support received than runaway males. Here we may be seeing the effects of the gay adolescents' sense of marginality.

Are Social Supports and Risk Behaviors Related?

Having friends who use alcohol and drugs appears to be associated with runaways engaging in sexual risk behaviors, reflecting a pattern of multiple problem behaviors described earlier. Among runaways, we found significant correlations between the number of youths' sexual partners and sexual encounters with number of friends who use alcohol and friends who use drugs. Each correlation was moderate, at about $r = .3$.

Having friends who engage in unprotected sexual intercourse was also correlated with having family and school stressors (r about .2). A disturbing trend was that satisfaction with one's support in the domains of intimacy and socialization was inversely related to condom use (r about .2), i.e., the more satisfied youths were with support, the less likely they were to report condom use. These data point to the role of sexuality in the youth's social life. Clearly, the quality and the type of support received, as well as the norms of the support network, are relevant to youth's understanding and behavior regarding sexual risk.

Conclusion

Runaway and gay adolescents comprise two highly stressed groups, reporting four times the number of events as does the typical adolescent.

Runaways must cope with issues of survival, as well as attempting to resolve problematic home and living situations. Gay youths have to come to terms with feelings and sexual desires typically punished by society, seek friendships with others who share their orientation, and cope with the anticipated and actual responses of family and other important heterosexuals to disclosure or discovery of the youngsters' sexual orientation. These data suggest that youths need help for coping with life stressors, which may include self-management techniques and improving the kinds of social support that keep them on a healthier "track."

The high rates of unprotected sexual intercourse, alcohol and drug use, and emotional distress document the need for interventions with these youths. Given the high rates of stressful life events, it is logical that runaway youths experience high rates of emotional distress (e.g., Robertson, 1989; Shaffer & Caton, 1984) as do gay male youths (Ramefedi, 1987a; Roesler & Deisher, 1972). Although these adaptations are understandable in light of the stresses they experience, it is critical for the youths to reduce their risk behavior. Schinke, Schilling, Palleja, and Zayas (1987) have demonstrated the effectiveness of behaviorally based preventive programs for helping ethnic-minority adolescents to reduce high risk sex and drug behavior and to manage stress. This might be a useful approach to help runaway and gay youths. However, the youth must also be convinced there is a need for intervention, and our data suggest that many of the youth do not have this level of perceived need.

Our preliminary analysis shows that although peers most frequently provide support, these youths do not sever family ties; on the contrary, family members were often sources of support. Unexpectedly, runaway and gay youths perceive their social support systems as adequate, an issue that calls for more detailed study. Runaways were also more satisfied with support received than gay youths. This was surprising, because gay youths have more stable home situations and have more stable peer networks than do runaways. This, however, may be an important effect of gays' sense of stigma.

We also found that many gay adolescents were disclosing their sexual orientation to friends and family. Approximately half of these disclosures were rated by gay youths as positive experiences and half as negative. This finding suggests that a homosexual youth cannot predict or control others' reactions to their disclosures, a significant source of chronic stress. Gay youths failure to disclose this identity results in the stress of shielding an intimate aspect of the self from heterosexuals and worrying about the heterosexuals' reactions to discovery or future disclosure of their sexual orientation.

One of the intriguing issues we soon hope to explore concerns the main and moderating relationships between stressful life events, social supports, and sexual risk behaviors. As we noted earlier, there seems to be variation within each of the groups in the quality of their lives and adaptation. Future analyses will seek to understand the reasons for these divergences in functioning and continue to document the ways in which runaway and gay adolescents are two populations in need of professional attention and services.

Acknowledgments

This work was supported by Center Grant 5-P50-MH43520 to the HIV Center for Clinical and Behavioral Studies from the National Institute of Mental Health and the National Institute on Drug Abuse, Anke A. Ehrhardt, Principal Investigator. We also wish to acknowledge the contributions of Jon Bradley, Elizabeth Grace, Ron Henderson, Joyce Hunter, A. Damien Martin, Alfonso Siverls, and Jan St. Hill.

Note

1.   For the undesirable or negative events, base rates were computed, reflecting the percentage of youths within each of the three groups who had experienced the event in the last 3 months. Comparisons of percentages between groups (runaway males vs. runaway females, and runaway males vs. gay males) were tested for significance with the z test, using the arcsine transformation. For social supports, the means for the three samples were tested with ANOVA. If F was significantly different, then pairwise comparisons, using the t test, were performed between runaway males and females and between runaway and gay males. Not all pairwise comparisons of percentages and means were performed. We decided a priori only to compare male and female runaways, and runaway and gay males. These comparisons allowed us to detect sex differences among runaways. Comparing runaway and gay males allowed us to control for gender while permitting runaway/nonrunaway status and sexual orientation to vary.

References

Alers, J.O. (1978). *Puerto Ricans and health: Findings from New York City*. New York: Hispanic Research Center.

Barrera, M., Jr. (1981). Social support in the adjustment of pregnant adolescents: Assessment issues. In B.H. Gottlieb (Ed.), *Social network and social support* (pp. 69–96). Beverly Hills, CA: Sage.

Bassuk, E., & Rosenberg, L. (1988). Why does family homelessness occur: A case-control study. *American Journal of Public Health, 78,* 1097–1101.

Berlin, I.N. (1980). Opportunities in adolescence to rectify developmental failures. In S.C. Feinstein, P.L. Glovacchini, J.G. Looney, A.Z. Schwartzberg, &

A.D. Sorosky (Eds.), *Adolescent psychiatry: Developmental and clinical studies* (Vol. VIII, pp. 231–243). Chicago, IL: University of Chicago.

Biglan, A., Wendler, C., Ary, D., Noell, J., Ochs, L., French, C., Hood, D., & Wirt, R. (1989). *Social and behavioral factors associated with high risk sexual behavior among adolescents.* Unpublished manuscript. Oregon Research Institute, Eugene, OR.

Bock, R.D., & Moore, E.G.L. (1986). *Advantage and disadvantage: A profile of American youth.* Hillsdale, NJ: Erlbaum.

Bucy, J., & Obolensky, N. (1990). Runaways and homeless youth. In M.J. Rotheram-Borus, J. Bradley, & N. Obolensky (Eds.), *Planning to live: Evaluating and treating suicidal teens in community settings* (pp. 333–353). Tulsa, OK: University of Oklahoma Press.

Chelimsky, E. (1982). The problem of runaway and homeless youth. In *Oversight Hearing on Runaway and Homeless Youth Program.* House of Representatives, Subcommittee on Human Resources, Committee on Education and Labor, Washington, DC.

Children's Defense Fund. (1988). *A children's defense budget FY 1989: An analysis of our nation's investment in children.* Washington, DC: Author.

Council on Scientific Affairs. (1989). Health care needs of homeless and runaway youths. *Journal of the American Medical Association, 262,* 1358–1361.

Daley, S. (1988). New York City street youth: Living in the shadows of AIDS. *New York Times,* November 14, pp. B1, B4.

D'Augelli, A.R. (1989). Lesbians' and gay men's experiences of discrimination and harassment in a university community. *American Journal of Community Psychology, 17,* 317–321.

DHHS. (1984). U.S. Department of Health and Human Services. Office of Human Development Services Administration for Children, Youth and Families. *Runaway youth centers: FY 1984 report to Congress.* Washington, DC.

Fagan, T. (1987). Testimony presented before the Select Committee on Children Youth and Families. U.S. House of Representatives Select Committee on Children, Youth and Families. *The crisis in homelessness: Effects on children and families.* Report of hearing February 24, Washington, DC.

Furstenberg, F.F. (1987). Race differences in teenage sexuality, pregnancy, and adolescent childbearing. *The Milbank Quarterly, 65* (Suppl. 2), 381–403.

Harding, R. (1986). Gay youths are six times more likely to commit suicide. *The Washington Blade,* May 16, p. 1.

Hermann, R.C. (1988). Center provides approach to major social ill: Homeless urban runaways, 'throwaways.' *Journal of the American Medical Association, 260,* 311–312.

Hersch, P. (1988). Coming of age in the city streets. *Psychology Today,* January, 28–37.

Hunter, J., & Schaecher, R. (1990). Teenage suicide: Lesbian and gay youth. In M.J. Rotheram-Borus, J. Bradley, & N. Obolensky (Eds.), *Planning to live: Evaluating and treating suicidal teens in community settings* (pp. 297–316). Tulsa, OK: University of Oklahoma Press.

Jessor, R., & Jessor, S.L. (1977). *Problem behavior and psychosocial development—A longitudinal study of youth.* New York: Academic Press.

Johnson, J.H., & McCutcheon, S.M. (1980). Assessing life stress in older children and adolescents: Preliminary findings with the Life Events Checklist. In I.G. Sarason & C.D. Spielberger (Eds.), *Stress and anxiety* (Vol. 6, pp. 111–125). New York: Wiley.

Kellog, P. (1978). Breaking up. In G. Vida (Ed.), *Our right to love: A lesbian resource book* (pp. 55–56). Englewood Cliffs, NJ: Prentice-Hall.

Manoff, S.B., Gayle, H.D., Mays, M.A., & Rogers, M.F. (1989). Acquired immunodeficiency syndrome in adolescents: Epidemiology, prevention and public health issues. *Pediatric Infectious Disease Journal, 8,* 309–314.

Martin, A.D. (1982). Learning to hide: The socialization of the gay adolescent. In S.C. Feinstein, J.G. Looney, A.Z. Schwartzberg, & A.D. Sorosky (Eds.), *Adolescent psychiatry: Developmental and clinical studies* (Vol. 10, pp. 52–65). Chicago, IL: University of Chicago Press.

Martin, A.D., & Hetrick, E.S. (1988). The stigmatization of the gay and lesbian adolescent. *Journal of Homosexuality, 15,* 163–183.

Meyer-Bahlburg, H.F.L., Ehrhardt, A.A., Exner, T.M., & Gruen, R.S. (1988). *Sexual Risk Behavior Assessment Schedule—Youth Baseline Interview.* Program of Developmental Pyschoendocrinology, New York State Psychiatric Institute, NY.

National Network of Runaway and Homeless Youths. (1985). *To whom do they belong?* Washington, D.C.: Author.

Newcomb, M.D., Huba, G.J., & Bentler, P.M. (1981). A multi-dimensional assessment of stressful life events among adolescents: Derivation and correlates. *Journal of Health and Social Behavior, 22,* 400–415.

Paroski, P.A. (1987). Health care delivery and the concerns of gay and lesbian adolescents. *Journal of Adolescent Health Care, 8,* 188–192.

Price, V. (1987). Runaways and homeless street youth. In The Boston Foundation (Ed.), *Homelessness: Critical issues for policy and practice* (pp. 24–28). Boston, MA: The Boston Foundation.

Remafedi, G. (1987a). Adolescent homosexuality: Psychosocial and medical implications. *Pediatrics, 79,* 331–337.

Remafedi, G. (1987b). Male homosexuality: The adolescent's perspective. *Pediatrics, 79,* 326–330.

Robertson, M.J. (1989). *Homeless youth: An overview of recent literature.* Paper presented at the National Conference on Homeless Children and Youth, Institute for Policy Studies at the Johns Hopkins University, Washington, DC.

Roesler, T., & Deisher, R.W. (1972). Youthful male homosexuality: Homosexual experience and the process of developing homosexual identity in males aged 16 to 22 years. *Journal of the American Medical Association, 219,* 1018–1023.

Rotheram-Borus, M.J., & Koopman, C. (1991). Sexual risk behaviors, AIDS knowledge, and beliefs about AIDS among runaways. *American Journal of Public Health,* in press.

Rotheram-Borus, M.J., Koopman, C., & Bradley, J. (1989). Barriers to successful AIDS prevention programs with runaway youth. In J.O. Woodruff, D. Doherty, & J.G. Athey (Eds.), *Troubled adolescents and HIV infection: Issues in prevention and treatment* (pp. 37–55). Washington, DC: CASSP Technical Assistance Center, Georgetown University Child Development Center.

Rotherman-Borus, M.J., Meyer-Bahlburg, H.F.L., Koopman, C., Rosario, M., Exner, T.M., Henderson, R., Matthieu, M., & Gruen, R.S. (1990). *Lifetime sexual behaviors among runaway males and females*. (Unpublished manuscript.)

Rothman, J., & David, T. (1985). *Status offenders in Los Angeles County: Focus on runaway and homeless youth (A study and policy recommendations)*. School of Social Welfare, University of California at Los Angeles.

Schinke, S.P., Schilling, R.F., Palleja, J., & Zayas, L.H. (1987). Prevention research among ethnic-racial minority group adolescents. *The Behavior Therapist, 10,* 151–155.

Schneider, S.G., Farberow, N.L., & Kruks, G.N. (1989). Suicidal behavior in adolescent and young adult gay men. *Suicide and Life-Threatening Behavior, 19,* 381–394.

Shaffer, D., & Caton, D. (1984). *Runaway and homeless youth in New York City: A report to the Ittleson Foundation*. New York: The Ittleson Foundation.

Shane, P.G. (1989). Changing patterns among homeless and runaway youth. *American Journal of Orthopsychiatry, 59,* 208–214.

Solarz, A.L. (1988). Homelessness: Implications for children and youth. *Social Policy Report, 3*(4). Washington, DC: Society for Research in Child Development.

Stricof, R., Novick, L.F., Kennedy, J., & Weisfuse, I. (1988). *Seroprevalence of adolescents at a homeless facility*. Paper presented at the American Public Health Association Conference, Boston, MA.

Strommen, E.F. (1989). "You're a what?": Family member reactions to the disclosure of homosexuality. *Journal of Homosexuality, 18,* 37–58.

Sullivan, T., & Schneider, M. (1987). Development and identity issues in adolescent homosexuality. *Child and Adolescent Social Work, 4,* 13–24.

Swearingen, E.M., & Cohen, L.H. (1985). Measurement of adolescents' life events: The Junior High Life Experiences Survey. *American Journal of Community Psychology, 13,* 69–85.

Troidan, R.R. (1988). Homosexual identity development. *Journal of Adolescent Health Care, 9,* 105–113.

Turner, C.F., Miller, H.G., & Moses, L.E. (Eds.) (1989). *AIDS: Sexual behavior and intravenous drug use*. Washington, DC: National Academy Press.

William T. Grant Foundation. (1988). *The forgotten half: Pathways to success for America's youth and young families*. Washington, DC: Youth and America's Future: The William T. Grant Commission on Work, Family and Citizenship.

Yates, G., MacKenzie, R., Pennbridge, J., & Cohen, E. (1988). A risk profile comparison of runaway and non-runaway youth. *American Journal of Public Health, 78,* 820–821.

Zelnik, M., & Kantner, J.F. (1980). Sexual activity, contraceptive use and pregnancy among metropolitan-area teenagers: 1971–1979. *Family Planning Perspectives, 12,* 230–237.

10

Childhood Victimization: Risk Factor for Delinquency

Cathy Spatz Widom

Stress has been studied from a variety of perspectives, and with different subject populations, from young children to the elderly. Stress researchers have also examined the role of a number of different types of stress, investigating the effects of psychosexual stressors (such as divorce or death of a parent) as well as stressful physical or medical conditions (such as surgery or trauma due to accidents or fire). In this chapter, the focus is on three forms of childhood victimization—physical abuse, sexual abuse, and neglect—as stressors.

Much has been written about the hypothesized relationship between child abuse, neglect, and later delinquency (Widom, 1989b). Despite widespread attention and writing on this topic, a 1984 national conference was held to examine whether child abuse represented a "prelude to delinquency?" (Gray, 1986). The conference concluded with a call for research that clarifies the link between child abuse and neglect and later delinquency. This chapter describes research, begun in 1986, which was explicitly designed to examine the link between child abuse and neglect and later delinquent, adult criminal, and violent criminal behavior. The focus here is on the period of adolescence and on officially recorded delinquent behavior.

Child Abuse, Neglect, and Delinquency

A number of studies have examined the relationship between child abuse and neglect and delinquency (for reviews, see Garbarino & Plantz, 1986; Gray, 1986; Widom, 1989b). Generally, in prospective studies that follow up individuals who had been abused or neglected as children earlier in their lives, the incidence of later delinquency has been reported as between 10 and 17%. Of the three prospective studies (Alfaro, 1981; Bolton, Reich, & Gutierres, 1979; McCord, 1983), two lacked control groups (nonabused comparisons). In contrast to the prospective studies, retrospective studies identify a sample of delinquent youths, and utilize a reverse records check to determine the incidence of abuse or neglect in the delinquent's backgrounds. In these retrospective studies, estimates of abuse generally range from 9 to 29%. Most studies of delinquents report that the majority were *not* abused as children. In at least one study (McCord, 1983), rejected children had the highest rates of delinquency.

Methodological problems, however, have limited our confidence in these findings (Widom, 1989b). Only two of the reverse records check studies used control groups (Glueck & Glueck, 1950; Lewis & Shanok, 1977). Without appropriate control groups and improved methodology, any conclusions remain highly ambiguous. Control groups are critical since it is otherwise impossible to determine what percentage of youths *not* referred for child abuse subsequently became delinquent or were referred to the juvenile court. As Newberger, Newberger, and Hampton (1983) pointed out:

> Left open in the discussion, and unfortunately not susceptible to definitive analysis . . . , is the extent to which the preferential selection of poor children both for reporting for maltreatment and for delinquency may have affected the perceived association and the extent to which poverty per se may have determined both problems. (p. 263)

Retrospective studies, in particular, also face threats to validity in terms of inaccuracies in recording and other biases. Many of these studies represent after-the-fact analyses of preexisting records or depend on the retrospective recall of the subjects for information. For example, Kratcoski (1982) abstracted information about abuse experiences by reading case summaries written by psychologists or social workers. These findings may be distorted since in many of the files the psychologists or social workers who interviewed the youths never brought up issues about parent relationships, missing the chance to uncover possible abuse. Furthermore, the parents had rarely been officially charged with child abuse. In some instances, determinations about whether abuse had occurred had to be made many years later by the researchers (McCord, 1983).

Child Abuse, Neglect, Violent Criminal Behavior

Several studies involving delinquents (Alfaro, 1981; Geller & Ford-Somma, 1984; Gutierres & Reich, 1981; Hartstone & Hansen, 1984; Jenkins, 1968; Kratcoski, 1982) have examined the link between abuse and neglect and violent criminal behavior. However, findings are contradictory. Some provide support for the relationship (Geller & Ford-Somma, 1984; Lewis et al., 1979, 1985); in others, abused and nonabused delinquents did not differ (Kratcoski, 1982); and in at least one study, abused delinquents were less likely to engage in later aggressive crimes (Gutierres & Reich, 1981). Fagan et al. (1983) found low incidences of both child abuse and parental violence among violent juvenile offenders compared with nationwide rates. Each of these studies has methodological problems, not the least of which is the lack of normal comparison groups providing baseline data.

In past research, abuse and neglect have typically been treated as one category of childhood victimization and rarely have the consequences of abuse *and* neglect been examined separately. This is particularly true in regard to the work on delinquency. Many studies that examine the relationship between child abuse and neglect and delinquency consider physical abuse only, omitting questions about neglect (in self-report surveys) or cases involving neglect. This is surprising since in most estimates of the incidence of child maltreatment, the incidence of neglect is much larger than that of abuse, with neglect reports outnumbering abuse reports by a factor of 2:1 (American Humane Association, 1984; Friedrich & Einbender, 1983).

In sum, despite widespread belief in the relationship between child abuse and neglect and later delinquency, conceptual and methodological limitations have substantially restricted our knowledge of the long-term consequences of early childhood victimization (Widom, 1989b). The purpose of the present research was threefold: (1) to identify a large sample of substantiated and validated cases of child abuse and neglect from approximately 20 years ago, (2) to establish a matched control group of nonabused children, and (3) to determine the extent to which these individuals and the matched control group subsequently engaged in delinquent and adult criminal and violent criminal behavior. At present, this research involves (and is limited to) the collection, tabulation, and analysis of existing official records.

Building on past work, this research was designed to incorporate a number of methodological improvements. These included a relatively unambiguous operational definition of abuse and neglect, a prospective design, separate abused and neglected groups, a large sample to allow for subgroup comparisons and to allow for conclusions with respect to violent criminal behavior, a control group matched as closely as possible for age, sex, race, and approximate social class background, and assessment of the long-term consequences of abuse and neglect beyond adolescence or juvenile court into adulthood.

Design of the Study

This research is based on a matched cohorts design (Leventhal, 1982). In this design, both groups are free of the outcome in question (violent or delinquent behavior) at the time they are chosen for the study and, because of matching, are assumed to differ only in the (risk) attribute to be examined (having experienced child abuse or neglect). Abused and neglected children were matched with nonabused and neglected children and followed prospectively into adolescence and young adulthood. Since it is not possible to randomly assign subjects to groups (and obviously this could not be done), the assumption of equivalency for the groups is an approximation.

In studies of the relationship between child abuse and neglect and later delinquency or criminality, it is important to avoid ambiguity in the direction of causality of the events. Specifically, cases occur where delinquency precedes abuse and/or neglect or delinquency may actually lead to abuse or neglect. Thus, to minimize this likelihood and to maximize the likelihood that the temporal direction is clear (that is, abuse or neglect leads to delinquency or criminality), abuse and neglect cases were restricted to those in which children were less than 11 years of age at the time of the abuse or neglect.

The decision was made to use official arrest records for the dependent variable for a number of reasons. Arrest records are relatively easy to locate and reasonably complete information on arrests in official records can be collected retrospectively (Blumstein, Cohen, & Farrington, 1988). Results of self-report studies and research using official records have been fairly consistent in terms of the correlates of crime (Hirschi, 1969). Although self-reports are basically reliable and valid for relatively minor offenses, the more serious offenses are more efficiently revealed (and with fairly little bias) by some official data (Hindelang, Hirschi, & Weis, 1981). Arrest records were also chosen because interviewing a large number of abused and neglected cases would be extremely costly.

Compared to a good survey by interviewers, a register study such as the one described here tends to be much less expensive per case (Schulsinger, Mednick, & Knop, 1981).

In comparisons of delinquent or violent behavior, it is also difficult to judge what portion of the differences is due to the experience or factors under study and what portion is due to being labeled a delinquent or violent offender. Our research does not totally avoid this problem, but by use of a prospective design, with data collection started at the point of abuse and/or neglect and before the onset of delinquency and violent behavior, the problem is minimized.

Abuse and Neglect Cases

All cases of physical and sexual abuse and neglect processed during the years 1967 through 1971 in the county juvenile court (situated in a metropolitan area in the midwest) and validated and substantiated by the court were initially included. Abuse and neglect cases from the *adult* criminal courts were also included. In these cases, a criminal charge was filed against the adult defendant. During 1967 through 1971, there were 140 cases (physical and sexual abuse and neglect) processed in adult criminal court in which the victim was 11 years of age or less. After 2623 abuse and neglect petitions were examined, a total of 908 cases were retained for this study (see Widom, 1989a for a complete description of the design and details of criteria for inclusion and exclusion of cases).

Physical abuse refers to cases in which an individual had "knowingly and willfully inflicted unnecessarily severe corporal punishment" or "unnecessary physical suffering" on a child or children (e.g., striking, punching, kicking, biting, throwing, or burning). *Sexual abuse* refers to a variety of charges, ranging from relatively nonspecific charges of "assault and battery with intent to gratify sexual desires" to more specific and detailed charges of "fondling/touching in an obscene manner," sodomy, incest, and so forth. *Neglect* refers to cases in which the court found a child to have no proper parent care or guardianship, to be destitute, homeless, or to be living in a physically dangerous environment. The neglect petition reflects the judgment that the behavior represents a serious omission by the parents—beyond acceptable community and professional standards at the time to provide needed food, clothing, shelter, medical attention to children, and protection from hazardous conditions.

Matched Control Group

One of the critical elements of this research design is the establishment of a control group, matched as closely as possible on the basis of sex, age, race, and appropriate family socioeconomic status during the time period under study (1967 through 1971). To accomplish this matching, the sample of abused and neglected cases was divided into two groups on the basis of age at the time of the abuse or neglect incident: under school age and over school age.

Initially, two control children were selected as potential matches for the abused or neglected child. This was done since one of the important elements of the design involves the assumption that the major difference between the abused/neglected group and the matched controls is in the abuse or neglect experience. Since this study is based on official records, it was important to check the official records to determine if the proposed control group subjects had been abused or neglected. If there was evidence that a potential control group subject had been officially abused or neglected, then he or she was excluded from our control group. This occurred in 11 cases.

Children who were *under school age* at the time of the abuse or neglect were matched with children of the same sex, race, date of birth ($\pm$ 1 week), and hospital of birth through the use of county birth record information. Of the 319 abused and neglected children under school age, there are matches for 229 (72%).

For children *of school age*, elementary school records for the same time period were used to find matches with children of the same sex, race, date of birth ($\pm$ 6 months) and the same class in elementary school during the years 1967 through 1971. Busing had not been implemented and the elementary schools were composed of students from small, socioeconomically homogeneous neighborhoods. Out of 589 school age children, there were matches for 438, representing about 74% of the group. Overall, there were 667 matches (73.7%) for the abused and neglected children.

Demographic Characteristics of the Groups

Among the abused and neglected group, there are about equal numbers of males and females (49 vs. 51%) and more whites than blacks (67 vs. 31%). The mean age for the abused and neglected subjects is currently 25.69 (SD = 3.53). The majority of the sample are between the ages of 20 and 30 (85%), with about 10% under age 20 (the youngest is 16) and 5% older than 30 (the oldest is 32).

The controls are well matched to the abused and/or neglected subjects in terms of age, sex, and race. Controls are equally divided between males and females. The racial composition of the group is quite similar to that of the abused and neglected group, although slightly more of the controls are black (35%). Their mean age is 25.76 (SD = 3.53, range = 16–33).

Data Collection

Detailed information about the abuse and/or neglect incident and family composition and characteristics was obtained from the files of the juvenile court and probation department, the authority responsible for cases of abused, neglected, or dependent and delinquent children. Juvenile court and probation department records were also examined for the control subjects. Detailed delinquency and detention information was recorded for both groups.

Dependent Variables

This paper focuses on *juvenile delinquency*, defined as any arrest for offenses committed while the person was less than 18 years of age. In addition to *any arrest as a juvenile*, offenses were categorized into one of six types: violent, property, alcohol, drug, order, and sex. *Violent* crimes include arrests for robbery, assault and battery, battery with injury, battery, aggravated assault, manslaughter/involuntary manslaughter/reckless homicide, murder/attempted murder, rape/sodomy, and robbery and burglary with injury. *Property* crimes include theft/shoplifting, burglary/attempted burglary, breaking and entering, possession of stolen property, larceny, arson, fraud/forgery, and embezzlement. *Alcohol* offenses include public intoxication and driving while intoxicated, and *drug* offenses referred to violations of the controlled substance act. *Order* offenses include criminal mischief/vandalism/trepassing, disorderly conduct, visiting a common nuisance, resisting arrest/fleeing a police officer, and vagrancy. *Sex* offenses include arrests for prostitution, incest, child molestation, rape, assault and battery with intent to gratify, peeping, public indecency, criminal deviant conduct, and contributing to the delinquency of a minor. *Status* offenses refer to those that are exclusively juvenile offenses (not criminal for an adult) and include runaway, truancy, ungovernability (incorrigibility), violation of curfew, and illegal possession of alcohol.

Research Questions

In an attempt to begin to clarify the linkage between child abuse and neglect and delinquency, the findings are organized around five research questions:

1. Is childhood victimization a risk factor for delinquency?
2. Does the amount of increased risk vary by the sex and race of the victimized child?
3. Does childhood abuse and neglect increase risk for all kinds of delinquent behavior or is it restricted to certain kinds?

4. Do victims of sexual abuse become juvenile sex offenders and prostitutes?
5. Do victims of physical abuse become violent juvenile offenders?

Findings

Is Childhood Victimization a Risk Factor for Delinquency?

Table 1 presents the findings on childhood victimization and involvement in officially recorded delinquency and compares the abused and neglected group with the control group. As can be seen in Table 1, abused and neglected children are at significantly increased risk for delinquency compared to the controls (26 vs. 17%). Abused and neglected children also begin their official criminal activity approximately one year earlier than the control subjects (16.5 vs. 17.3 years) and have approximately two times the number of offenses.

Even though these findings indicate that abused and neglected children have significantly increased risk of delinquency, in some ways these results are surprising. For some readers, the difference in delinquency between the abused and neglected children and the controls will be perceived as *only* 9% overall. Others, however, will focus on the fact that the majority of the abused and neglected children (74%) do not become delinquents. Interestingly, these findings are consistent with the previous literature in terms of the percentage who become delinquent and the majority who do not. However, the comparison with a matched control group provides a new perspective on these percentages. Are all abused

Table 1. Childhood Victimization and Involvement in Officially Recorded Delinquent Activity

	Abused/neglected (N = 908)	Controls (N = 667)	p
Any juvenile offense (%)	26.0	16.8	***
Number of juvenile offenses			
M	.87	.47	***
SD	2.07	1.36	
Age at any first offense			
M	16.49	17.31	*
SD	3.86	3.87	
n	370	197	

*p < .05.
**p < .01.
***p < .001.

and neglected children, regardless of sex and race, at increased risk for delinquency?

Does the Amount of Increased Risk Vary with the
Sex and Race of the Victimized Child?

Figure 1a presents the increased risk associated with abuse and neglect by the sex and race of the children. The first breakdown by *sex* reveals that, within each sex, being abused and neglected makes a difference in increased risk. For females, the risk is increased from 11 to 19% [$x^2(1) = 8.66, p < .01$] and for males it is increased from 22 to 33% [$x^2(1) = 11.38, p < .001$].

Similarly, the breakdown by *race* indicates that, within each race, being abused and neglected increases the risk for delinquency, although the increased risk seems to be stronger for blacks. For black children, being abused and neglected doubles the risk for delinquency [38 vs. 19%, $x^2(1) = 21.29, p < .001$]. For whites the difference is significant [21 vs. 15%, $x^2(1) = 5.36, p < .05$], but of smaller magnitude. This pattern becomes more dramatic on inspection of the *interaction of race and sex* on rates of officially recorded delinquency (see the bottom portion of Figure 1b). Here, 51% of abused and neglected black males have arrests for delinquency compared to about 20–26% of all other groups of males. Similarly, black abused and neglected females have much higher rates of delinquency (26%) than all other females (10–16%).

In a log linear analysis fitting models to any juvenile record, sex, race, and abuse/neglect versus control group status were all significant factors. Calculating the odds ratios from these individual coefficients, the odds are increased by a factor of 2.17 for males versus females, 1.91 for blacks versus whites, and 1.89 for abused/neglected versus controls.

Does Childhood Abuse and Neglect Increase Risk for
All Kinds of Delinquent Behavior or Is It
Restricted to Only Certain Kinds?

Table 2 presents the frequency of arrests for specific offenses for the abused and neglected group versus controls. Childhood abuse and neglect do *not* increase risk significantly across all types of offenses. Rather, the increased risk associated with childhood victimization is primarily with property crimes and status offenses such as runaway, truancy, and ungovernability.

Table 2 also presents specific juvenile offenses by sex. To the extent that childhood victimization is a prelude to delinquency, it has been suggested (Gray, 1986) that the "symptoms" of the females would be runaway, street prostitution, and mental health problems. The current

Sex, Race, and Abuse/Neglect

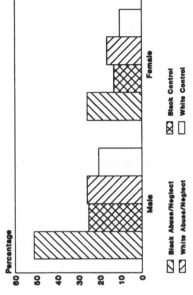

☒ Abuse/Neglect ☐ Controls

Figure 1a. Frequency of juvenile arrest.

Interaction

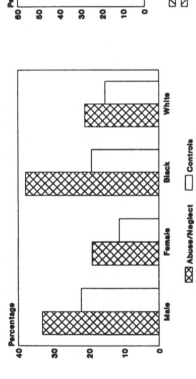

☒ Black Abuse/Neglect ☒ Black Control
☒ White Abuse/Neglect ☐ White Control

Figure 1b. Frequency of juvenile arrest.

Table 2. Comparison of Types of Juvenile Offenses For Abuse/Neglect and Control Groups by Sex[a] (in Percentages)

Juvenile offense	Total Sample		Males		Females	
	Abuse/neglect (N = 908)	Controls (N = 667)	Abuse/neglect (N = 443)	Controls (N = 334)	Abuse/neglect (N = 465)	Controls (N = 333)
Violent	4.2	2.8	6.5	5.4	1.9	.3*
Property	14.3	8.5***	21.2	12.6***	7.5	4.5*
Status	14.2	7.2***	16.0	8.4**	12.5	6.0**
Drugs	1.7	1.2	12.4	9.9	3.2	1.5
Alcohol	1.4	1.8	2.9	1.8	.4	.6
Order	7.7	5.7	2.5	2.7	.4	.9
Sex	1.3	1.0	2.5	1.8	.2	.3

[a]Significance levels based on χ^2; Yates correction used when cells have less than 5.
   *$p < .10$.
  **$p < .05$.
 ***$p < .01$.

findings indicate that, as adolescents (that is, before the age of 18), abused and neglected females do become runaways, but they also engage in theft, vandalism, and violence against others. Specifically, abused and neglected females are more likely to be arrested for property and status offenses than the matched control group females, *and* there is a surprising trend for the abused and neglected females to have higher rates of arrest for violent offenses. Interestingly, abused and neglected males are more likely to be arrested for property and status offenses as juveniles, as compared to the controls, but they do *not* differ on violence.

Do Victims of Sexual Abuse Become Juvenile Sex Offenders and Prostitutes?

Based on past literature (Browne & Finkelhor, 1986; Greenwald, 1970; James, 1976; Silbert & Pines, 1981), one would expect that victims of sexual abuse are more likely to become juvenile prostitutes and sex offenders. The results of the present study indicate that abused and neglected children in general are significantly more likely to be runaways than the control children (5.8 vs. 2.4%). However, there does *not* appear to be a "direct causal link" between childhood victimization, becoming a runaway, and in turn becoming an adult prostitute. Of the 69 runaways in this sample (this includes 53 abused and neglected cases as well as 16 controls), five have adult arrests for sex crimes, but *none* has arrests for prostitution.

To further examine the consequences of sexual abuse for delinquency, victims of sexual abuse were divided into two groups: *sexual abuse only* ($n = 125$) (those who, according to the official records, suffered only sexual abuse) and *sexual abuse plus* ($n = 28$) (those who suffered sexual abuse plus physical abuse or neglect). Because those who were sexually abused were predominantly female (although by no means exclusively so), it would be inappropriate to compare their rates of delinquency to rates for the entire control group. Figure 2, therefore, illustrates the rates of delinquency for each offense type (any, status, runaway, property, order, violent, and sex) for the two sexual abuse groups (sexual abuse only and sexual abuse plus) and their matched controls ($n = 100$). Across most offense types (except property and order), the *sexual abuse plus* group had the highest rates of delinquent activity. For runaway arrests, the difference reached significance ($p < .05$) and for status and sex crimes, it approached significance ($p < .10$). Some victims of sexual abuse become juvenile sex offenders and runaways. However, there does not appear to be a direct linkage between early childhood sexual abuse and arrests as an adolescent for runaway and arrests as adult for prostitution.

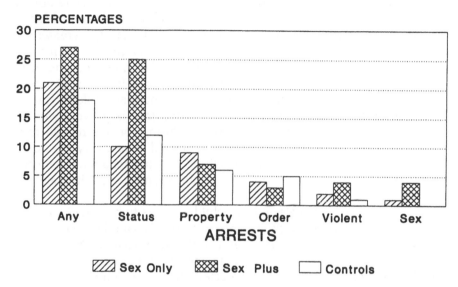

Figure 2. Patterns of juvenile offending: sexual abuse and control groups.

Do Victims of Physical Abuse Become Violent Juvenile Offenders?

Based on the "cycle of violence" hypothesis (Widom, 1989b,c), one would expect that childhood victims of violence would be at increased risk for becoming violent juvenile offenders. Table 3 presents rates of arrest for juvenile violent offenses by type of childhood victimization experienced. Overall, children who were *neglected* had the highest rates of juvenile violence. This was also true for neglected *males*, although both these differences did not reach customary levels of significance. Interestingly, the pattern for *females* was different from the males and significant. The *physically abused females* had the highest rates of juvenile arrests for violent offenses, compared to the other females who had been sexually abused or neglected and the controls. Findings such as these illustrate the complex nature of the relationship between child abuse and neglect and later delinquency and reinforce the need for careful disentangling of these effects.

Discussion and Conclusion

Childhood victimization is a risk for delinquency in adolescence. In fact, being abused or neglected increases a child's chance of having a juvenile record by a factor of almost two (1.89) over children who were not officially abused and/or neglected. Even for individuals with a low risk of offending, being abused or neglected as a child significantly increases risk.

For girls, who are generally at low risk for delinquency, their risk of offending increased from 11 to 19%. Interestingly, abused and/or neglected females were at greater risk of being arrested for a violent juvenile offense than control females. Since a similar increased risk for juvenile violence was not found in males, this difference is provocative. It is possible that this represents a spurious finding, or one related to increased surveillance of abused and neglected females by the justice system. However, these findings illustrate why further attention must be paid to the antisocial consequences of abuse and neglect in males and females.

Being abused and neglected as a child appears to have had a particularly strong effect on black children within this sample. Being abused and/or neglected increased risk significantly for black and white children; however, for blacks, the differences were more dramatic. Among black males, half of the abused and neglected children had arrests as adolescents in contrast to 25% of the controls. For black females, the corresponding figures were 26 versus 13%. Smaller differences were found among white males (26 vs. 21%) and among white females (17 vs. 11%).

Since the present findings are based on official records and since official records overrepresent minority groups, the most obvious explanation for the higher rates of arrest among blacks is that these results reflect bias and

Table 3. Do Victims of Physical Abuse Become Violent Juvenile Offenders?

Type of abuse/neglect	N	Overall[a]	Males[b]	Females[c]
		Percent with arrest for juvenile violence		
Neglect	609	5.3	8.4	1.4
Physical abuse	76	3.9	2.1	6.9
Physical abuse and neglect	70	—	—	—
Sexual abuse	125	1.6	—	1.9
Sexual abuse plus	28	3.6	—	4.3
Controls	667	2.8	5.4	0.3

[a] $\chi^2(5) = 9.92$, $p < .10$.
[b] $\chi^2(5) = 8.97$, ns.
[c] $\chi^2(5) = 12.52$, $p < .05$.

discrimination within the criminal justice system. However, this explanation does not seem to explain the difference *within blacks* and the smaller differences within whites.

Another possible explanation is that parental violence is more severe among blacks than whites or that nonwhites are more physically abusive with their children and within their homes than whites. To the extent that this research can address these issues, however, our data indicate that this is not the case. Within whites, approximately 20% suffered physical abuse, compared to the percentage for blacks which was less than 9%. Blacks suffered more neglect, relative to whites in our sample.

Furthermore, based on data from the National Study on the Incidence and Severity of Child Abuse and Neglect (NCCAN, 1981) and the National Study on Child Neglect and Abuse Reporting (AHA, 1984), the percentage of black and white children reported for child abuse and neglect appears to be representative of the United States population at large. If anything, black families were characterized by more neglect and slightly less physical and sexual abuse (as found in this study), whereas white families were characterized by more abuse or combined abuse/neglect. Thus, racial bias in official reports showing more blacks being reported for abuse or neglect was not found in the NCCAN and AHA studies.

Our further possibility is that still another type of discriminatory treatment by the system might be at work here. If we postulate a justice system that expects and tolerates higher levels of violence among black families, then it is possible that abused and neglected black children in our sample were subjected to more extreme victimization than white children *before* coming to the attention of the officials at the time. If this were the case, only the most extreme cases of physical abuse in black families would have been reported to the authorities. Thus, these cases would not be comparable to cases of physical abuse from white families. Unfortunately, the present data do not permit examination of this question. However, given these findings about what appear to be differential effects on black and white children, future research should systematically examine this question considering the range of possible explanations.

The present findings illustrate and reinforce the importance of examining separately the effects of different types of child maltreatment. In the past, most of the research conducted has focused on physical and sexual abuse, with relatively little attention paid to neglect. The current findings suggest that neglect by itself (life threatening omission of food, clothing, shelter, and medical attention) may have serious long-term negative consequences. Here, the large group of neglected children had the highest rates of arrests for violence as juveniles. It may be that the accumulation of stressful experiences associated with neglect, presumably occurring over a long period of time, produces as devastating consequences for young children, similar to those produced through direct victimization of children by physical abuse. Given that the number of cases of child neglect far outweigh those for physical abuse in national statistics, these findings may be of relevance to forecasts of future violent behavior. There are also implications from these findings for the prevention of further abuse and violent behavior. Although the task of preventing episodic explosive outbursts of physical abuse by parents or caretakers may appear enormous and exceedingly difficult, the prevention of severe neglect appears, at least in principle, more malleable. Thus, the implication for prevention strategies may differ depending on the type of abuse or neglect. Clearly, it is time to examine these questions more thoroughly.

The current practice of treating abused and neglected children together, or eliminating one type of child victim from the study, may obscure other important differences and reveal only a partial portrait of the consequences of childhood victimization. Different patterns of delinquent behavior were found across the two groups of sexually abused children up through the age of 18. In another paper focusing exclusively on the sexual abuse cases (Ames & Widom, 1988), the picture that emerged for adult criminal behavior differed yet again. In early adulthood, the *sexual abuse plus* victims no longer stand out with the highest rates of offending. There is also some evidence that the sexual abuse only group may have alcohol and drug problems manifest as adult arrests. Together these findings suggest the potential usefulness of differentiating between childhood sexual abuse victims who have been *sexually abused only* and those who may have been physically *and* sexually abused or neglected *and* sexually abused.

Pagelow (1984) has noted that a growing number of professionals who work with status offenders or delinquents are increasingly recognizing that "many runaway children are not running *toward* something, but rather are running *away* from something—a home life in which they were subject to abuse, particularly sexual abuse" (p. 49). Perhaps much of the runaway behavior associated with child abuse is adaptive behavior for the abused child. Perhaps the long-term consequences are different for sexually abused children who run away as opposed to those who remain in abusive homes. In the future, we need to explore not only consequences as a function of type of abuse (including cases involving multiple forms of abuse), but also the role of in-home versus out-of-home perpetrator and variations in forms of coping.

This research also illustrates the importance of examining the consequences of stress in a temporal (and preferably longitudinal) perspective. In the case of the sexually abused child who runs away, as suggested above, delinquent behavior seen during adolescence may be an adaptive response to a crisis situation. For these children, one might speculate that the long-term consequences may actually be less traumatic than for those child victims who do not manifest "acting-out" as adolescents.

At the same time, the effects of early abusive experiences may be manifested in ways not related to delinquency or criminality. One possible explanation for the lack of a more substantial relationship between childhood victimization and later delinquency may lie in more subtle manifestations of emotional damage such as depression, withdrawal, or, in the extreme, suicide (Green, 1978). Thus, it is important to examine alternative, and perhaps more subtle, manifestations of the consequences of early childhood victimization.

Very likely, there are multiple pathways by which early abusive or neglectful experiences are linked with later disorders. Child abuse may not cause delinquency directly. Rather, this outcome may be an indirect by-product of these early experiences. Rutter's (1983) discussion of ways in which early stressful experiences may be linked to disorders some years later provides a useful analogy. A number of possible pathways are suggested briefly below.

First, abuse and neglect might lead to immediate sequellae, which then have an irremediable effect on the subsequent development of the child; and these, in turn, would be related to later outcomes. For example, some forms of physical abuse (battering) or severe neglect (dehydration, diarrhea, and failure to thrive) may lead to developmental retardation, which, in turn, may affect school performance, the likelihood of truancy, and so on.

Second, abuse and/or neglect may lead to changed environments or family conditions, which, in turn, may later predispose one to delinquency. In this way, antisocial behavior may result not so much from the abuse or neglect but as a result of the chain of events subsequent to the abuse or neglect. For example, being taken away from one's biological parents and placed in foster care—as a result of abuse or neglect—may be associated with deleterious effects.

Third, the experiences of early abuse and neglect may lead to bodily changes, which, in turn, relate to the development of delinquent behavior. As a result of being beaten continually, a child might become "desensitized" to future painful or anxiety-provoking experiences, as proposed in the television violence literature (Slaby & Quarforth, 1980). This desensitization, in turn, might influence the child's later behavior, making him or her less emotionally and physiologically responsive to the needs of others. On the other hand, this might also work to protect the individual in later life by the development of certain "steeling" effects to overcome stress and adverse life events.

Fourth, early abuse or neglect may lead directly to altered patterns of behavior, the results of which might become manifest only some years later, although in place during early childhood. Abuse or neglect may encourage the development of certain styles of coping, which might be less than adaptive. For example, these early experiences might lead to the development of impulsive behavioral styles, which, in turn, are related to deficiencies in problem-solving skills or inadequate school performance, which, in turn, predispose those affected towards delinquency.

Child abuse and neglect are definite risk factors for delinquency. However, the pathway from childhood victimization to delinquency is far from inevitable. Future research must be directed at understanding the processes involved in how these early stressful life experiences increase risk for later delinquent and ultimately adult criminal behavior.

Specifically, we need to compare the development of childhood victims who do and do not succumb. In attempting to unravel these complex interactions, the challenge will be to design research that will incorporate some combination of internal and external factors, recognizing that an individual's behavior (deviant and prosocial) occurs in a social context. Future research will require more complex models of these relationships, including individual and family as well as neighborhood and community variables, in the search for possible mechanisms for the intergenerational transmission of abusive and violent behavior.

Acknowledgments

This research was supported by grants from the National Institute of Justice (86-IJ-CX-0033), Indiana University Biomedical Research Committee (SO7 RR07031), and the Talley Foundation (Harvard University). Points of view are those of the author and do not necessarily represent the position of the United States Department of Justice. The author wishes to thank Ashley Ames, Jeffrey Lindsay, Beverly Rivera, and Brian Tshanz for their help with the data collection, Beverly Ross for her assistance with the analysis, and Joan McCord for her wisdom in her role as consultant to the project.

Note

1. The findings presented here should be treated cautiously and generalization to different samples should be avoided. The abuse and neglect cases studied here are those where agencies have intervened, and those cases processed through the system. These cases were dealt with before most states had adopted mandatory child abuse reporting laws, and before the Federal Child Abuse Treatment and Prevention Act was passed. Many cases of abuse and neglect were not reported, and those reported are more likely to be biased toward the lower

mandatory child abuse reporting laws, and before the Federal Child Abuse Treatment and Prevention Act was passed. Many cases of abuse and neglect were not reported, and those reported are more likely to be biased toward the lower end of the socioeconomic spectrum. Thus, one cannot generalize from these findings to unreported cases of abuse and neglect, such as those cases handled unofficially by private medical doctors. Similarly, because of our exclusions, these findings are not generalizable to abused and neglected children who were adopted in early childhood.

References

Alfaro, J. (1981). Developmental considerations in the definition of child maltreatment. In R. Rizley & D. Cicchetti (Eds.), *Developmental perspectives on child maltreatment: Vol. II. New Directions for child development* (pp. 1–31). San Francisco: Jossey-Bass.

American Humane Association (1984). *Trends in Child Abuse and Neglect: A National Perspective.* Denver, CO: Author.

Ames, M.A., & Widom, C.S. (1988). *Childhood sexual abuse and later delinquent and criminal behavior.* Paper presented at the annual meeting of the American Society of Criminology, Chicago, Illinois, 9–13 November, 1988.

Blumstein, A., Cohen, J., & Farrington, D.P. (1988). Criminal career research: Its value for criminology. *Criminology, 26,* 1–35.

Bolton, F.G., Reich, J., & Gutierres, S.E. (1979). Delinquency patterns in maltreated children and siblings. *Victimology, 2,* 349–359.

Browne, A., & Finkelhor, D. (1986). Impact of sexual abuse: A review of the research. *Psychological Bulletin, 99,* 66–77.

Fagan, J., K.V. Hansen, & M. Jang (1983). Profiles of chronically violent delinquents: Empirical test of an integrated theory. In J. Kleugel (Ed.), *Evaluating juvenile justice* (pp. 91–119). Beverly Hills, CA: Sage.

Friedrich, W.H., & Einbender, A.J. (1983). The abused child: A psychological review. *Journal of Clinical Child Psychology, 12,* 244–256.

Garbarino, J., & Plantz, M.C. (1986). Child abuse and juvenile delinquency: What are the links? In J. Garbarino, C. Schellenbach, & J. Sebes (Eds.), *Troubled youth, troubled families* (pp. 27–39). New York: Aldine de Gruyter.

Geller, M., & Ford-Somma, L. (1984). *Violent homes, violent children. A study of violence in the families of juvenile offenders.* New Jersey State Department of Corrections, Trenton. Division of Juvenile Services. Prepared for National Center on Child Abuse and Neglect. Washington, February.

Glueck, S., & Glueck, E. (1950). *Unraveling juvenile delinquency.* Cambridge, England: Cambridge University Press.

Gray, E. (1986). *Child abuse: Prelude to delinquency?* (Findings of a research conference conducted by the National Committee for Prevention of Child Abuse). Washington, D.C.: U.S. Government Printing Office.

Green, A.H. (1978). Self-destructive behavior in battered children. *American Journal of Psychiatry, 135,* 579–582.

Greenwald, H. (1970). *The elegant prostitute*. New York: Ballantine.

Gutierres, S., & Reich, J. A. (1981). A developmental perspective on runaway behavior: Its relationship to child abuse. *Child Welfare, 60*, 89–94.

Hartstone, E., & K. Hansen (1984). The violent juvenile offender: An empirical portrait. In R. Mathias, P. DeMuro, & R.S. Allison (Eds.), *Violent juvenile offenders: An anthology* (pp. 82–112). San Francisco: National Council on Crime and Delinquency.

Hindelang, M.J., Hirschi, T., & Weis, J.G. (1981). *Measuring delinquency*. Beverly Hills, CA: Sage.

Hirschi, T. (1969). *Causes of delinquency*. Berkeley: University of California Press.

James, J. (1976). Motivations for entrance into prostitution. In L. Crites (Ed.), *The female offender: A comprehensive anthology*. Lexington, MA: D.C. Heath.

Jenkins, R.L. (1968). The varieties of children's behavioral problems and family dynamics. *American Journal of Psychiatry, 124*, 1440–1445.

Kratcoski, P. C. (1982). Child abuse and violence against the family. *Child Welfare, 61*, 435–444.

Leventhal, J.M. (1982). Research strategies and methodologic standards in studies of risk factors for child abuse. *Child Abuse and Neglect, 6*, 113–123.

Lewis, D.O., & Shanok, S. (1977). Medical histories of delinquent and nondelinquent children: An epidemiological study. *American Journal of Psychiatry, 134*, 1020–1025.

Lewis, D.O., S. Shanok, J. Pincus, & G. Glaser (1979). Violent juvenile delinquents: Psychiatric, neurological, psychological, and abuse factors. *Journal of the American Academy of Child Psychiatry, 18*, 307–319.

Lewis, D.O., Moy, E., Jackson, L.D., Aaronson, R., Restifo, N., Serra, S., & Simos, A. (1985). Biopsychological characteristics of children who later murder: A prospective study. *American Journal of Psychiatry, 142*, 1161–1167.

McCord, J. (1983). A forty-year perspective on effects of child abuse and neglect. *Child Abuse and Neglect, 7*, 265–270.

National Center on Child Abuse and Neglect (1981). *Study findings: National study of the incidence and severity of child abuse and neglect* (DHHS publication no. OHDS 81-30325). Washington, D.C.: U.S. Government Printing Office.

Newberger, E.H., Newberger, C.M., & Hampton, R.L. (1983). Child abuse: The current theory base and future research needs. *Journal of the American Academy of Child Psychiatry, 22*, 262–268.

Pagelow, M.D. (1984). *Family violence*. New York: Praeger.

Rutter, M. (1983). Stress, coping, and development: Some issues and some questions. In N. Garmezy & M. Rutter, (Eds.), *Stress, coping and development in children*. New York: McGraw-Hill.

Schulsinger, F., Mednick, S. A., & Knop, J. (1981). *Longitudinal research: Methods and uses in behavioral sciences*. Boston: Martinus Nijhoff.

Silbert, M., & Pines, A. (1981). Sexual child abuse as an antecedent to prostitution. *Child Abuse and Neglect, 5*, 407–411.

Slaby, R.G., & Quarforth, G.R. (1980). Effects of television on the developing child. In B.W. Camp (Ed.), *Advances in behavioral pediatrics* (Vol. 1.). Greenwich, CT: JAI Press.

Widom, C.S. (1989a). Child abuse, neglect, and adult behavior: Research design and findings on criminality, violence, and child abuse. *American Journal of Orthopsychiatry, 59,* 355–367.
Widom, C.S. (1989b). Does violence beget violence? A critical examination of the literature. *Psychological Bulletin, 106,* 3–28.
Widom, C.S. (1989c). The cycle of violence. *Science, 244,* 160–166.

11

Psychoactive Substance Use and Adolescent Pregnancy: Compounded Risk among Inner City Adolescent Mothers

Hortensia Amaro and Barry Zuckerman

Introduction

Two major public health problems affecting adolescents today are adolescent pregnancy and use of illicit drugs. Individually, pregnancy and parenting during adolescence and use of illicit drugs place adolescents at increased risk for psychosocial problems and jeopardize optimal development (Zuckerman, Amaro, & Beardslee, 1987). Although both of these topics have received substantial empirical attention, little information is available regarding the prevalence and patterns of drug use among pregnant and parenting adolescents, the impact of drug use on the psychosocial outcomes of adolescent mothers, or the role of social relationships in the cooccurrence of these problems (Amaro & Zuckerman, 1990).

Experimentation with drug use is extremely common among adolescents. Prevalence of drug use in adolescents differs markedly for various drugs, with legal drugs having a higher frequency of use than illegal drugs. In the past, it was more common for males than females to use cigarettes, alcohol, and marijuana. However, the sex ratio on substance use is changing so as to narrow the gender gap. In the 1986 National Cohort Study of High School Seniors (Johnston, O'Malley, & Bachman,

1987), lifetime prevalence for cocaine (19.2% for males and 14.3% for females), marijuana (53.3% for males and 48.2% for females), alcohol (92.3% for males and 90.6% for females), and cigarettes (65.9% for males and 68.9% for females) was similar for males and females. The 30-day prevalence for cocaine (7.2% for males and 5.1% for females), marijuana (26.8% for males and 20% for females), alcohol (69% for males and 61.9% for females), and cigarettes (27.9% for males and 30.6% for females) also indicate similar rates of drug use among male and female adolescents. While these prevalence rates do not reflect continued or regular drug use, it is unusual for an adolescent to try an illicit drug or alcohol only once; a high proportion of adolescents who ever try these substances will use them again.

Although existing studies document drug use in adolescent females, they tell us little about drug use in parenting adolescents. To date, none of the major studies on drug use among adolescents provide data on drug use among pregnant adolescents or adolescent mothers. Applying existing prevalence rates of substance use to adolescent mothers raises various problems.

First, these surveys may underrepresent substance use among adolescents, since some of them exclude teens who are not in school and who may be more involved in drug use. Second, drug use may be affected, either increased or decreased, by the pregnancy experience, health education during pregnancy, and responsibilities or frustrations of the parenting role. Thus, it is not possible to estimate reliably the prevalence of drug use among teenage mothers based on current estimates on prevalence of drug use among the general population of adolescent females.

There are several reasons to suspect that drug use may be a more common problem among adolescent mothers than among adolescents who do not get pregnant and have children. Problem proneness behavior theory (Jessor & Jessor, 1977) suggests that adolescents who engage in one problem behavior (e.g., sexual intercourse) are also more likely to engage in other problem behaviors (e.g., drug use), and that problem behaviors are considerably stable from adolescence to young adulthood (Jessor, 1983). Several studies have indicated that adolescents who are sexually active are more likely to also engage in drug use than those who are not sexually active (Jessor & Jessor, 1977; Jessor, 1983; Kandel, 1982; Elliot & Morse, 1987; Hundleby, Carpenter, Ross, & Mercer, 1982; Kandel, Single, & Kessler, 1976). In fact, the antecedents and correlates of drug use and adolescent pregnancy are strikingly similar, suggesting that these problems may often coexist (Amaro & Zuckerman, 1990). Finally, the demands and challenges of early motherhood are charged with environmental and economic stressors coupled with few psychological and social resources (Furstenberg, 1976). Adolescent mothers who lack strategies for coping with potentially overwhelming and prolonged stress may use drugs as a coping response (Kandel, 1982; Paton, Kessler, & Kandel, 1977).

Considering the risk posed by adolescent pregnancy and adolescent drug use individually, the combined effect of pregnancy, parenthood, and drug use on adolescent development and outcomes is potentially serious. Thus, adolescent mothers who use drugs may be a subgroup of adolescent mothers who are at greater risk for negative outcomes than other mothers and who perhaps account for a substantial proportion of the observed negative outcomes in this population.

With the exception of our present investigation, we are not aware of any studies assessing drug use among adolescent mothers beyond the pregnancy period. Two studies that have assessed drug use among adolescents during pregnancy present conflicting results. One study reported more cigarette smoking and alcohol and drug abuse among pregnant teenagers than older pregnant women (Merrit, Lawrence, & Naeye, 1980). Another study (Zuckerman, Hingson, Alpert, Dooling, Kayne, Morelock, & Oppenheimer, 1983) investigated illicit substance use in a sample of inner city, poor, and largely Black and Hispanic adolescents and adult women. Data from that study indicated that a similar number of adolescents and adult women used cigarettes and marijuana during pregnancy. However, adolescents were less likely than adult women to report use of alcohol and other psychoactive drugs. The conflicting results of these two studies on drug use during pregnancy among adolescents may reflect different samples or different assessment procedures, including the use of interview versus clinical data, and retrospective versus prospective data.

In this chapter, we review our previously published work on drug use during pregnancy among adolescents and present preliminary findings on the social context of drug use among adolescent mothers 1 year postpartum.

Prevalence and Patterns of Substance Use among Adolescents during Pregnancy

In previous publications we have reported findings on the prevalence and patterns of drug use during pregnancy (Amaro, Zuckerman, & Cabral, 1989; Zuckerman, Amaro, & Cabral, 1989; Zuckerman, Frank, Hingson, Amaro, Levenson, Kayne, Parker, Vinci, Aboagye, Fried, Cabral, Timperi, & Bauchner, 1989). Since the methods are described in detail in these references, only a brief review of methods is provided here.

Participants were consecutively recruited in the Women's and Adolescent Prenatal Clinics of Boston City Hospital from July 1984 to June 1987. Eligible women were interviewed during the prenatal and immediate postpartum period. The interview protocol employed questions developed for this study to measure self-reported drug use, experience of violence, demographic characteristics, and other attitudinal factors, as well as validated measures for depression (Radloff, 1977; Schoenbach, Kaplan, Wagner, Grimson, & Miller, 1983), life stress (Sararson, Johnson, & Siegel, 1978), and social support (Norbeck, Lindsey, & Carrieri, 1981a,b). At the time of each interview, urine was obtained and assayed for marijuana and cocaine metabolites by Enzyme Mediated Immunoassay Technique (EMIT). Positive findings were reconfirmed.

Participants were classified as marijuana or cocaine users if any urine sample was positive for metabolites of these drugs or if they reported using these drugs during the time period under study. The use of other drugs was ascertained by self-report elicited in the interview.

The sample of this study consisted of 253 adolescents (aged 19 years and younger) and 761 adult women who perceived prenatal care and delivered at Boston City Hospital. The majority of eligible patients agreed to participate (87%) and according to information abstracted from maternal medical records, no significant differences existed between participants and nonparticipants in race, age, parity, or in the use of illicit or licit drugs. The demographic profile of study participants reflects the characteristics of patients served at Boston City Hospital. The majority were recipients of Medicaid (52%), North American Black (47%), foreign-born Black (19%), or Hispanic (18%), and single (78%). Approximately one-fourth of participants were between 13 and 19 years of age.

Table 1 shows the prevalence of lifetime use and use during pregnancy of psychoactive substances. The lifetime use of cigarettes and alcohol in the adolescent sample is somewhat lower than that reported in the National Study of High School Seniors (Johnston, O'Malley, & Bachman, 1987). However, the use of marijuana and cocaine is more prevalent in this sample than among girls in the High School Seniors Survey. These differences in prevalence of drug use are difficult to interpret because the national sample is composed of white high school seniors, whereas the sample in this study representing a broader age spectrum, is composed primarily of Blacks and Hispanics and includes adolescents who are not in school. As will be discussed in more detail in the following section, the assessment of drug use also differed in the two studies, thereby rendering comparisons difficult.

The overall use of all substances was lower during the pregnancy period than the reported lifetime use. However, a substantial proportion of adolescents and adults reported use of alcohol (53.4 vs. 63.1%), marijuana (31.6 vs. 27.5%) and cocaine (13.4 vs. 19.2%) during pregnancy (see Table 1).

Adolescents differed from adults in the age at onset of use of drugs (see Table 2). The majority of adolescents between 17 and 19 years of age who had ever used legal or illegal substances had done so by the time they were 16. On the other hand, most adult women first used these substances when they were 17 or older. The earlier age at onset of use among the younger cohort is important because earlier substance use has been

Table 1. Prevalence of Psychoactive Substance Use

Substance	Adolescents (n = 253)	Adults (n = 761)	
	Percent		p
Lifetime use:			
Cigarettes	57.5	57.0	0.89
Alcohol	82.2	88.4	0.01
Marijuana	61.3	55.9	0.14
Cocaine	20.2	29.3	0.005
Opiates	0.4	6.6	0.0002
Other drugs	10.3	22.1	0.0001
Use during pregnancy:			
Cigarettes	45.5	43.8	0.64
Alcohol	53.4	63.1	0.006
Marijuana	31.6	27.5	0.20
Cocaine	13.4	19.2	0.04
Opiates	0.4	5.5	0.0009
Other drugs	1.6	2.8	0.30

All comparisons were conducted using Chi-square analyses

Table 2. Percent Who Ever Used Licit and Illicit Substances by Age 16

Substance used	Age of subject			
	17–19 (n = 82)	20–29 (n = 227)	> 30 (n = 65)	
	Percent			p
Cigarettes	82.0	62.6	37.9	0.0001
Alcohol	75.9	47.9	31.5	0.0001
Marijuana	79.9	49.4	19.2	0.0001
Cocaine	46.7	8.7	2.4	0.0001

All comparisons were conducted using Chi-square analyses

associated with more pronounced negative outcomes and is a risk factor for subsequent acceleration into heavier drug use (Kandel, 1982).

These results suggest that drug use is common among both adolescent and adult pregnant women, with adult women having a greater lifetime use. We have also shown that adult women have a greater quantity and frequency of use of alcohol, cocaine, and opiates during pregnancy (Amaro & Zuckerman, 1990). However, adolescents and adults did not differ in the prevalence of cigarette or marijuana use prior to or during the pregnancy. Since onset occurs at an earlier age, it is likely that drug use among these adolescents will increase with age (Kandel, 1982). If this occurs, they may ultimately surpass the prevalence, quantity, and frequency of substance use of the adult women.

Validity of Self-Reported Drug Use

A key methodological limitation of previous research on drug use among adolescents and adults is the common use of self-report as a measure of drug use and the questionable validity of this method. As we have previously shown for marijuana use in pregnancy (Hingson, Zuckerman, Amaro, Frank, Kayne, Sorenson, Mitchell, Parker, Morelock, & Timperi, 1986), merely informing women that their urine will be tested for drug metabolites results in higher self-report of illicit drug use, while legal drug use is unchanged. In addition, the use of a urine screen identifies women who deny use through self-report. Thus, self-report alone has been shown to underestimate use of drugs in pregnant adult women.

Although clinicians are well aware of the limitations of assessing drug use among adolescents through self-report (Macdonald, 1984; DuPont, 1983; Committee on Adolescence, 1983), there is a lack of research on the extent of denial of drug use among adolescents compared to adults and whether the rate of denial is different for different drugs. In order to explore these questions, we conducted analyses with data from our study of drug use during pregnancy described in the previous section. The goals of the analyses were (1) to determine the number of pregnant adolescents who deny either marijuana or cocaine use but who have positive assay results for the metabolites of these drugs, and (2) to compare the rate of denial between pregnant adolescents and pregnant adults (Zuckerman, Amaro, & Cabral, 1989).

Of the pregnant adolescents, 90 (30%) either reported using marijuana or had at least one positive urine assay result for marijuana during pregnancy. Eleven of these adolescents (12%) denied marijuana use throughout pregnancy, but had a positive urine assay result for marijuana metabolites. Forty adolescents (12%) either had a positive urine test result or reported cocaine use during pregnancy. Of these, 14 (35%) denied cocaine use during pregnancy, but had at least one positive urine assay result. One hundred and two adolescents used one or both of these illicit drugs, and 25 (23%) denied use but had a positive urine assay result for one or both drugs. There was no statistically significant difference between adolescent and adult pregnant women in the percentage who had a positive urine assay result for marijuana but denied use (see Table 3). Although not statistically significant ($p < .08$), adolescents may be more likely than adults to deny cocaine use.

The results of this study provide important preliminary information regarding the prevalence of denial of illicit drug use among pregnant adolescents. The different rate of denial for marijuana and cocaine use among adolescents may indicate that adolescents have drug-specific attitudes and perceived social norms about the acceptability of marijuana and cocaine use, which leads them to admit use for marijuana but to deny use of cocaine. Moreover, adolescents and adults may have different perceptions of the acceptability of reporting cocaine use. A better understanding of adolescent attitudes, beliefs, and perceived social norms about the use of these substances could prove useful in the design of prevention and intervention programs.

Psychosocial Profile of Drug Using Pregnant Adolescents

In addition to the differences in drug use between adolescent and adult pregnant women, drug use among pregnant adolescents is associated

Table 3. Comparison of rates of deniers of illicit drug use between adolescent and non-adolescent women who used drugs during pregnancy

	Percent of (n)		
	Adolescent Users	*Adult Users*	*p*
Marijuana deniers	12% (of 90)	17% (of 247)	0.33
Cocaine deniers	35 (of 40)	20 (of 181)	0.08
Marijuana and/or cocaine deniers	25 (of 102)	23 (of 300)	0.76

Marijuana and cocaine use was determined by a positive urine assay and/or self reported use of these drugs.
Percentage of deniers for each drug was calculated from the number of users for each drug shown in parentheses.
All analyses were conducted using Chi-square analyses.

with a profile of risk factors. Our findings (Amaro, Zuckerman, & Cabral, 1989) indicate that compared to nondrug users, pregnant adolescents who use drugs were more likely to have a history of elective abortion (33 vs. 16.3%, $p < .003$) and venereal diseases (37.5 vs. 18.4%, $p < .001$), report more negative life events in the previous year ($p < .006$), violence during pregnancy (24 vs. 9%, $p < .002$), and have a male partner who used marijuana (68.6 vs. 30.3%, $p < .0001$) or cocaine (37.4 vs. 9.0%, $p < .0001$).

Since social support is generally considered a protective factor against poor social and behavioral outcomes for mothers and children, we expected nonusers to report having more social support than girls who were using drugs. However, we found no differences in the amount of social support reported. Instead, the difference between these two groups appears to be related to the *source* of the support. Among drug users, the male partner provided a larger portion of the social support received than among nonusers (11.6 vs. 6.8%, $p < .05$). Since partners of drug using adolescents are more likely to be drug users themselves, their support may provide a context for continued drug use that places the adolescent mother at greater risk of drug use and violence (Amaro, Fried, Cabral & Zuckerman, 1990). In view of the demonstrated role that male partners play in women's initiation and progression into drug use and addiction (Kandel, 1984; Hser, Anglin & McGlothlin, 1987; Anglin, Hser, & McGlothlin, 1987; Rosenbaum, 1981), it is possible that adolescent mothers who have drug using partners and who already use drugs themselves are at great risk for continued and escalated drug use and drug abuse. In summary, these findings suggest that drug use, whether as a marker or a mechanism, is associated with social and medical outcomes that may have a negative impact on the health of the mother and her child.

The Social Context of Drug Use among Adolescent Mothers: Preliminary Findings

Since previous studies with nonpregnant and nonparenting adolescents have demonstrated that peer and adult relationships exert an important influence on adolescents' drug use (Kandel, 1980; 1984; Jessor, Chase, & Donovan, 1980; Wills, 1986; Gfroerer, 1987), we were interested in whether the social context of support from friends among adolescent mothers may involve support for drug use. In order to explore this and other questions, we are conducting a study that investigates (1) adolescent mothers' patterns of drug use up to 1 year after delivery, (2) the social factors associated with drug use among adolescent mothers, and (3) the reproductive, educational, and psychological outcomes associated with drug use among adolescent mothers and their children. In this section, we present preliminary findings on perceived social norms and drug use in the adolescent mother's social network.

Participants are adolescents who register for prenatal care at Boston City Hospital. Interviews are conducted at four points in time: on registration at prenatal care, within 48 hours of delivery, at 6 months postpartum, and at 12 months postpartum. At the time of each interview, drug use is assessed by self-report and urine assay. At the last interview, a developmental assessment of the participant's study infant is conducted.

At the 6 month postpartum follow-up interview, we asked participants to rate the degree to which individuals in their social network approve or disapprove of their actual or potential drug use. The adolescent rated their perceived social norms on a 5 point scale (Table 4 shows responses dichotomized into approving/don't care vs. disapproving responses). In addition, we asked participants to report current drug use among family, friends, and partner. For the purposes of this analysis adolescents who self-reported drug use or who had a positive urine assay for drugs during pregnancy or postpartum were compared to nondrug users.

Very few adolescents, regardless of their own drug use, reported that their mother approved (or didn't care about) of their drug use or herself used marijuana or cocaine. No adolescent reported approval of drug use by the father. However, girls who used drugs were more likely than girls who did not use drugs to report that their mother and/or father were current users of marijuana and cocaine.

Adolescent mothers who used drugs were more likely than nonusers to report that their siblings and friends approved of their use of alcohol, marijuana, and cocaine. Drug-using adolescent mothers were also more likely than nonusers to have siblings and friends who were users of these substances. However, between one-fourth and one-third of adolescent mothers who do not use drugs have siblings or friends who use marijuana, placing them in an environment of heightened risk.

Partners of drug users were also more likely to be perceived by adolescent mothers as approving of their drug use. The partners of drug-using girls were also more likely to be current users of alcohol, marijuana, and cocaine.

Thus, siblings, friends and partners of adolescent mothers who use drugs provide a social context of support for drug use. The profile that emerges in these analyses suggests that adolescent mothers who use drugs are exposed to a social context which differs significantly from that of adolescent mothers who do not use drugs. These findings are not surprising; after all, many studies of nonpregnant or nonparenting adolescents have found that peers exert a significant effect on drug use among adolescents (Kandel, 1980, 1984; Jessor et al., 1980; Wills, 1986;

Table 4. Adolescent Mothers' Perception of Social Network Support
for Drug Use by Drug Use Status

	Drug Users % (n = 34)	Nonusers % (n = 49)
Mother approves/ Doesn't care		
Alcohol	5	0
Marijuana	5	3
Cocaine	3	0
Mother uses		
Alcohol	46	28
Marijuana	9	3
Cocaine	5	0
Father approves/ Doesn't care		
Alcohol	0	0
Marijuana	0	0
Cocaine	0	0
Father uses		
Alcohol	30	54
Marijuana	20	4
Cocaine	11	0
Siblings approve/ Don't care		
Alcohol	43	17
Marijuana	35	9
Cocaine	21	9
Siblings use		
Alcohol	64	32
Marijuana	57	23
Cocaine	21	9
Friends approve/ Don't care		
Alcohol	71	31
Marijuana	43	14
Cocaine	14	7
Friends use		
Alcohol	80	51
Marijuana	82	35
Cocaine	19	3
Partner approves/ Doesn't care		
Alcohol	25	3
Marijuana	25	0
Cocaine	10	0
Partner uses		
Alcohol	75	36
Marijuana	65	12
Cocaine	5	0

Gfroener, 1987) and studies of women's initiation into drug use have established that male partners play a significant role in women's initiation into drug use (Kandel, 1984; Hser, Anglin, & McGlothlin, 1987; Anglin, Hser, & McGlothlin, 1987; Rosenbaum, 1981).

The implications of drug use and the social context of drug use have additional consequences for adolescent mothers. First, adolescent mothers in this sample already face a series of risks to optimal development and outcomes. The environmental and social impact of poverty and minority status place them at greater risk of early and repeat pregnancy, dropping out of school, unemployment, and depression. Drug use and its associated social context compound this risk. Second, in addition to the risks of in utero drug exposure (Zuckerman et al., 1989), the risks associated with drug use in the adolescent mother postnatally have implications to the development and well-being of the child. We are presently investigating these concerns.

Summary

Findings from our research indicate that drug use in our sample of adolescent mothers is as common if not more common than in the general adolescent population and that drug use is associated with increased risk for stress, exposure to violence, and having a male partner who is a drug user. Siblings and friends, who often serve as sources of social support for the adolescent mother, are also sources of support for continued drug use. Drug use in the adolescent mother, male partner, siblings, and friends may be associated with increased risks for negative outcomes for the mother such as repeat pregnancy and school dropout, and adverse consequences for the child such as injuries and poor growth development, among other variables.

Male partners, friends, and siblings play an important role in adolescents' social relationships. Yet, when individuals who are the primary sources of social support engage in drug use and support drug use in the adolescent mother, the social support they provide may increase drug use and as a result other risks associated with drug use in the adolescent mother. These findings suggest that interventions targeted at reduction of drug use among adolescent mothers need to address the social context of drug use and intervene with the adolescent mother as well as with those in her immediate social support network.

Further, since drug use may be a self-medicating response that adolescent mothers employ to cope with stressful situations and social relationships, programs to reduce drug use in this group should teach adolescent mothers alternative coping mechanisms for coping with stress.

Acknowledgments

This work is supported by grants from the National Institute of Drug Abuse (NIDA-R01DA03508), William T. Grant Foundation, The Harris Foundation, and Academic Training Program in Behavioral Pediatrics funded by the Bureau of Health Care Delivery and Assistance, Maternal and Child Health Branch (Grant MCJ-009094).

The authors thank Gabrielle Lozez, Elva Perez Trevino, Claudia Caicedo, Julie Skoler, and Isolde Gornemann for conducting the interviews and Rose Dobosz for coding of the data. We also thank Dr. Ralph Timperi and Laura Hennigan who were responsible for conducting the urine assays, and Pat Schofield for her help in preparing the manuscript.

Paper presented at Adolescent Stress, Social Relationships, and Mental Health Research Conference, University of Massachusetts, Boston, MA. Portions of this chapter are reprinted from *Pediatrics*, 1989, *84*(1), and *Journal of Pediatrics*, 1989, *115:* 812–815, 144–151. Copyright © 1989 by Pediatrics. Reprinted by permission, Copyright © 1989, Journal of Pediatrics.

References

Amaro, H., Fried, L.E., Cabral, H. & Zuckerman, B. (1990). Violence during pregnancy and substance use. *American Journal of Public Health, 80*(5), 575–579.

Amaro, H., & Zuckerman, B. (1990). Drug use among adolescent mothers. In A.R. Stiffman & R.A. Feldman (Eds.), *Advances in Adolescent Mental Health, Volume IV, Sexual Activity, Childbearing and Childrearing.* London: Jessica Kingsley Pubs., pp 203–221.

Amaro, H., Zuckerman, B., & Cabral, H. (1989). Drug use among adolescent mothers: A profile of risk. *Pediatrics, 84*(1), 144–151.

Anglin, D., Hser, Y., & McGlothlin, W. (1987). Sex differences in addict careers. II. Becoming addicted. *American Journal of Drug and Alcohol Abuse, 13*(1,2), 59–71.

Committee on Adolescence. (1983). The role of the pediatrician in substance abuse counseling. *Pediatrics, 72,* 251–252.

DuPont, R.L. (1983). Teenage drug use: Opportunities for the pediatrician. *J Pediatrics, 102,* 1003–1007.

Elliot, D.S., & Morse, B.J. (1987). *Delinquency and drug use as risk factors in teenage sexual activity and pregnancy.* Paper presented at the Convention of the American Psychological Association, August 31.

Furstenberg, F.F. (1976). *Unplanned parenthood: The social consequences of teenage childbearing.* New York: Macmillan.

Gfoerer, B.A. (1987). Correlation between drug use by teenagers and drug use by older family members. *American Journal of Drug and Alcohol Abuse, 13*(1,2), 95–108.

Hingson, R., Zuckerman, B., Amaro, H., Frank, D., Kayne, H., Sorenson, J.R., Mitchell, J., Parker, S., Morelock, S., & Timperi, R. (1986). Maternal marijuana use and neonatal outcome. Uncertainty posed by self reports. *American Journal of Public Health, 76,* 667–669.

Hser, Y., Anglin, D., & McGlothlin, W. (1987). Sex differences in addict careers. I. Initiation of use. *American Journal of Drug and Alcohol Abuse, 13*(1,2), 33–57.

Hundleby, J.D., Carpenter, R.A., Ross, R.A.J., & Mercer, G.W. (1982). Adolescent drug use and other behaviors. *Journal of Child Psychology and Psychiatry, 23*(1), 61–68.

Jessor, S., & Jessor, R. (1977). *Problem behavior and psychological development: A longitudinal study of youth.* New York: Academy Press.

Jessor, R. (1983). The stability of change: Psychosocial development from adolescence to young adulthood. In D. Magnisson & V. Allen (Eds.) *Human Development: An international perspective.* New York: Academic Press.

Jessor, R., Chase, J.A., & Donovan, J.E. (1980). Psychosocial correlates of marijuana use and problem drinking in a national sample of adolescents. *American Journal of Public Health, 70*(6), 604–613.

Johnston, L.D., O'Malley, P.M., & Bachman, J.G. (1987). National trends in drugs use and related factors among American high school students and young adults, 1985–86. Rockville, MD: National Institute on Drug Abuse (DHHS Publication No. (ADM) 87-1535).

Kandel, D., Single, E., & Kessler, R.D. (1976). The epidemiology of drug use among New York State high school students: Distribution, trends and change in rates of use. *American Journal of Public Health, 66,* 43–53.

Kandel, D.B. (1980). Developmental stages in adolescent drug involvement. In D. Lettieri (Ed.), *Drug Theories,* (pp. 120–127). Washington, D.C.: U.S. Government Printing Office.

Kandel, D.B. (1982). Epidemiological and psychosocial perspectives on adolescent drug use. *Journal of the American Academy of Child Psychiatry, 21,* 328–347.

Kandel, D.B. (1984). Marijuana users in young childhood. *Archives of General Psychiatry, 41,* 200–209.

MacDonald, D. (1984). I. Drugs, drinking and adolescence. *American Journal of Diseases in Children, 138,* 117–125.

Merritt, T.A., Lawrence, R.A., & Naeye, R.I. (1980). The infants of adolescent mothers. *Pediatric Annals, 9,* 200–220.

Norbeck, J.S., Lindsey, A.M., & Carrieri, V.L. (1981a). Further development of the Norbeck social support questionnaire: Normative data and validity testing. *Nursing Research, 32*(1), 4–9.

Norbeck, J.S., Lindsey, A.M., & Carrieri, V.L. (1981b). The development of the Norbeck social support questionnaire: Normative data and validity testing. *Nursing Research, 32*(5), 264–268.

Paton, S., Kessler, R., & Kandel, D. (1977). Depressive mood and adolescent illicit drug use; A longitudinal analysis. *Journal of Genetic Psychology, 131,* 267–289.

Radloff, L.S. (1977). The CES-D Scale: A self-report depression scale for research in the general population. *Applied Psychology Measurement, 1,* 385–401.

Rosenbaum, M. (1981). *Women on heroin.* New Brunswick, NJ: Rutgers University Press.

Sararson, I.G., Johnson, J.H., & Siegel, J.M. (1978). Assessing the impact of life changes: Development of the life experiences survey. *Journal of Consulting and Clinical Psychology, 46,* 932–946.

Schoenbach, V.J., Kaplan, B.H., Wagner, E.H., Grimson, R.C., & Miller, F.T. (1983). Prevalence and self-reported depressive symptoms in young adolescents. *American Journal of Public Health, 73*(11), 1281–1287.

Wills, T.A. (1986). Stress and coping in early adolescence: Relationships to substance use in urban school samples. *Journal of Health Psychology, 5*(6), 503–529.

Zuckerman, B.S., Amaro, M., & Beardslee, W.R. (1987). Mental health of adolescent mothers: The implications of depression and drug use. *Journal of Developmental and Behavioral Pediatrics, 8,* 111–116.

Zuckerman, B.S., Amaro, H., & Cabral, H. (1989b). The validity of self-reported marijuana and cocaine use among pregnant adolescents. *Journal of Pediatrics, 115,* 812–815.

Zuckerman, B.S., Frank, D.A., Hingson, R., Amaro, H., Levenson, S., Kayne, H., Parker, S., Vinci, R., Aboagye, K., Fried, L.E., Cabral, H., Timperi, R., & Bauchner, H. (1989a). Effects of maternal marijuana and cocaine use on fetal growth. *New England Journal of Medicine, 320,* 762–768.

Zuckerman, B.S., Hingson, R., Alpert, J.J., Dooling, E., Kayne, H., Morelock, S., & Oppenheimer, E. (1983). Neonatal outcome—Is adolescent pregnancy a risk factor? *Pediatrics, 71,* 489.

12

Stress in Mentally Retarded
Children and Adolescents

Gary N. Siperstein and Melodie Wenz-Gross

Introduction

Since the groundbreaking work of Piaget in the 1930s, developmental psychologists have continued to revise their view of the child. Contemporary developmental theory now describes the young child as a complex, active perceiver—one who experiences and comprehends far more than was previously thought. In particular, we now know that the young child is extremely sensitive and experiences a wide range of emotions. However, we recognize that this more competent child is also more vulnerable. Not surprisingly, we have learned that children experience stress at a younger age and are also subject to a wider range of childhood disorders such as depression and anxiety.

In addition, we now recognize that today's children are burdened by a wider range of societal pressures. For instance, they spend much more time, and at much younger ages, in the care of extraparental adults, often sharing adult attention with 10 to 15 other children. Divorce rates have steadily increased and two-career parents have less time and energy to devote to their children. Further, drugs, sexuality, and AIDS have become evident even at the elementary school level. Overall, as children grow, they are faced with adult concerns and pressures at a much younger age and thus have greater opportunity to experience stress. In light of this new view of children as burdened with greater familial and social demands, developmental and social psychologists have now begun to consider the effects of stress in children.

As a result of growing interest in stress in childhood and adolescence, researchers have made progress in studying the various stressors, stress reactions, and mediators of stress in children and adolescents. Recently, researchers also have begun to look at children "at risk" for stress (e.g., Seifer & Sameroff, 1987). These groups include children whose parents are suffering from depression, schizophrenia, or other mental disorders, children from economically deprived backgrounds, and children who have lost a parent. However, one group of children and adolescents who are potentially "at risk" has not yet been included in the study of stress. The children and adolescents we refer to are those with developmental disabilities, particularly mental retardation. We believe this population is potentially "at risk" because they may experience more stress, and have fewer resources to deal with that stress than do average children. Our goal in this chapter is to draw attention to the mildly mentally retarded child and adolescent, and to stimulate research and clinical interest in examining the stressors they face and the ways in which we may help to alleviate that stress.

In the following discussion, we will focus our attention on children with mild mental retardation, specifically those considered as having mild cognitive delays (IQ~55–75). We have chosen to focus on these children for several reasons. First, children with mild cognitive delays are often less visible because those outside of the field of mental retardation generally conceive of mental retardation in its more severe forms. Further, those within the field have become more concerned with the moderately to severely mentally retarded because they are increasingly being placed in more public independent living arrangements. As a result, those with mild mental retardation, who comprise the highest percentage of children with mental retardation (over 60%), have been largely ignored.

Lastly, children with mild mental retardation are perhaps the most vulnerable because they are integrated more fully into society and are exposed to greater social demands, labels, and stigmas. These social stigmas and stereotypes can be damaging because children with mild mental retardation are quite aware of them, despite the mistaken perception that they are oblivious. In fact, Budoff and Siperstein (1982) found that mentally retarded children were as negative toward other children labeled mentally retarded as were nonretarded children, suggesting that they had internalized the stigma. These children not only perceived themselves as mentally retarded, but were also aware that others labeled them as such. Unfortunately, the misconception that these children are unaware of other's perceptions persists. To quote a nonretarded eleventh grade boy in a study of students' and teachers' perceptions of mentally retarded children (Siperstein & Bak, 1980):

> Mentally retarded people are not able to comprehend what life really is. They are unable to function as normal people because of brain disease or damage. I know this from viewing them doing their menial tasks and from books I have read. They got that way because of a lack of air during birth, thus their brain [is] damaged, or because of freak mutations like too many chromosomes—just one extra will do it. They are outwardly obvious, that is, they have cloudy haircuts, outdated clothes and cheap eyeglasses. They feel nothing. They haven't the capabilities to understand what they are. (p. 207)

This stereotype of the mentally retarded as being unaware, "feeling nothing," or being "unable to understand what they are" is not new. In fact, historically, mentally retarded individuals have been perceived as being incapable of appreciating society's expectations, or of experiencing depression, anxiety, guilt, or unworthiness (Gardner, 1967). Yet studies conducted with mentally retarded adolescents suggest they are aware of their differences and the rejection they generate from family and peers (Wayment & Zetlin, 1989; Zetlin & Turner, 1985). Far from being incapable of experiencing depression or anxiety, mentally retarded children have been shown to be more depressed and anxious than nonretarded children (Cullinan, Epstein, Matson, & Rosemier, 1984). For these and other reasons that we will elaborate, we feel the mildly mentally retarded child is at substantial risk for experiencing stress.

Stressors of Mentally Retarded Children and Adolescents

Family Stress

One way to begin to look at mentally retarded children's experience of stress is to see them as they are perceived—that is, as a stressor. Although researchers and clinicians have been concerned about stress in families with mentally retarded children, they have focused almost exclusively on the impact of these children on the family. For instance, research shows that mentally retarded children impact negatively on parental mental health. Mothers of mentally retarded children show greater depression, more preoccupation with the child, more possessiveness, but also less enjoyment and less of a sense of maternal competence (Cummings, Bayley, & Rie, 1966). Fathers have also been shown to be more depressed, to have lower self-esteem, and less interpersonal satisfaction (Cummings, 1976). Further, parents of mentally retarded children have been shown to have MMPI profiles that suggest problems with impulse control and aggressiveness, similar to parents with emotionally disturbed children (Erikson, 1969; Miller & Keirn, 1978).

Researchers have also shown that mentally retarded children affect the relationship between parents. Specifically, parents with mentally retarded children report significantly less marital satisfaction than parents without a mentally retarded child (Friedrich & Friedrich, 1981). Further, they have found that the stress presented by raising a mentally retarded child is chronic, with periods of greater and lesser stress as the child grows into adulthood. Some of the periods of heightened stress occur when parents first learn that their child is disabled, when developmental milestones are late or not attained, and when the parents must make decisions regarding independent living situations and care of the individual when they are no longer able to do so themselves. The financial strain, disruption of family routines, social stigma, and limitations on social outlets that often plague parents raising a disabled child have also been enumerated (for a review, see Crnic, Friedrich, & Greenberg, 1983).

What, if any, are the effects of this stressful family climate on the mentally retarded child? Can it be that the mentally retarded child is unaffected by the familial strain caused by his/her mental retardation? There is a growing body of evidence that points to a reciprocal influence between mentally retarded children and their home environment (e.g., Nihira, Mink, & Meyers, 1985). This research documents a relationship between various environmental variables, such as family harmony, quality of parenting, and family cohesion, and the overall emotional adjustment of both mildly and moderately retarded adolescents.

We contend that the stressful family climate created by the presence of a mentally retarded child may, in turn, become a stressor for the mentally retarded child. This argument is supported by research on the relationship between familial environment and stress in nonretarded children. Recent evidence indicates that the most detrimental kinds of stressors in childhood are those that are chronic and that involve the family, such as marital discord, maternal depression or psychiatric disorder, and parental rejection (see Rutter, 1981; Garmezy, 1984). Further, these stressors are known to affect children of all ages, even preschoolers who may be too young to comprehend the meaning or nature of the stress (Wallerstein, 1984). These familial stressors, which are among the most difficult for nonretarded children, are even more prevalent in families with mentally retarded children. Thus, we can assume that if the families of mentally retarded children are stressed, the mentally retarded child will also be stressed.

School Stress

Although there are many stressors that could affect the mentally retarded child and adolescent within the school, we would like to focus on those environmental stressors created by school policies. As mentally retarded children move into the public schools, they are often main-streamed into regular classroom settings because of the federal mandate to educate disabled children in the least restrictive environment. As a result of these policies, children with disabilities have come, once again, to be viewed as a stressor, both to educators within the classroom and to administrators in the educational system. In fact, mildly mentally retarded children can be seen as the most difficult to educate because of the questions raised regarding how much integration should take place and at what age. Unfortunately for the child, these school policies also often produce inconsistent learning environments, unpredictable transi-tions, and social isolation, as well as inadvertently contributing to de facto labeling. Thus, educators are stressed, and in turn, the child is stressed both indirectly (as a result of the stress of the teacher) and directly (through the number of changes the child must adjust to on a daily basis).

For example, many mainstreamed children are moved from one class to another, spending minimal parts of the day or week in regular class-rooms. Thus, they are never fully integrated into the normal routine of these classrooms. As a result, many regular education teachers are uncomfortable with mainstreaming and see the mentally retarded child as an impediment to teaching and to behavior management in the classroom. Research shows that teachers rate these children as disturbing and disapprove of their placement in regular classrooms (Horne, 1983). They also have been found to show more negative affect toward the child with learning problems than toward those without (Siperstein & Goding, 1985). Thus, teachers often perceive the mentally retarded child as a source of stress and respond with negative attitudes and affect. Research on nonretarded children indicates that not only are children aware of negative teacher expectancies and attitudes, but they are negatively affected by them as well (Brophy, 1983). We assume that mildly mentally retarded children, who are subjected to greater teacher negativity than nonretarded children, will be similarly affected. Thus, once again we contend that these children are not only a source of stress to those around them, but are also reciprocally stressed.

The nature of these school policies, which determine the child's place-ment and level of integration, may also serve as a source of stress. Many times these integration policies are dictated by convenience more than by the needs of the child. In a recent longitudinal study, Siperstein (1990) found that children were sometimes integrated one year but not the next. This move back into a segregated classroom after being integrated often results in the child experiencing a sense of failure.

Siperstein (1990) also found that sometimes children were moved back two grades or ahead two grades from one year to the next. For example, a child might be moved from fifth grade back to third, or ahead to junior high or even high school, depending on the available programming. As a result, these children are sometimes integrated with children younger than themselves, other times with children older. This may create problems for the child in adjusting to the educational and social demands of the classroom setting and may further contribute to the child's social isolation with peers. Most nonretarded children are consistently with their agemates who are physically and developmentally their equivalents. The mentally retarded child, when placed with younger or older children, may not only be cognitively and socially different, but may also be physically ahead of or behind his/her classmates. Finally, sometimes these children are integrated along with other mentally retarded children, other times alone. Being the only mentally retarded child in an integrated classroom contributes to social isolation because mentally retarded children are generally rejected or ignored by their nonretarded peers (Bak & Siperstein, 1987).

As is evident, mentally retarded children's school environments are often full of unpredictable, uncontrollable, and seemingly questionable transitions. Unpredictability and lack of control have both been shown to lead to the perception of threat and symptoms of distress (see Lazarus & Folkman, 1984). Further, research on nonretarded children shows that even regular, predictable school transitions can be stressful (Felner, Primavera, & Cauce, 1981). However, during these transitions most nonretarded children stay with the same peers during the greater part of the school day and from one year to the next. The transitions that mentally retarded children face are not only predictable, but are isolating in that they are thrust on the individual child rather than occurring as part of an entire peer group transition (e.g., the normal transition to junior high). We contend then that the combination of these nonnormative transitions and teachers' negative responses toward mentally retarded children in the regular classroom may place these children at substantial risk for stress.

Peer Stress

I'm nicer when you know me.
Even when the people don't know you they make fun of you?

Yeah.
—12 year-old mentally retarded boy playing with a nonretarded "friend"
during an experimental situation.

The lack of stability created by integration policies is compounded by other policies that segregate mentally retarded children in ways that label them and contribute to problems with peers. For instance, sometimes these children ride to school on special buses or eat lunch at separate time periods. One mentally retarded child, in a personal interview, stated that he wished he could be dropped off his special needs bus before it reached the school so that he would not have to face the harassment associated with being on this bus. In fact, in a recent study Wayment and Zetlin (1989) found that adolescents with mild mental retardation reported conflict with others (e.g., with peers) and social injustices (e.g., being teased) as the most frequently named stressors.

Thus, the stress created by integration and segregation policies contributes to and is further potentiated by stress within the peer network. Although mentally retarded children have been found to form friendships with other retarded children (Siperstein & Bak, 1989), these friendships may also be compromised by the integration policies and the lack of environmental stability outlined above. Further, neglect and rejection from nonretarded peers, which start at an early age, become a chronic omnipresent fact of life by middle childhood and adolescence.

Peer rejection and social isolation can be devastating to the child's self-concept, adjustment, and developing social skills, which in turn, may further isolate him/her. Research on mentally retarded children shows that as a result of this rejection these children experience greater loneliness than their nonretarded peers (Luftig, 1988). Further, when given the choice, they choose to be with other retarded children (Siperstein, Brownley, & Scott, 1989), further isolating them from their nonretarded peers. Thus, mentally retarded children show that they are aware of this rejection and they no doubt experience stress in relation to it.

In sum, children with mild mental retardation face many stressors, at home, at school, and with peers. Some of these stressors arise out of the stress created in others because of the child's disability, while others arise from school policies and social stigmas over which the child has little influence. It is our contention that mentally retarded children are not only aware of these stressors, but are negatively impacted by them.

Unfortuntely the impact of these stressors has not been directly examined. However, research has shown that children with mental retardation exhibit greater depression, anxiety, and behavior problems than do nonretarded children (Cochran & Cleland, 1963; Rutter, Tizard,

Yule, Graham, & Witmore, 1976). These problems have been associated with stress in nonretarded populations. For instance, stress has been associated with emotional problems (e.g., anxiety and depression), poor grades and school adjustment problems, and behavioral problems (O'Grady & Metz, 1987; Rutter, 1981; Sterling, Cowen, Weissberg, Lotyezewski, & Boike, 1985). Given the above portrait, we may conclude that these problems are related to stress in retarded children and adolescents as well.

Internal and External Resources for Dealing with Stress: Coping Skills and Social Support

In considering the resources mentally retarded adolescents have for dealing with stress, we are limited in our discussion and in the conclusions we can draw by a general lack of data on the coping resources available to the mentally retarded child. However, we will attempt to speculate on these resources by drawing from research on nonretarded groups as it may apply to mentally retarded children.

Internal Resources: Coping Skills

One factor that may serve to compound the challenges mentally retarded children face in the family, at school, and with peers is their coping style. Two main types of coping have been studied in relation to stress: emotion-focused and problem-focused coping. Emotion-focused coping strategies function to control the negative affect associated with stressful situations. Alternatively, problem-focused coping strategies function to change the situation.

Lazarus and Folkman (1984) hypothesize that stressful situations that are within one's control (e.g., school failure, peer difficulties) require the use of more problem-focused strategies, while those outside of one's control (e.g., medical procedures) require the use of more emotion-focused strategies. Research has demonstrated that emotion-focused and avoidant strategies tend to be efficacious over the short-term, but in the long run, problem-focused coping is associated with more positive adaptation (see Suls & Fletcher, 1985 for a review). Further, research suggests that although both emotion-focused and problem-focused strategies are necessary in successfully coping with stress, flexibility in the use of these strategies is most important (Compas, 1987). Other factors which seem to contribute to effective coping are high self-esteem, an internal locus of control (Garmezy, 1984), and good problem solving skills (Spivack & Shure, 1982).

Research on nonretarded children show that they tend to use more active, problem-focused coping (Band & Weisz, 1988). In fact, Compas, Malcarne, and Fondacaro (1988) found that nonretarded children who were less able to generate and use problem-focused coping experienced more emotional and behavioral problems. However, even as young as age 6, nonretarded children varied their strategies depending on the stressor (Band & Weisz, 1988). Problem-focused coping was used most for stressors such as peer difficulties and school failure. Emotion-focused coping was used more for problems outside of their control, such as medical procedures.

Children with mental retardation, on the other hand, tend to exhibit inflexibility, emotional simplicity, and an external locus of control (Webster, 1970). They also tend to give up rather than persevere in achievement situations in which they may fail. Further, Wayment and Zetlin (1989) found that adolescents with mild mental retardation use more passive and emotion-focused coping strategies than nonretarded adolescents. In fact, mentally retarded children in general tend to show a passive response to new situations and in interactions with nonretarded peers. These types of situations (achievement situations, peer interactions, etc.) may be seen as requiring more active, problem-focused coping strategies. Therefore, in general, the coping strategies used by mentally retarded children may not be effective in mediating many of the stresses they face.

External Resources: Social Support

Another factor which may interfere with the mentally retarded child's ability to deal with stress is limited social support. In research on nonretarded children, social networks and social supports have been shown to be effective buffers against stress (O'Grady & Metz, 1987) and to be important to both development (Hartup, 1989) and to psychological health and adjustment (Furman, 1987).

In theory, social support buffers stress in a number of ways, including enhancing self-esteem, providing cognitive reinterpretation of stressful situations, enhancing affect and coping, and decreasing the likelihood of the occurrence of stressful events (Shumaker & Brownell, 1984; Thoits, 1986). Therefore, social support from family, peers, and others may help children manage stress by regulating emotion, developing coping skills, and improving self-esteem.

At present there are very few studies of social networks and perceptions of support in mentally retarded children and adolescents. However, in a recent study of mentally retarded adolescents' social relationships, Siperstein and Bak (1989) began to look at social networks by examining friendships inside and outside of the classroom. They found that mentally retarded adolescents named a wide range of people as important, including parents and other adults in the school and community. They also found that these adolescents frequently formed friendships with other mentally retarded peers, but much less frequently with nonretarded peers (Bak & Siperstein, 1987). Whether or not these relationships are a source of support for these adolescents was not examined. In another recent study of how mentally retarded adolescents deal with their social challenges, Wayment and Zetlin (1989) found that girls often turned to adults for help while boys turned to peers. However, at present we know little about the role that these relationships play in mediating stress. We also lack knowledge of younger mentally retarded children's resources for support.

The above studies, while limited, serve as a starting point and highlight the importance and complexity of the mentally retarded child's social network and social support. Given that mentally retarded children may be more dependent on others than nonretarded children and may have fewer adaptive coping skills, social support could potentially play an even more crucial role in their ability to deal with stress.

Studies of social support in nonretarded children and adolescents show that children seek different types of support from different network members. In general, children turn to peers most often for companionship, emotional support, and intimacy. Same-sex friendships, in particular, play increasingly important roles with age. But even for children as young as age 4, friendships play an important supportive role. Parents are the other main source of support and are turned to most often for affection, enhancement of worth, and reliable and instrumental aid.

Other relationships, such as those with siblings, extended relatives, neighbors, and teachers, are also important but seen to play less significant roles. For instance, grandparents are turned to for enhancement of worth and affection. Older siblings are perceived as a source of instrumental aid and closely spaced same-sex siblings are frequently a source of companionship and intimacy. Further, girls tend to form more intense relationships and to report more intimacy, affection, and enhancement of worth in their best friendships than do boys (Buhrmester & Furman, 1987; Furman & Buhrmester, 1985; Reid, Landesman, Treder, & Jaccard, 1989; Wenz-Gross, 1990).

To what extent can the above findings be generalized to mentally retarded children? As was reviewed in the previous section, the families of mentally retarded children are often stressed. Research demonstrates that when a family is under stress, those within the family system are in need of support themselves and have little to offer others within that system (Atkinson, Liem, & Liem, 1986). In fact, parents of mentally retarded children have been shown to be overprotective, angry, and rejecting toward their child (Ricci, 1970). Therefore, the stress that is present in the family of the mentally retarded child and the ways in which that stress affects the parent–child relationship may not only limit the amount of support available from parents, but may increase stress for the mentally retarded child.

Further, the lack of stability in the school system combined with the low social status these children have with their nonretarded peers may further limit the amount of support available from the school and peer network. However, mentally retarded children and adolescents may seek support from less typical sources (e.g., neighbors, siblings, grandparents) or from a few key individuals on whom they rely heavily. Overall, it would appear that mentally retarded children and adolescents may have more limited resources for support, which may contribute to their lack of coping skills and exacerbate the amount of stress experienced as well.

Developmental Issues in the Study of Stress in Mentally Retarded Children and Adolescents

Because it is our goal to stimulate research and clinical interest in stress and mentally retarded children and adolescents, we would like to propose a framework that may guide the future study of stress in this population. In this effort, we will first define stress as it may apply to the mentally retarded child. We will then explore some of the developmental issues that may be important in the study of stress in these children.

Stress has been defined and measured in many ways. Some define stress in terms of a stimulus, as in life events or stressors (Holmes & Rahe, 1967). Others define it in terms of a response, as in the resulting distress or physical reactions one might show to certain stressors (Selye, 1979). We believe that the best way to conceptualize stress in children with mental retardation is in terms of the interaction between the individual and the environment, and, specifically, between environmental demands and individual resources. Lazarus and Folkman (1984) state:

> Psychological stress is a particular relationship between the person and the environment that is appraised by the person as taxing or exceeding his or her resources and endangering his or her well-being. (p. 19)

This definition is particularly relevant for children with mental retardation because it is precisely this lack of fit between demands and resources that defines their disability and places it in bold relief. Although it is normal for everyone to experience this lack of fit at times, coping with discrepancies between environmental demands and individual resources is part of the mentally retarded child's everyday experience.

One aspect of this definition that deserves further attention is that of the individual's appraisal of threat or endangerment. The child's appraisal of an event as demanding or threatening will depend, in part, on his or her understanding of the threat. For instance, Maccoby (1984) states in regard to stress in the young child,

> we cannot be humiliated by failure to handle problems whose solutions are someone else's responsibility; we cannot be distressed by anticipating other's contemptuous or critical reactions to our weaknesses if we are not aware of others' probable reactions and if our egos are not yet invested in appearing strong and competent. (p. 219)

However, the above quote does not imply that young children (or children with limited cognitive abilities) do not experience stress. Rather, it argues for the examination of stress within a developmental framework.

Examining stress within a developmental framework requires that we keep in mind the child's developmental level (i.e., the child's social, emotional, and cognitive competence) and the tasks that need to be negotiated at that level (e.g., separation in early childhood). Together, the child's developmental competence and investment in related tasks will provide the lens through which certain events are viewed as stressful. At each developmental level, there are several tasks that need to be negotiated. Each task remains important to the child throughout development, but diminishes in importance relative to new emerging developmental issues (Cicchetti & Schneider-Rosen, 1986). As the child strives to accomplish these developmental tasks, certain classes or types of stressors will come into focus. The child will be more vulnerable to stressors related to those areas in which developmental investment is greatest (Maccoby, 1984).

In the following sections, we will briefly review some of the normative developmental tasks of early and middle childhood and adolescence as they relate to the child's appraisal of stress within each period. We will then speculate on the types of stressors that may be developmentally relevant to the mentally retarded child at different ages. Research demonstrates that mentally retarded children pass through the same stages of development in the same order but at a slower rate, and with a lower ceiling (see Morgan, 1986 for a review). Thus, we can assume that mentally retarded children will face the same developmental tasks at a later chronological age than their nonretarded peers.

However, the nature and timing of mentally retarded children's experience of stress are not expected to be precisely predicted by developmental level due to the forces of their experience in chronological years (i.e., a mildly mentally retarded child with the cognitive abilities of a 6-year-old will have lived 3 or 4 years longer than the nonretarded 6-year-old). This review stands then as a rough guide rather than a blueprint. Further, we must keep in mind that the nature of the mentally retarded child's experience subjects them to stressors most nonretarded children do not have to face (e.g., school policies, social stigma). Therefore, the actual taxonomy of stressors may be very different for mentally retarded children. Until future research addresses these issues, however, we feel the developmental framework provides a logical starting point from which to theoretically approach the study of stress in mildly mentally retarded children and adolescents.

Early Childhood

In early childhood, separation is one of the major developmental tasks to be negotiated (Cicchetti & Schneider-Rosen, 1986). Toddlers will view even brief separations from primary care-givers as particularly stressful because of the developmental importance of the attachment relationship at that age. If separations are excessive (in frequency and duration), they may cause considerable behavioral disturbance and long-term difficulties (Bowlby, 1969). Similarly, the birth of a sibling, which changes the nature of the parent–older child relationship, will constitute a significant threat at this age. Thus, family stressors will be particularly salient for children at this time.

We may expect that the mildly mentally retarded child will begin to deal with separation issues at a later age and take a longer period of time to master them. Thus, the mildly mentally retarded child may still be negotiating separation issues at the time he/she is starting school, exacerbating this stress for these children. In addition, mildly mentally retarded children are often not diagnosed as such until they begin school. Parents of these children may react to this diagnosis with increased parental conflict and either rejection or overprotection of the child. This may compound the stress of entering school at this time and further complicate the mastery of this developmental task.

Middle Childhood

In middle childhood, the development of peer relations is a primary developmental task (Cicchetti & Schneider-Rosen, 1986). Thus, peer conflicts will be viewed as particularly stressful because of their developmental salience. In addition, in middle childhood, children are developing a sense of self-efficacy, of right and wrong, and of the psychological aspects of self and others. Empathy and perspective-taking become more advanced and complex. This allows the child to compare him/herself to others, and to be more greatly affected by other's evaluations. Thus, excessive peer rejection, unpopularity, school failure, or unrealistic expectations from parents and teachers would be particularly stressful at this time.

In terms of mildly mentally retarded children, we know that they are faced with peer rejection and isolation from a young age, with this rejection increasing as they progress into the upper grades. Unfortunately, it is in the upper grades that we may expect these children to begin negotiating the developmental tasks relating to peer relationships, self-efficacy, and perspective-taking. Thus, although these children are subjected to peer rejection from an early age, it may not be until late childhood or adolescence that they feel the full force of this negative peer evaluation. As a result, considerable social stress may be generated at a time when they are also going through the bodily and hormonal changes of puberty. Their placement in classrooms with younger or older children may create additional stress due to the lack of physical synchrony (with younger children) or social synchrony (with older adolescents). Together, these factors may interfere with their mastery of these developmental tasks. Further, if the establishment of self-efficacy and peer relationships is compromised, the development of active coping skills, an internal locus of control, and peer social supports may also be compromised, leaving the mentally retarded adolescent with few resources to deal with the stress.

Adolescence

As the nonretarded child grows into adolescence, the major tasks involve developing identity and life goals, independence from family, and deepening intimate relationships within friendships and with the opposite sex (Compas & Wagner, this volume). Cognitively, adolescents have a greater capacity for abstract thinking. Physically, adolescents are changing rapidly and often unevenly. Socially, they are developing new roles with new expectations. Also, adolescents move from the relatively stable and protected environment of the elementary school to the constantly changing middle or junior high school. The timing of these changes becomes important (e.g., pubertal changes coinciding with school transition, pubertal changes occurring earlier or later than peers, see Petersen, Kennedy, & Sullivan, this volume). Thus, there are many opportunites for challenge and many areas vulnerable to stress. However, among the most salient may be developing a sense of identity and long-term goals (e.g,, getting into college), establishing independence (e.g., dealing with parental overprotectiveness), and developing intimate relationships (e.g., losing a boyfriend or girlfriend, managing sexual intimacy).

The mildly mentally retarded adolescent would not be expected to face many of these developmental tasks until late adolescence or early adulthood, if at all. Some may never reach a developmental level in which they become stressed by such things as existential identity and long-term goals. However, as they graduate from high school and enter adulthood, most mildly retarded adolescents would be expected to establish some level of independence. In this regard, they may face conflicting role expectations from parents (who may encourage dependence) and society (who may push toward greater independence). Most mildly mentally retarded adolescents would also be expected to have some of the same desires for a normal life as do their nonretarded peers. Their awareness of their limitations in this regard may produce considerable stress. In addition, parental overprotectiveness and their more limited social networks may also make it difficult to develop intimate relationships and establish their independence.

For example, in a retrospective study of mildly mentally retarded adolescents' transition to adulthood, Zetlin and Turner (1985) found that stresses related to independence, parental overprotectiveness, future goals, and lack of intimate relationships were most frequently mentioned. Specifically, many felt that parents were overly intrusive and restrictive, treated them like children, made decisions for them, and prevented them from experiencing normal social situations and activities. They became frustrated at seeing younger siblings and peers surpass them, realizing that achieving normative life goals—dating, getting a job, moving out on their own—would be hindered by their cognitive limitations. Parents also reported worrying about their mentally retarded adolescent's sexuality, lack of judgment, and possible pregnancy. Many tried to discourage dating or went along on arranged dates as chaperons. Some arranged to have their adolescent sterilized. Thus, it appears that these adolescents faced similar types of stressors as many nonretarded adolescents (e.g., identity, life goals, independence, and sexuality). However, these stresses occurred at a later age and were compounded by their disability, and by parental restrictiveness and overprotectiveness.

To summarize, in terms of the mildly mentally retarded child's experience of stress, we may expect that stresses related to family stress, parental rejection, and separation or loss (particularly in relation to parents and family) will be particularly salient in the preschool to middle childhood years. Thus, entering school and facing school transitions during the school day may be particularly stressful for these children at this age. Stresses related to peer rejection and school failure may take on more significance in later childhood and early adolescence. These stresses may be compounded by pubertal changes. Finally, stresses related to parental overprotectiveness and lack of intimate relationships may be most significant in later adolescence and early adulthood. Although many mildly retarded children may never reach an advanced level of cognitive development, socially they still face many of the challenges of adolescence.

Conclusion

In this chapter, we have tried to dispel the myth that mentally retarded children and adolescents are unaware of, and unaffected by the social pressures and stigmas associated with their disability. Such a characterization is no longer tenable or acceptable. We have described the ways in which the realities of mentally retarded children's lives at home, in school, and with their peers place them "at risk" for stress. We also have suggested a developmental framework to guide future research on stress in this population.

Studies are needed to directly examine the heuristic value of such a framework. Employing both cross-sectional and longitudinal designs, we need to track the impact of developmental tasks concerning separation, peer group pressure, etc. Further, we need to assess the presence of nonnormative events and their potential to elicit stress. There are scales presently available that hierarchically list the stress-inducing events that can occur in a child's or adolescent's life (for example, loss of a pet or separation of parents). To what extent this hierarchy of nonnormative life events holds true for mentally retarded children or adolescents is not clear.

We also need to understand the resources these children employ to deal with stress in their lives. Although we know that mentally retarded children use more passive coping strategies than nonretarded children, we have yet to fully examine the appropriateness of these strategies given their unique circumstances. For instance, it may be that their use of passive strategies is more adaptive given the amount of rejection they face everyday. In addition, mentally retarded children may have more limited resources for social support. We need to explore who these children rely on given that the typical sources of support for children (e.g., family and peers) are often sources of stress.

With a better understanding of the stressors that plague the mentally retarded child, and the resources available to deal with these stressors, we may begin to develop programs to help alleviate the negative impact of stress in their lives. Programs may be developed to inform parents of the signs of stress in their mentally retarded child, and to reduce that stress for both themselves and their child. Further, school policies that increase stress may be redesigned with greater sensitivity to the needs of mentally retarded students. Finally, programs may be introduced that increase mentally retarded children's coping skills and opportunities for supportive peer interaction.

In addition to the conceivable benefits this line of research has for mentally retarded individuals, it has potential benefits for the field of stress and coping as well. Because of the combined effects of mentally retarded individuals' cognitive delays and their potential for experiencing significant stress related to their disability, this group offers a unique opportunity to examine stress and its mediators developmentally. Since the child's cognitive ability is central to their appraisal of stressful events, it is important to consider both their chronological age and their developmental level. The fact that mentally retarded children's developmental level lags behind their chronological age allows us to tease apart the relationship between cognitive level (mental age) and experience (chronological age) in the child's perception of and reaction to various stressors.

For instance, certain events may be stressful for nonretarded adolescents at particular ages (e.g., opposite sex relationships and body image). However, we do not know how much of their appraisal of these stressors is due to cognitive abilities and how much is due to their experience within their social environment. Mentally retarded adolescents will have the physical development of their nonretarded peers, and some of the social pressures as well. However, their cognitive development will resemble that of a much younger child. Therefore, the relationship between cognition, social experience, and appraisal of and response to stress may be explored. Thus, knowledge of stress and its mediators in mildly mentally retarded children would, in turn, contribute to our understanding of stress and development in nonretarded children.

In conclusion, we believe that the mentally retarded child and adolescent represents a population "at risk" for significant stress. Identifying the sources and mediators of their stresses will not only enhance the lives of these individuals, but will contribute to the field of stress and coping as well.

Acknowledgements

This chapter was made possible in part by funding from the National Institute for Child Health and Human Development Grant HD14772-07.
Special thanks to Kate Sullivan for editorial assistance.

References

Atkinson, T., Liem, R., & Liem, J. H. (1986). The social costs of unemployment: Implications for social support. *Journal of Health and Social Behavior, 27,* 317–331.

Bak, J. J., & Siperstein, G. N. (1987). Perceived similarity as a factor effecting change in children's attitudes toward mentally retarded peers. *American Journal of Mental Deficiency, 91,* 524–531.

Band, E. B., & Weisz, J. R. (1988). How to feel better when it feels bad: Children's perspectives on coping with everyday stress. *Developmental Psychology, 24*(2), 247–253.

Bowlby, J. (1969). *Attachment and loss, Volume 1. Attachment.* New York: Basic Books.

Brophy, J. E. (1983). Research on the self-fulfilling prophecy and teacher expectations. *Journal of Education and Psychology, 75,* 631–661.

Budoff, M., & Siperstein, G. N. (1982). Judgements of EMR students toward their mentally retarded peers: Effects of label and academic competence. *American Journal of Mental Deficiency, 86,* 367–371.

Buhrmester, D., & Furman, W. (1987). The development of companionship and intimacy. *Child Development, 58,* 1101–1113.

Cicchetti, D., & Schneider-Rosen, K. (1986). An organizational approach to childhood depression. In M. Rutter, C. E. Izard, & P. B. Read (Eds.), *Depression in young people* (pp. 71–134). New York: Guilford Press.

Cochran, U. L., & Cleland, C. C. (1963). Manifest anxiety of retardates and normals matched as to academic achievement. *American Journal of Mental Deficiency, 67,* 539–542.

Compas, B. E. (1987). Coping with stress during childhood and adolescence. *Psychological Bulletin, 101,* 393–404.

Compas, B. E., Malcarne, V. L., & Fondacaro, K. M. (1988). Coping with stressful events in older children and young adolescents. *Journal of Consulting and Clinical Psychology, 56*(3), 405–411.

Crnic, K. A., Friedrich, W. N., & Greenberg, M. T. (1983). Adaptation of families with mentally retarded children: A model of stress, coping and family ecology. *American Journal of Mental Deficiency, 88*(2), 125–138.

Cullinan, D., Epstein, M. H., Matson, J. J., & Rosemier, R. A. (1984). Behavior problems of mentally retarded and nonretarded adolescent pupils. *School Psychology Review, 13*(3), 381–384.

Cummings, S. T. (1976). The impact of the child's deficiency on the father: A study of fathers of mentally retarded and of chronically ill children. *American Journal of Orthopsychiatry, 46,* 246–255.

Cummings, S. T., Bayley, H., & Rie, H. (1966). Effects of the child's deficiency on the mother: A study of mothers of mentally retarded, chronically ill and neurotic children. *American Journal of Orthopsychiatry, 36,* 595–608.

Erickson, M. T. (1969). MMPI profiles of parents of young retarded children. *American Journal of Mental Deficiency, 73,* 728–732.

Felner, R. D., Primavera, J., & Cauce, A. M. (1981). The impact of school transitions: A focus for preventive efforts. *American Journal of Community Psychology, 10,* 277–290.

Friedrich, W. N., & Friedrich, W. L. (1981). Psychosocial assets of parents of handicapped and nonhandicapped children. *American Journal of Mental Deficiency, 85,* 551–553.

Furman, W. (1987, April). *Social support, stress, and adjustment in adolescence.* Paper presented at the biennial meeting of the Society for Research in Child Development, Baltimore.

Furman, W., & Buhrmester, D. (1985). Children's perceptions of the personal relationships in their social networks. *Developmental Psychology, 21,* 1016–1024.

Gardner, W. I. (1967). Occurrence of severe depression reactions in the mentally retarded. *American Journal of Psychiatry, 124,* 142–144.

Garmezy, N. (1984). Stressors of childhood. In N. Garmezy & M. Rutter (Eds.), *Stress, coping, and development in children* (pp. 43–84). New York: McGraw-Hill.

Hartup, W. W. (1989). Social relationships and their developmental significance. *American Psychologist, 44,*(2), 120–126.

Holmes, T. H., & Rahe, R. H. (1967). The social readjustment rating scale. *Journal of Psychosomatic Research, 11,* 213–218.

Horne, M. (1983). Attitudes of elementary classroom teachers toward mainstreaming. *Exceptional Child, 30,* 93–98.

Lazarus, R. S., & Folkman, S. (1984). *Stress, appraisal, and coping.* New York: Springer.

Luftig, R. L. (1988). Assessment of the perceived school loneliness and isolation of mentally retarded and nonretarded students. *American Journal of Mental Retardation, 5,* 472–475.

Maccoby, E. E. (1984). Social-emotional development and response to stressors. In N. Garmezy & M. Rutter (Eds.), *Stress, coping, and development in children* (pp. 217–234). New York: McGraw-Hill.

Miller, W. H., & Keirn, W. C. (1978). Personality measurement in parents of retarded and emotionally disturbed children: A replication. *Journal of Clinical Psychology, 34,* 686–690.

Morgan, S. B. (1986). Autism and Piaget's theory: Are the two compatible? *Journal of Autism and Developmental Disorders, 16,* 441–457.

Nihira, K., Mink, I. T., & Meyers, C. E. (1985). Home environment and development of slow-learning adolescents: Reciprocal relations. *Developmental Psychology, 21*(5), 784–794.

O'Grady, D., & Metz, J. R. (1987). Resilience in children at high risk for psychological disorder. *Journal of Pediatric Psychology, 12,* 3–23.

Reid, M., Landesman, S., Treder, R., & Jaccard, J. (1989). "My family and friends": Six- to twelve-year-old children's perceptions of social support. *Child Development, 60,* 896–910.

Ricci, C. S. (1970). Analysis of child-rearing attitudes of mothers of mentally retarded, emotionally disturbed and normal children. *American Journal of Mental Deficiency, 74,* 756–761.

Rutter, M. (1981). Stress, coping and development: Some issues and some questions. *Journal of Child Psychology and Psychiatry, 22*(4), 323–356.

Rutter, M., Tizard, J., Yule, W., Graham, P., & Whitmore, K. (1976). Research report: Isle of Wight studies, 1964–1974. *Psychological Medicine, 6,* 313–332.

Seyle, H. (1979). *The stress of life* (rev. ed.). New York: Van Nostrand Reinhold.

Seifer, R., & Sameroff, A. J. (1987). Multiple determinants of risk and invulnerability. In E. J. Anthony & B. J. Cohen (Eds.), *The invulnerable child* (pp. 51–69). New York: Guilford Press.

Shumaker, S. A., & Brownell, A. (1984). Toward a theory of social support: Closing conceptual gaps. *Journal of Social Issues, 40,* 11–36.

Siperstein, G. N. (1990). *The stability of mentally retarded children's social status in mainstreamed classrooms.* In preparation.

Siperstein, G. N., & Bak, J. J. (1980). Students' and teachers' perceptions of the mentally retarded child. In J. Gottlieb (Ed.), *Educating mentally retarded persons* (pp. 207–230). Baltimore: University Park Press.

Siperstein, G. N., & Bak, J. J. (1989). Social relationships of adolescents with moderate mental retardation. *Mental Retardation, 27,* 5–10.

Siperstein, G. N., Brownley, B., & Scott, C. K. (1989). *Social interchanges between mentally retarded and nonretarded friends.* Paper presented at the biennial meeting of the Society for Research in Child Development, Kansas City.

Siperstein, G. N., & Goding, M. J. (1985). Teachers' behavior toward LD and non-LD children: A strategy for change. *Journal of Learning Disabilities, 18*(3), 139–144.

Spivak, G., & Shure, M. B. (1982). The cognition of social adjustment: Interpersonal cognitive problem-solving thinking. In B. B. Lahey & A. E. Kazdin (Eds.), *Advances in clinical child psychology* (Vol. 5, pp. 323–372). New York: Plenum Press.

Sterling, S., Cowen, E. L., Weissberg, R. P., Lotyczewski, B. S., & Boike, M. (1985). Recent stressful life events and young children's school adjustment. *American Journal of Community Psychology, 13*(1), 87–98.

Suls, J., & Fletcher, B. (1985). The relative efficacy of avoidant and nonavoidant coping strategies: A meta analysis. *Health Psychology, 4,* 249–288.

Thoits, P. A. (1986). Social support as coping assistance. *Journal of Consulting and Clinical Psychology, 54,* 416–423.

Wallerstein, J. S. (1984). Children of divorce: Stress and developmental tasks. In N. Garmezy & M. Rutter (Eds.), *Stress, coping, and development in children* (pp. 265–302). New York: McGraw-Hill.

Wayment, H. A., & Zetlin, A. (1989). Coping responses of adolescents with and without mild learning handicaps. *Mental Retardation, 27*(5), 311–316.

Webster, T. G. (1970). Unique aspects of emotional development in mentally retarded children. In F. J. Menolascino (Ed.), *Psychiatric approaches to mental retardation* (pp. 3–54). New York: Basic Books.

Wenz-Gross, M. (1990). *Developmental changes in young children's perceptions of social support.*

Zetlin, A. G., & Turner, J. L. (1985). Transition from adolescence to adulthood: Perspectives of mentally retarded individuals and their families. *American Journal of Mental Deficiency, 6,* 570–579.

IV

Editors' Overview

Strategies for Intervention

In this final section of the volume authors Elias and Gottlieb present chapters that analyze the complexities of prevention and intervention. Much of the research on the etiology of distress and disorder emphasizes the importance of moderating factors, especially coping abilities and social supports, that account for significant variation in individual responses to stress. In these discussions of interventions we see a parallel focus on strategies to enhance both coping ability (Elias) and the supportive functions of social ties (Gottlieb), with both papers providing considerable insight into the critical parameters in formulating and enacting effective interventions. Here, we will highlight some important features of the papers, and underscore the common ground that emerges from examining these two lines of intervention for youth at risk.

* * * *

The paper by Elias focusses on school-based programs, specifically a program in social decision making and problem solving skills designed to help all students adapt to the challenges and demands associated with the transition from elementary to middle school. The extensive research on this important transition documents both the many different kinds of stressors and negative outcomes that occur during these early adolescent years (see Simmons & Blyth, 1987). The Improving Social Awareness-Social Problem Solving Project is a curriculum intervention aimed at

257

alleviating the stress of two broad classes of problems: initial transition difficulties (many associated with changes in routine), and more long-term, socially-mediated difficulties (including coping with peer pressure and a new school culture). Elias does not characterize this project as a program in coping effectiveness, but the emphasis on decision-making and problem solving skills suggests the relevance of an underlying stress and coping perspective.

Interestingly, the data on the program's effectiveness establishes that the intervention—which occurs early in the fifth and sixth grades while students are still at the elementary level—must be supplemented with modifications in the middle school environment to support the in-coming students. This coupling of a pre-transition individual-centered curriculum program with post-transition changes at the institutional level highlights the need for a long term perspective and demonstrates the interplay of individual and institutional levels in this model.

Gottlieb's paper on the concept of social support as a basis for intervention strategies directs attention to reaching different groups of at-risk youth, including: bereaved adolescents, chronically ill youth, those whose parents are separated or divorced, victims of domestic sexual abuse, and teenage parents. In much of the discussion of the social situation of these youth there is the assumption that the supportive intervention should be understood as involving the giving of emotional support to compensate for deficiencies within the primary group. This is not, however, Gottlieb's position. He instead argues that a "developmentally valid appreciation of social support" requires that modes to address these and other problems must take as their point of departure the significant developmental role of social relationships and supports at this time in life.

For example, Gottlieb illustrates this developmentally sensitive appreciation of social support with data showing that supportive interventions are most successful in groups where there is a mutuality of aid rather than a unidirectional transmission of help. This demonstrates the importance of peer support processes that are nonstigmatizing—which is a particularly salient issue for this age group—and which are conducted in what Elias calls the "grammar" that adolescents can understand. Furthermore, while Gottlieb recognizes that the "network is the crucible in which self regard is formed," (p. 286) he does not limit the consideration of support processes to the esteem–bolstering function of support that is often described in the literature. He notes that very little is known about what actually constitutes support in so-called support groups, but proposes that much of the communication may also promote the acquisition of valuable cognitive and interpersonal skills.

This possibility suggests to the reader that the social support strategies described by Gottlieb may share much with the socially mediated decision making program described by Elias. In fact, it is Gottlieb's thesis that a developmentally informed understanding of intervention should not entertain the notion of a polarity between personal resourcefulness (e.g., problem solving coping efforts) and social support, that is, coping that is socialized and sustained through social exchange. This is a significant point because it suggests the need to see the common theoretical territory of coping and social support research (Thoits, 1986), and that both concepts are part of a larger systems perspective that requires attention to individual and social levels of analysis. On this point, also, Gottlieb and Elias take a similar position. While Elias points to the importance of the organizational system, including: students, schools, families, mental health facilities, and the university (through its researchers), he also speaks to a systems perspective on the intervention itself. Specifically, he argues that no amount of intervention to promote resilience in individuals will show a significant effect "where we have not [also] been able to reduce stressors" (p. 237).

Gottlieb similarly argues that social support research and interventions must be embedded in the institutional realities that both place youth at risk and shape the nature and effectiveness of the resources available to them. On this point, his own studies of the availability of adult guidance and mentoring within the high school setting show that school adults are less responsive to the needs for support of lower income youth, the group most in need of the attention of these significant others. Thus, while social support interventions are usually understood as individual-centered, these findings provide compelling evidence of the work that is needed in the institutional arena.

References

Simmons, R. S., & Blyth, D. (1987). *Moving into adolescence: The impact of pubertal change and school context*. Hawthorne, N.Y., Aldine.

Thoits, P. A. (1986). Social support as coping assistance. *Journal of Consulting and Clinical Psychology, 54,* 416–423.

13

A Multilevel Action-Research Perspective on Stress-Related Interventions

Maurice J. Elias

The burgeoning interest in stress-related research and intervention is shared by professionals from a variety of disciplines, as well as policy makers and those charged with the efficient operation of business and educational settings. This chapter will examine a specific subset of this interest, namely systematic, programmatic stress-related interventions based in educational settings. Much of what will be presented generalizes to other types of organizational settings and is derived from theory, research, and practice that extends beyond the schools. However, educational settings will be the focus to allow issues to be addressed in sufficient detail to provide clear direction for specific applications.

First, a review of stress-related interventions as discussed in the context of traditions from the preventive mental health and social competence promotion fields will be presented. Then, using the decade-long, ongoing, school-based Improving Social Awareness–Social Problem Solving (ISA-SPS) Project as an example, structural and process considerations inherent in developing stress-related interventions will be illustrated. Specifically, an action-research model with persons and environments as dual foci will be emphasized with a focus on coping with stress-related transitions from elementary school to middle school. The chapter concludes with a discussion of the tensions inherent in managing an action-research enterprise and some thoughts about how training programs can better prepare researchers and practitioners for working in an action-research context.

Stress-Related Interventions from a Prevention/Social Competence Promotion Perspective

In an important book summarizing a major conference, researchers at the National Institute of Mental Health concluded that the link of "life stress" to psychopathology was so clearly supported in the literature that the focal question had become, "How is life stress related to adverse health consequences?" (Goldman & Goldston, 1985). For the purpose of clarifying this and subsequent points, it is useful to provide a working definition of stress and related terms as will be used in this chapter:

> Stressors—stressful environmental changes, particularly circumstances requiring changes in patterns and routines
> Stress—hypothesized psychological and physiological changes within the organism in consequence of the stressor
> Stress responses—the behavioral, psychological, and physiologic responses of the organism in the attempt to cope and adapt
> Adverse health consequences—increased susceptibility to physical illness or emotional disorders (Klerman & Weissman, 1985, p. 56).

Most prevention researchers and theorists subscribe to a model of psychopathology that includes stressors as a causative or moderating influence, interacting with personal dispositions and factors in the social environment (Dohrenwend & Dohrenwend, 1985). Accordingly, early theorists and planners of preventive interventions articulated a strategy that suggested programs be targeted at reduction of stressors and/or promotion of positive responses to stress (Bloom, 1979; Price, Ketterer, Bader, & Monahan, 1980). This strategy has been elaborated at the individual level by Albee (1982) and at the environmental level by Elias (1987; Elias & Branden, 1988). Albee's work reflected the input of President Carter's Commission on Mental Health and Mental Illness and is summarized in the following equation:

$$\frac{\text{Incidence of behavioral and emotional disorder}} = \frac{\text{stress} + \text{physical vulnerability}}{\text{coping skills} + \text{social support} + \text{self-esteem}}$$

It suggests that *individual* risk of psychopathology is exacerbated by the presence of debilitating stress and physical handicaps and is reduced to the extent to which a person possesses coping skills, a positive sense of self, and perceives the existence of support in one's social world.

The environment-centered analogue to this equation focuses on risk of psychopathology in a *population*:

$$\text{Likelihood of disorder in a population} = \frac{\text{stressors} + \text{risk factors in the environment}}{\underset{\text{practices}}{\text{socialization}} + \underset{\text{resources}}{\text{social support}} + \underset{\text{for connectedness}}{\text{opportunities}}}$$

Here, the emphasis is on reducing the presence of harmful stressors or handicapping conditions in the environment by instituting changes in organizations and institutions, i.e., the operation of settings, not the characteristics of individuals. Psychopathology is less likely to occur in a *population* to the extent that there are socialization practices that teach and promote social competence, supportive resources available in the environment, and opportunities available to people to form constructive, positive social bonds and identities connected with mainstream societal values.

The interdependent nature of these equations broadens the boundaries of what might be considered as stress-related intervention. Indeed, stress-related problems abound. Schools engender considerable and often debilitating stress in the service of advancing students' academic abilities (Elias, 1989). Individuals now live with the threat of AIDS and amidst constant media disclosures about harmful substances in our food, our water, our beverages, and our atmosphere. The acknowledgment of cultural diversity brings with it the pressures of adapting to a variety of norms and standards. Finally, there are pressures to engage in premature sex, to smoke or take drugs, or just to survive living within a dysfunctional family. Stress accompanies all of these conditions, and there is mounting evidence that these conditions also are accompanied by an unacceptably high incidence and prevalence of adverse health consequences (Irwin, 1987; London, 1987; William T. Grant Commission on Work, Family, and Citizenship, 1988).

The preventive mental health field acknowledges the role of stress management, stress reduction, and stress relief procedures as viable intervention strategies. However, both equations implicitly identify a variety of mediating influences on the extent to which gains from such interventions are sufficient to improve mental health.

A Multilevel, Action-Research Perspective

In recent years, intervention theorists and practitioners have come to question the structure of many mental health and prevention programs (Weissberg, Caplan, & Sivo, 1989). There has been a concern that programs that prove to be successful as demonstration projects are not organizationally configured in a way that ensures their continuity, adaptive flexibility to changing circumstances in the host setting and broader social environment, and linkages with ongoing service delivery systems (Elias, 1987; Price, Cowen, Lorion, & Ramos-McKay, 1988; Stolz, 1984; Weissberg et al., 1989). The predominant fate of innovative interventions is, quite simply, a rapid demise following the demonstration period (Commins & Elias, in review; Huberman & Miles, 1984; Yin, 1984). Indeed, literature about our most promising programs (e.g., Price et al., 1988; Zins & Forman, 1988) is based on demonstration models and far less on ongoing, operative programs. The technology of practice has been neglected, and this neglect has occurred at the peril of finding many of our social and mental health problems undiminished despite massive expenditures of resources (Fishman & Neigher, 1982; Stolz, 1984; William T. Grant Commission on Work, Family, and Citizenship, 1988).

A reconceptualization of what it means to conduct an "intervention" is occurring. It is fueled by detailed examinations of the expected lines of transmission from delivery of an intervention to desired long-term effects. One such examination is aided by analogies with sophisticated medical research. No longer can it be assumed that interventions, as a rule, lead to permanently internalized changes—an implicit assumption in many intervention models. Rather, as in medical transplant research and practice, it is assumed that an intervention involves preparation of the "host," the host environment, and surrounding resources. Further, it is assumed that monitoring must occur constantly and changes will be made in an ongoing manner to ensure continued health. The implanting of a new organ is not expected to result in health. There are dynamic forces at biological, psychological, interpersonal, and broader social levels which comprise the pathway from implant to health.

No doubt, other analogies occur to the reader. With regard to stress-related interventions, however, the medical analogy allows several points to be derived:

1.   Successful interventions are likely to be those with a multilevel focus, i.e., with explicit components at both the person and environment levels.

2.   Successful interventions are likely to be designed with key aspects of the person and environment levels, as defined in the prevention equations presented earlier, explicitly addressed.

3.   Successful interventions are likely to conceptualize the operation of those components over time, particularly as relates to program goals.

4.   Successful interventions are likely to follow an action research model (Elias & Clabby, in press; Price & Politser, 1980; Price & Smith, 1985; Sarason, 1978; Weissberg et al., 1989) and have explicit procedures for addressing the "lines of transmission" mentioned earlier.

Out of concern for the gap between demonstration projects and ecologically adaptive interventions that will continue to fulfill their purposes despite changes in the implementation environment, Weissberg et al. (1989) have developed and refined a set of tasks to guide intervention development and operation (see Table 1). These tasks do not have discrete starting and ending points; their unfolding has been described as anything from chaotic to spiralling to cyclic (Munoz, Snowden, & Kelly, 1979). Nevertheless, Weissberg et al. (1989) have challenged those interested in intervention and intervention-related research to reconceptualize the meaning, form, and implications of their work. Further, they have articulated a new starting point for intervention work, from which more refined paradigms will, no doubt, develop.

The remainder of this chapter will provide an example of a program of stress-related intervention and research conducted along the parameters in Table 1. The emphasis will be on the action-research process and on the multifaceted considerations that shaped the program and the products and influenced team members. General principles for operating focused, ongoing joint intervention and research programs will be advanced, and implications for future work in the field, particularly professional training, will be discussed.

Establishing an Initial Focus: Reduction of Difficulties Resulting from Stressful Transition to Middle School

The Improving Social Awareness–Social Problem Solving (ISA-SPS) Project began in 1979 when the University of Medicine and Dentistry of New Jersey-Community Mental Health Center at Piscataway (UMDNJ-CMHC) chose to respond to President Carter's Commission on Mental Health and Mental Illness' challenge to develop primary prevention programs. A review of the Commission's report and available literature suggested that Spivack and Shure's (1974) work in interpersonal-cognitive problem solving would provide a practical model for a preventive effort. An elementary school-level program involving an educator-clinician from UMDNJ-CMHC (John Clabby) co-leading classroom problem-solving discussions twice per week with regular education classroom teachers was outlined, and a sample lesson was developed for presentation to school personnel.

A local elementary school principal (Thomas Schuyler) with whom the UMDNJ-CMHC had a positive relationship was approached about participating. During the initial negotiations, several needs of the school system became apparent: (1) given a high divorce rate and a growing delinquency rate, many children had stress-related problems that were interfering with their learning and the smooth academic functioning of the classroom; (2) parents were apprehensive about their children moving from elementary to middle school—they perceived the latter as leading to what could be labeled "negative stress responses" and "ad-

Table 1. Key Tasks Underlying Successful, Enduring Interventions[a]

1. Program conceptualization	1a. Use existing theory, research, and intervention information at both person and environment levels to specify main program concepts, assumptions, and goals
2. Program design	2a. Identify and review potentially appropriate intervention materials and practices
	2b. Examine these for developmental appropriateness and cultural relevance and modify as necessary
	2c. Prepare explicit training materials and procedures and guidelines for implementation
3. Program implementation	3a. Conduct a pilot study and adapt the intervention to recipients, implementers, and ecological realities
	3b. Fine-tune implementer training and supervision procedures
	3c. Develop a system to ensure high quality implementation
	3d. Develop contacts at various organizational and community levels to ensure ongoing support of the intervention and resources needed to carry it out
4. Program evaluation	4a. Select valid, viable approaches to measure extent and quality of implementation, changes in focal attitudes, knowledge, skills, relationships, and mediating factors
	4b. Design an appropriate, time-framed data gathering and analysis system
5. Program diffusion	5a. Conceptualize how the program can be carried out elsewhere, by others, with varying degrees of involvement by the program developers
	5b. Produce transportable materials and clear and specific training and replication guidelines
	5c. Determine procedures for minimal program evaluation in new sites and provide relevant materials and training

[a]Adapted from Weissberg et al. (1989).

verse health consequences" on the part of their children; and (3) assurance of careful accountability to the Board of Education and Superintendent of Schools was a necessary feature of any program activity to be initiated in the schools. The latter need raised evaluation research goals to an equivalent level as program/action goals, and necessitated a reconsideration of the team needed to carry out the project and the approach the project would use.

To find someone with particular expertise in assessment of social problem solving and behavioral and emotional adjustment, John Clabby consulted Spivack and Shure directly. They recommended a faculty member in the Psychology Department at Rutgers University, within the catchment area of the UMDNJ-CMHC, who had an extensive background in these areas (the author). After several meetings involving members of this core team (UMDNJ-CMHC Educator-Clinician, school principal, university faculty member), a set of questions evolved that began to frame the ISA-SPS Project's action-research goals:

1. How do social decision-making and problem-solving skills act to moderate the impact of interpersonal and life stressors?
2. What contributions do social decision-making and problem-solving skills make to children's social and academic functioning?
3. What elements of the school and family environments influence social decision-making and problem-solving abilities and their behavioral expression?
4. How can social decision-making and problem-solving skills be conveyed to children most effectively? How does this vary according to developmental level, cultural and ethnic background, and childrens' level of psychosocial competence?
5. What kinds of linkages are necessary among and within the collaborating systems to forge an enduring action/research partnership?

Defining the Ecology of a School-Base Problem

Because the focal problem—ameliorating difficulties encountered by children entering middle school—was clearly defined, it was possible to set appropriate expectations about what would be necessary for problem resolution. It was humbling to examine the existing literature and find that the problem of transition to middle school was rarely discussed, particularly in terms of its behavioral and emotional impact. An analysis of the stressors involved in the transition was made, using children, teachers, and administrators as sources of data. Over 20 discrete stressors were uncovered, ranging from remembering one's locker combination to resisting peer pressure to use alcohol or drugs. The range and perceived severity of these stressors were considerable and affected a broad population of children, including those who had shown satisfactory patterns of adjustment during elementary school. In addition, there was evidence that stressors operated on children entering middle school in two waves: (1) initial transition difficulties, centering around adapting to many new routines; and (2) longitudinal difficulties, centering around peer pressure and acculturation into a middle school social system (Elias, Gara, & Ubriaco, 1985).

Typically, attempts at preparing children for transitions involve showing elementary school "seniors" the new physical layout, having them oriented by a principal or guidance counselor, and perhaps having them meet students at different levels of the middle school population who could answer questions and provide reassurance that some of the children's more frightening expectations were unfounded. These short-term interventions, taking place just before the summer vacation, seem to be effective only in some aspects of initial transition difficulties, such as finding the school, locating rooms, feeling overwhelmed by the physical size of the school and learning of the existence of new routines, such as using lockers, changing classes at fixed intervals, and having a variety of teachers (and more male teachers, usually). From the action-research perspective outlined earlier, a reconsideration of what constituted an appropriate intervention to alleviate undesirable stress related to middle school entry was necessary. The resulting task, that of equipping children with a set of generalized cognitive and behavioral coping skills that would be retained throughout the first year in middle school, was an initial objective. Complementing this person-level focus was a concern with having an impact on key socialization practices in three environments: elementary school, middle school, and the home. Based on an analysis of the problem from a child and systems perspective, several assumptions were identified as cornerstones of project planning:

1.   An effective skills training program should be instituted at least 2 years before middle school transition.
2.   Because of the developmental level of children in fourth, fifth, and sixth grade (i.e., in transition from concrete to formal operations), it could not be assumed that they would learn, integrate, and generalize a set of cognitive strategies to a sufficient extent that would allow them to spontaneously use these strategies without external reminders.
3.   Many parents had apprehensions about middle school that they transmitted to their children and that these could act in a powerful way to counteract reassuring messages from other sources (i.e., teachers, administrators, other children).
4.   The core components of any program directed toward the children

must focus on *children and environments* as a unit of intervention, that is, successful coping for most children would occur to the extent to which they develop their social decision-making and problem-solving competencies and the extent to which school, family, and peer environments in which they interact support the use of those competencies.

Structure of the Action-Research Team

Within this conceptualization of the problem were guidelines for organizing the action-research team. Over the initial 3 years of the project, a series of intervention tasks and target populations were identified, corresponding to the assumptions just enumerated. Research/evaluation tasks also were identified: (1) *formative*, including assessing and providing feedback on appropriate formats, strategies, and structures for interventions; (2) *summative*, including a determination of the extent to which intended and unintended outcomes were attained; (3) *impact*, including a focus on how the functioning of larger organizational units (e.g., school system, local parent–teacher organizations, UMDNJ-CMHC, neighborhoods) was affected by combined aspects of the interventions; and (4) *feedback and modification*, including methods for using formative and summative evaluation information to modify action/research activities. For each of these tasks, primary responsibility or leadership roles were specified, to enhance efficiency and accountability.

The organization of an action-research team is an intricate and important task with profound implications for the nature and outcome of work undertaken. An action-research team must build and maintain external linkages between its own structure and those of a variety of organizations and groups. These linkages enable the action-research team to acquire information about the phenomena being studied and the properties of the primary environments and populations toward which intervention is targeted, assemble resources necessary to implement and evaluate interventions within an action-research cycle, and disseminate relevant findings and procedures. The task of building these linkages can seem overwhelming, as well as quite abstract. For this reason, successful action-research projects tend to concentrate initial entry into one focal system and label this effort as a "pilot" (Elias & Clabby, 1984). Additionally, the approach of the team is couched in the grammar of that system and contains a concrete vehicle around which collaboration can occur. Each organizational system has its own grammar and basic structural units. Sarason (1982) has insightfully documented what he calls the "culture of schools"; within that culture, the most appropriate vehicle for action-research is the *curriculum*. Curricula are powerful organizational building blocks within school systems. They are the foundation of educational planning, and time, resources, funds, and effort are distributed first to mandated curriculum units, secondarily to "important" curricula, and lastly to "programs" and other short-term, noncurricular activities.

The ISA-SPS Curricular Intervention

In the case of the ISA-SPS Project, team activities are organized around the development of a 2-year curriculum appropriate for both regular and special education students in fourth and fifth grade, the 2 years prior to middle school entry. The details of action-research decision making which guided curriculum development are described elsewhere (Elias & Clabby, in press). However, what evolved was a tripartite strategy for building students' social competence: (1) *skill building in self-control and group participation and social awareness* was the first component, covering students' ability to follow directors, calm themselves when upset, start and maintain a conversation without being provoked by others (or provoking others) to lose self-control, give, receive, and obtain help, and build trusting, caring friendships; (2) *skill building in social decision making and problem solving,* involving students' learning an eight step affective and cognitive strategy to use when under stress and when they have to make choices or decisions or face problems; and (3) *promoting skill acquisition and application in the environment,* by training teachers, administrators, other school personnel, and parents in techniques to "dialogue" with children to elicit their thoughtful social decision making in social and academic domains and to prompt and cue them to use specific self-control and group participation skills. Over a period of 6 years, the curriculum was modified through action research feedback until curriculum in formative and summative evaluation finding consonant with program goals were attained.

Managing the Dialectic between Planful Research and Opportunities for Action

The enmeshment of action-research efforts within community-based settings exposes team members to all of the social forces that operate on those settings. Perhaps foremost is the crisis orientation of many such settings. Immediate problems generally must be solved and not studied at length. Meeting current demands and perhaps anticipating ones that might occur in the near future are most visibly reinforced. Most human service settings are not structured or budgeted around long-range planning or monitoring unintended negative effects of well-intentioned activities. Certainly the growing number of mandated educational programs has created a host of difficulties, while attempting to guarantee children's educational rights.

For action-research teams, a capacity to be responsive to ongoing issues that affect host systems is therefore a necessity for carrying out viable interventions. Where these issues can be anticipated, the team is better able to preserve the integrity of its work, as well as capitalize on changing conditions to extract new knowledge. These conditions, however, set up a dialectic between planful research and pressing opportunities for action. "Keeping the ship on course" when there are several collaborating systems with differing mandates and internal operating principles requires exceptional working relationships. Within the ISA-SPS Project team, the core systems are studies in contrast:

1. *School system:* this system does not recruit its target group, but instead continually receives children and has responsibility for them for over a decade; it is organized in a tight multilevel hierarchy and is subject to the wishes of local citizens, parents, county, and state officials and federal economic and social policy; its preference is for goal-oriented, well-documented curriculum programs that are easily implemented and relatively inexpensive; its value is basic academic skills.

2. *CMHC:* this system must recruit clients, particularly those that can pay or who are eligible for third party reimbursements; its mandate increasingly emphasizes short-term programs, and it therefore depends on "volume" for success; its organization varies, depending on whether it is relatively free-standing or associated with a larger institution, such as a medical hospital; the system tends to be dominated by professionals and to be very attuned to the demands of its funding sources; its preference is for discrete programs that are responsive to crises, provide positive public relations, and are income-generating; its value is remediation of diagnosable psychological disorder.

3. *University:* this system also must recruit clients, generally those within a narrow age range and with an ability to pay; it is organized in a loose hierarchy that affords bottom-level professional personnel considerable freedom of movement, and is subject to market forces, government regulations, and prevailing academic norms, in proportion to the nature of its funding and its status within the academic community; its preference is for written products appearing with noticeable frequency in prestigious outlets (such as professional journals); its values are, paradoxically, less based on client outcomes than centered on gathering significant new knowledge.

Four Principles of Action-Research Partnership

Reconciling differences of this magnitude are beyond the boundaries of any single project. However, through the ISA-SPS Project, four principles for forging an enduring working relationship have been formulated:

1.   The core group of the action-research team must contain members of the participating systems with decision-making power; this allows meetings to run efficiently and reduces interference due to bureaucratic hurdles within particular systems. Within the ISA-SPS Project, going strictly "through channels" has consistently led to costly delays that have endangered progress and placed considerable added stress on team members.

2.   The action-research team must contain members that have a thorough understanding of their own system and at least one of the other collaborating systems; the educator-clinician was a certified school psychologist, as well as a respected member of the CMHC; the elementary school principal was linked to a range of networks within the school system and community, including the CMHC; the Rutgers faculty member had spent several years working within both school and CMHC settings, perhaps offsetting a bit his junior status within the university. From this overlap comes a respect for the limits of what other systems can and cannot do. Plans can be concrete and the grammars of each system can be understood by others. Expectations can be realistic and framed within an attainable timeline. After 3 years, members of the core team had educated themselves and team members about their respective systems, thereby forging a working partnership that has continued over a decade, as of this writing.

3.   An action-research team benefits from having two sets of superordinate goals. The first centers around demonstrating the success of the intervention. For the ISA-SPS Project, it is the enhancement of children's well being, particularly upon entering middle school. This fits schools' values around improving academic and life-skills capabilities, meets the CMHC's mandates for prevention and remediation, and meets the university focus of understanding the factors affecting children's social competence and designing scientific approaches to enhancing that competence.

There is another set of goal structures that the ISA-SPS team has called "the happy convergence of mutual self-interest." Participation in this project achieves something unique for each individual system and makes a contribution to that system's functioning that is highly valued. For example, the CMHC has become involved in new sets of linkages with teachers, administrators, special educators, parents, and other professionals. Its role as a linking and capacity building agent in both remediative and preventive contexts represents a refocusing of the usual concern with discrete, short-term crisis-oriented service units. A school-based action-research project places the CMHC in an improved position to genuinely tap community wide needs, and not infer them largely from client flow profiles. Over the 10 years of operation of the ISA-SPS Project, the UMDNJ-CMHC has become viewed as a national leader in the prevention field (Clabby & Elias, 1990).

One concrete bit of learning that has emerged for the UMDNJ-CMHC has been the importance of attending to individuals' incentive structures for participating in project-related and CMHC-based activities. We have found that educators and parents face a host of stressors that serve to block altruistic motives to do or learn purely "for the children sake." Our training approaches with parents and teachers have evolved so that we begin by attempting to identify and relieve some of their predominant stressors, and *then* introduce new skills and approaches in ways that will allow parents and teachers to help children *and* reduce stress in home and school contexts. Where we have not been able to reduce stressors, recipients of our training have "heard" us but showed no significant, enduring behavioral change.

Participation in the ISA-SPS Project clearly has helped schools become less insular. New relationships with parents have been opened and problems that were "owned" by the schools and kept in-house are now being expressed. Middle school transition and special education services are two areas in which project-related systems analyses showed that without parental collaboration, the schools could not deliver services effectively. Such conclusions became obvious and almost "irresistible" once the problems were examined and discussed in the context of a child–environment unit. Additionally, the project's focus on a set of generalizable problem-solving thinking abilities filled an unmet and unspoken need. That is, there was no previously existing way to go beyond the "3 R's" and yet still retain a *curriculum, skills-based format.* Affective education and values clarification activities tended to be highly difficult to bring up to a board of education and defend on their academic relevance. Because the ISA-SPS team understood the grammar of the school and could translate freely from CMHC service delivery methods and University research data into that language, it was possible to create a "match" with the host environment.

Finally, the University also was in a position to make new linkages in ways that traditional research projects often do not achieve. Several hundred Rutgers students at all levels have had outlets to a range of learning experiences and potential career tracks. They have been exposed to a context for knowledge acquisition that is ecologically valid and application-oriented. Much disseminable learning has occurred and found its way into diverse professional and public forums (e.g., Clabby & Elias, 1986; Elias, 1989; Elias & Clabby, 1989; Elias, Ubriaco, & Gray, 1986). Studies initiated over the 10-year course of the ISA-SPS Project are summarized in Elias & Clabby (1989, in press). However, two points are particularly germane to the discussion of stress-related interventions. These are (a) the results of the intervention to reduce students' stress upon entry to middle school, and (b) interventions at the environmental level in middle school.

a. *Results of the intervention.* Students receiving no, partial, or full training by their teachers in social decision-making and problem-solving were compared upon entry into middle school. The focal measure was a survey of 28 middle school stressors covering peer relationships, conflicts with authority and older students, academic pressure, peer pressure for substance abuse, and logistical hassles, developed through county-wide surveys involving educators and students (Elias et al., 1985). Significant differentiations could be made between students receiving any intervention and no-treatment controls; further, on 24 of 28 stressors, students receiving full training reported fewer adaptational difficulties than those receiving partial training. Additional data analyses showed that students' levels of social decision-making and problem-solving skills mediated intervention outcomes (Elias, Gara, Ubriaco, Rothbaum, Clabby, & Schuyler, 1986).

b. *Interventions at the environmental level.* Observations were conducted in the middle school following students' transition. It became clear that the students were able to access their social decision-making skills when prompted by the guidance counselor, principal, or vice-principal, but their spontaneous use of their skills appeared to diminish as the year went on. This was reflected largely in guidance contacts and disciplinary records. Therefore, interventions were planned to improve socialization practices in the middle school and provide increased opportunities for students to use their thinking skills. Over a period of several years, a "middle school survival skills program" was developed, consisting of an organizational and study skills program for all students throughout their first year of middle school and an infusion of social decision making into the social studies curriculum, particularly around current events. Results indicate that it is beneficial and perhaps necessary to complement a skills-focused intervention at the elementary school level with supportive changes in the middle school environment if stress during the transition process is to be reduced in any ongoing manner (Elias & Clabby, in press; Haboush, 1988; Smith, 1989).

The happy convergence of the interests of multiple systems is an implicit principle that runs throughout successful action-research processes, embodied in the accomplishment of the tasks outlined in Table 1. Stress-related interventions almost invariably will encompass multiple systems and therefore will have to conceptualize and carry out procedures to ensure systems convergence.

The principle of the happy convergence of mutual self-interest also applies to the personal incentives of individual team members, for such things as novelty, stimulation, recognition, challenge, fun, redefining of professional role, and financial gain. This is another critical aspect of the development of an action-research team that often is not attended to until a valued individual has refused to participate or departed.

4. The final principle, that of *accountability*, supports the various research/evaluation components of the action-research team. Service systems and business, public, and private organizations have elevated the bottom line to the top of the list. If goals are not specified, evaluated, and met, it is unlikely that a program will be supported. As the cost of an intervention rises, scrutiny and doubt are mobilized. Good ideas are not sufficient entry credentials, as they had been at times in the past. The longitudinal intervention perspective outlined earlier was reflected in efforts to obtain and maintain the support of parents, administrators, school board members, and the children and teachers most closely involved in the work. Our formulation of the problem and intervention necessitated a program of action and research that would extend over a period of years. A comprehensive monitoring, evaluation, and feedback component to the project clearly was in everyone's apparent best interest.

Nevertheless, core action-research team members have engaged in a continuing effort to defuse the seemingly constant stress engendered by requesting participation in research and evaluation activities. The accountability issue has been managed effectively only to the extent to which there has been a happy convergence of how the three ISA-SPS partnering systems look at the need for data. The UMDNJ-CMHC is primarily interested in whether or not the interventions are working to improve competence and reduce distress. The school is most interested in the pragmatic, generic question of "what works best, for what, with whom, and can we afford it." The university is interested in "why" questions, as well as with understanding such things as implementer × approach × recipient interaction effects. To some degree, each system understands, respects, and values all of these questions. But research/evaluation reports written for each system would look quite different (and have!).

Toward Making Graduate Training More Congruent with an Action-Research Approach: A Key to Systems Change

The previous discussion has suggested some of the interrelated facets of developing and maintaining a stress-related intervention using an action-research approach. These concerns fall mainly within the realm of applied social and organizational psychology. It is clear that certain formal and informal structures must be set in place to study applied research questions in their naturalistic contexts. But where are the requisite administrative and planning skills learned? Action-research does not fit easily within the present mainstream of academic research training. Too often, research design is taught from a purely technical perspective. But all research is designed for a particular research environment. Studying the properties of that environment, learning its grammar, and assembling the needed resources for an action-research team requires a series of learned skills that one often acquires mainly through experience. More common, however, is the tendency to focus on research that can be kept under the tight experimental control of one or two researchers. Such efforts tend to be discrete and reflect the grammar of academic journal articles.

The stress-related problems outlined in the beginning of this article will not yield to simple, sterile, fragile, limited interventions. Research fueling interventions must be ambitious and reflect the ecology of application of those findings. Price (1983) raises the issue that there may be too many skills required for successful action-research to expect any one researcher to embody them all. For preventive interventions, he suggests that the minimal research team might require an expert at each of Weissberg et al.'s (1989) tasks (cf. Table 1). To better prepare research trainees for the kinds of roles they will have to occupy in the future, University training in disciplines conducting stress-related research and intervention must prepare researchers and practitioners for working within action-research formats. In a complementary way, administrators in training in education, human service, and business fields should be taught the importance of action-research approaches and learn how to help build and maintain action-research teams.

The problems engendered by stress in our society will not abate as a result of some specific "solution"; rather, they must be addressed through ongoing collaborative relationships with the capacity to provide information on program development, implementation, and effects. Universities can play a valuable role as the "glue" in such arrangements. But the grip will be stronger if members of many fields have been primed for an action-research bond.

Acknowledgments

I would like to acknowledge George Allen, Jack Chinsky, Steve Larcen, John Lochman, Howard Sellinger, Susan Zlotlow, George Howe, Larry

LaVoie, and Jim Dalton for their inspiration to do action research and their support of my early action research endeavors. I also thank the William T. Grant Foundation Consortium on the School-Based Promotion of Social Competence for many stimulating and practical action-research ideas. Finally, this manuscript could not have been completed without the gracious support of Pat Dooley, Ellen Elias, and the Schumann Fund for New Jersey.

References

Albee, G. W. (1982). Preventing psychopathology and promoting human potential. *American Psychologist, 37,* 1043–1050.

Bloom, B. (1979). Prevention of mental disorders: Recent advances in theory and practice. *Community Mental Health Journal, 15,* 179–191.

Clabby, J. F., & Elias, M. J. (1986). *Teach your child decision making,* New York: Doubleday.

Clabby, J. F., & Elias, M. J. (1990). Competence enhancement and primary prevention as core functions of CMHC'S: A case study and blueprint for the future. *Prevention in Human Services, 7,* 3–15.

Commins, W. W., & Elias, M. J. (in review). Institutionalization of mental health programs in organizational contexts: The case of elementry schools.

Dohrenwend, B. S., & Dohrenwend, B. P. (1985). Life stress and psychopathology. In H. Goldman & S. Goldston (Eds.), *Preventing stress-related psychiatric disorders.* (DHHS Pub. No. ADM 85-1366) (pp. 37–51). Rockville, MD: NIMH.

Elias, M. J. (1987). Establishing enduring prevention programs: Advancing the legacy of Swampscott. *American Journal of Community Psychology, 15,* 539–553.

Elias, M. J. (1989). Schools as a source of stress to children: An analysis of causal and ameliorative influences. *Journal of School Psychology, 27,* 393–407.

Elias, M. J., & Branden, L. R. (1988). Primary prevention of behavioral and emotional problems in school-aged populations. *School Psychology Review, 17,* 581–592.

Elias, M. J., & Clabby, J. F. (1984). Integrating social and affective education into public school curriculum and instruction. In C. Maher, R. Illback, & J. Zins (Eds.), *Organizational psychology in the schools: A handbook for professionals* (pp. 143–172). Springfield, IL: Charles C Thomas.

Elias, M. J., & Clabby, J. F. (1989). *Social decision making skills: A curriculum guide for the elementary grades.* Rockville, MD: Aspen.

Elias, M. J., & Clabby, J. (in press). *School-based enhancement of children and adolescents' social problem solving skills.* San Francisco: Jossey-Bass.

Elias, M. J., Gara, M., & Ubriaco, M. (1985). Sources of stress and support in children's transition to middle school: An empirical analysis. *Journal of Clinical Child Psychology, 14,* 112–118.

Elias, M. J., Gara, M., Ubriaco, M., Rothbaum, P. A., Clabby, J. F., & Schuyler, T. (1986). The impact of a preventive social problem solving intervention on children's coping with middle school stressors. *American Journal of Community Psychology, 14,* 259–275.

Fishman, D., & Neigher, W. (1982). American psychology in the Eighties: Who will buy? *American Psychologist, 37*, 533–546.

Goldman, H., & Goldston, S. (Eds.) (1985). *Preventing stress-related psychiatric disorders* (DHHS Pub. No. ADM 85-1366). Rockville, MD: NIMH.

Haboush, K. (1988). *An evaluation of student learning outcomes under a critical thinking social studies program.* Unpublished doctoral dissertation, Graduate School of Applied and Professional Psychology, Rutgers University, New Brunswick, NJ.

Huberman, M., & Miles, M. (1984). *Innovation up close: How school improvement works.* New York: Plenum.

Irwin, C. D., Jr. (Ed.) (1987). *Adolescent social behavior and health: New Directions for Child Development* (No. 37). San Francisco: Jossey-Bass.

Klerman, G., & Weissman, M. (1985). Affective responses to stressful life events. In H. Goldman & S. Goldston (Eds.), *Preventing stress-related psychiatric disorders* (DHHS Pub. No. ADM 85-1366) (pp. 55–76). Rockville, MD: NIMH.

London, P. (1987). Character education and clinical intervention: A paradigm shift for U.S. schools. *Phi Delta Kappan,* May, 667–673.

Munoz, R. F., Snowden, L. R., & Kelly, J. G. (1979). *Social and psychological research in community settings.* San Francisco: Jossey-Bass.

Price, R. (1983). The education of a prevention psychologist. In R. Felner, L. Jason, J. Moritsugu, & S. Farber (Eds.), *Preventive psychology: Theory, research, and practice* (pp. 290–296). New York: Pergamon.

Price, R., Cowen, E., Lorion, R., & Ramos-McKay, J. (Eds.) (1988). *14 ounces of prevention: A casebook for practitioners.* Washington, D.C.: American Psychological Association.

Price, R., Ketterer, R., Bader, B., & Monahan, J. (Eds.) (1980). *Prevention in mental health: Research, policy, and practice.* Newbury Park, CA: Sage.

Price, R., & Politser, P. (Eds.) (1980). *Evaluation and action in the social environment.* New York: Academic Press.

Price, R., & Smith, S. (1985). *A guide to evaluating prevention programs in mental health* (DHHS Pub. No. ADM 85-1365). Rockville, MD: National Institute of Mental Health.

Sarason, S. B. (1978). The nature of problem solving in social action. *American Psychologist, 33*, 370–380.

Sarason, S. B. (1982). *The culture of the school and the problem of change* (2nd ed.). Boston: Allyn & Bacon.

Smith, C. (1989). *Assessing student improvement in study skills: The role of the Organizational/Study Skills (O/S) program.* Unpublished ISA-SPS research report. New Brunswick, NJ: Rutgers University.

Spivack, G., & Shure, M. (1974). *The social adjustment of young children.* San Francisco: Jossey-Bass.

Stolz, S. B. (1984). Preventive models: Implications for a technology of practice. In M. Roberts & L. Peterson (Eds.), *Prevention of problems in childhood* (pp. 391–413). New York: John Wiley.

Weissberg, R., Caplan, M., & Sivo, P. (1989). A new conceptual framework for establishing school-based social competence promotion programs. In L. Bond & B. Compas (Eds.), *Primary prevention and promotion in the schools* (pp. 255–296). Newbury Park, CA: Sage.

William T. Grant Commission on Work, Family, & Citizenship. (1988). *The forgotten half: Pathways to success for America's youth and young families.* New York: William T. Grant Foundation.

Yin, R. (1984). *Case study research: Design and methods.* Beverly Hills, CA: Sage.

Zins, J. E., & Forman, S. G. (Eds.). (1988). Primary prevention: From theory to practice (Special issue). *School Psychology Review, 17*(4).

14

Social Support in Adolescence

Benjamin H. Gottlieb

This chapter examines selected characteristics of the immediate social environment in which adolescents participate, including its structural properties, the nature and meaning of the supportive provisions it communicates, and the processes that confer its protective effects as well as its more general salutary influence on personal development. In addition, the chapter considers strategies of marshalling, improving, and augmenting the support available to adolescents in particularly vulnerable circumstances. Since research on social support among adolescents is in a state of chrysalis, I include suggestions for basic and evaluation research aimed to improve our understanding of the nature and impact of social support in both the natural environment and in intervention programs.

The Relevance of Support to Adolescents

Recently awakened interest in the social networks and social support of adolescents has been spurred by a combination of forces occurring in the larger society and developments in several areas of scholarly inquiry. With respect to the former, the past decade has witnessed a set of alarming social trends among youth and their immediate families, including a precipitous rise in the incidence of marital disruption, school dropouts, teenage pregnancy, and alcohol and drug abuse. In *Turning*

Points, the Carnegie Council on Adolescent Development's (1989) recent report on the education of young teenagers, it is estimated that "of the 28 million girls and boys ages 10 to 17 in the United States, about 7 million may be extremely vulnerable to the negative consequences of multiple high-risk behaviors such as school failure, substance abuse, and early unprotected intercourse" (p. 27). Moreover, the proportion at risk is far exceeded among youth who are poor, members of racial or ethnic minorities, or recent immigrants.

Even more calamitous, during the first half of the past decade, the suicide rate more than doubled for youth between the ages of 10 and 14 (Waller, Baker, & Szocka, 1989). Among all adolescents in the United States, the suicide rate has increased 132% since 1961, compared to 22% in the general population (Holinger, 1978), making it the third leading cause of death (U.S. Bureau of the Census, 1982). Perhaps the single best indicator of the extent of turbulence in the social world inhabited by today's youth is the divorce rate; based on current statistics, it is predicted that 60% of children of all ages will spend at least some part of their childhood in a single-parent context (Norton & Glick, 1986). Again, the prediction for Black children is much higher (Hofferth, 1985). In short, at a time when youth are in peril of self-injurious behaviors, their family circumstances jeopardize their access to durable and consistent support.

In the scholarly community, a number of lines of research have shown promise of improving our understanding of the factors moderating the impact of these dislocations on the lives of children and adolescents. First, calling on a growing body of research on early life stressors and protective processes, Garmezy (1983) and Rutter (1983) have chronicled the psychiatric sequelae of several acute childhood stressors, highlighting both the protective and stress-inducing properties of the enveloping social fabric. Garmezy's (1983) review of a number of cross-cultural studies has led him to propose three factors that distinguish more resilient from more vulnerable youth: advantageous personality dispositions such as social responsiveness and autonomy, a supportive family milieu, and the presence of external support from peers and adult members of the community's institutions. Beardslee and Podorefsky's (1988) study of 18 male and female adolescents whose parents had major affective disorders is exemplary of the latter protective resource. Selected on the basis of their healthy functioning at initial assessment and an average of two and a half years later, 16 of the 18 adolescents described themselves as valuing close, confiding relationships and emphasized that these relationships were a central part of their lives. Nine of them specifically mentioned contacting an identified other person during episodes when their parent was acutely ill in order to make sense of the experience or to derive comfort. Although other factors also contributed to these adolescents' resilience, including constitutional strengths, and their self-understanding and self-regard, these factors are typically harder to alter than environmental resources or more exactly, the quality and availability of social support. It is for this reason that social support interventions hold such great promise in working with adolescents.

A second line of research has had a narrower focus on social skills and peer ties in childhood and early adolescence, linking various problems in this domain to concurrent maladjustment and psychiatric disorders in adulthood. Although there are wide variations in the methods and diagnostic criteria used to identify children with problems in social relations, Coie, Dodge, and Cappotelli (1982) state that about 12% of children are socially rejected; they receive relatively few nominations as being liked and relatively many as being disliked. Data derived from sociometric nominations reveal that the socially maladjusted children are either rejected, neglected, or are "controversial" because they are both highly liked and highly disliked (Coie & Dodge, 1983). Research on the risk status of children with problems in social relationships generally suggests that the rejected group's high levels of aggressive and inappropriate behaviors place them at risk for delinquency and school dropout. There is much more controversy about the links between the shy, withdrawn, and anxious behaviors of the neglected group and subsequent maladaptive outcomes (Asher, Markell, & Hymel, 1981).

From the perspective of those interested in social support, the emphasis of the preceding research on the popularity and social position of children and their influence on adjustment sheds little light on the qualitative aspects of relationships and on the processes implicated in the activation of social ties by and for youth in stressful circumstances. Furthermore, this literature has paid virtually no attention to the relationships among social competence, social support, and the character of social ties, particularly among youth in the middle years of adolescence.

However, two recent edited volumes signal an emergent interest in the supportive functions of adolescents' social networks (Belle, 1988b; Salzinger, Antrobus, & Hammer, 1988). Together, they begin to fill the gaps in knowledge about the structure of adolescents' social ties during the period extending from puberty to the late teens, about gender differences in the intimacy of these ties, and about the forms and meaning of social support during this developmental phase. Combined with a handful of studies published elsewhere, they also illuminate the impact of adolescents' social ties on their personal and social development. I will briefly review the main themes and findings of these studies, placing special emphasis on their relevance to the topic of social support.

Support and the Social Circles of Adolescents

As children enter the period of adolescence, peers make up a larger portion of their networks (Blyth & Traeger, 1988) but do not displace or supplant family ties (Hartup, 1983; Hunter & Youniss, 1982; Youniss, 1980). However, as Blyth and Traeger (1988) note, there is a transformation of relations with parents in both emotional and behavioral terms, peer relations taking priority over relations with family members with respect to particular psychosocial needs. For example, peers are uniquely capable of providing support for valued identities, shoring up or undermining self-esteem in particular domains (Harter, 1987), serving as targets of social comparisons along numerous dimensions of performance (Suls & Sanders, 1982), and meeting needs for a sense of belonging and community apart from family ties. Peer interaction provides opportunities for learning of the social skills involved in maintaining relationships that are achieved rather than ascribed, such as reciprocity. Above all, the commerce occurring daily among adolescents adds stability and continuity to their lives, and for some children compensates for a turbulent and disrupted family life.

In adolescence the composition and structure of the social network increasingly reflect the personal preferences and skills of youth rather than parental influences. Increased independence and mobility facilitate the establishment of relationships outside the home, leaving decisions about the extent of integration of family members and friends to the youth themselves. Accordingly, from early to late adolescence the degree of network integration across this boundary varies a great deal. For example, in their late teens college students may form a cluster of peer ties that is segregated from their family ties or they may selectively integrate college friends. In a fascinating prospective study tracing differences in the development of the support networks of first year college students who commuted and those who lived in residence, Hays and Oxley (1986) found a higher "density" in the networks of the dorm residents compared to the commuters; that is, a greater proportion of the dorm residents' networks was composed of mutual friends than of the commuters'.

As adolescents age, the greater latitude they have in the choice of friends and in the structuring of their networks is accompanied by greater stability and intensity of their ties, two factors that have an important bearing on the intimacy of their relationships. Moreover, with the maturation of cognitive skills in adolescence, there are increases in the capacity to observe and evaluate the self and an attendant increase in introspection and self-evaluation (Selman, 1980). Developmental changes in the ability to adopt perspectives on the self are in turn accompanied by increases in the capacity to take the perspective of others with respect to affective and motivational processes. As Berndt (1982) points out in his discussion of the influence of cognitive abilities on the nature and functions of friendships in early adolescence, "adolescents should be more able to understand their friends' thoughts and feelings and be more aware of the importance of mutuality and reciprocity in friendships" (p. 1448). A number of studies attest to these qualitative changes in the character of adolescents' peer ties, principally those investigating the intimacy of their close relationships. Since intimacy provides a basis for the exchange of certain types of social support, it is useful to review research on adolescents' perceptions of their intimate relationships.

Generally, intimate relationships provide opportunities to share personal thoughts and feelings, to be well known by others, and reciprocally, to have privileged knowledge of others' thoughts, feelings, and personalities (Berndt, 1982; Buhrmester & Furman, 1987; Sullivan, 1953). Investigations of this topic have relied on both indirect measures of intimacy, involving reports of close relationships and "chumships," and on ratings of the extent of exclusive, confiding communications with others.

Buhrmester and Furman's studies of developmental changes in the intimacy afforded by various relationships have contributed the most detail to this subject (Buhrmester & Furman, 1987; Furman & Buhrmester, 1985), spotlighting significant gender differences in the intimacy of different actors in the social fields of young adolescents. Specifically, among eighth graders, they observed marked gender differences in the self-reported intimacy of various relationships. Although boys and girls both rated their best same-sex friend as the most intimate relationship, the girls rated this relationship significantly higher than the next highest relationships with mothers, siblings, opposite-sex friends, and boyfriends. In contrast, eighth grade boys did not report a significantly more intimate relationship with their best same-sex friends than with their mother, father, and girlfriend. Moreover, there was a significant gender difference in the reported intimacy with fathers, boys rating this relationship among their most intimate ties. Developmental changes in the intimacy of boys' and girls' relationships with peers revealed that between the second and eighth grades, there is a steady increase in intimacy for girls but not for boys, leading Buhrmester and Furman (1987) to conclude that "it appears that male–male friendships never achieve the same level of intimate disclosure as female–female friendships" (p. 1111). However, a developmental shift experienced in common by boys and girls is for parents to become less important providers of companionship and intimacy in the middle years of adolescence.

Finally, there is a small literature on dimensions of relationships other than intimacy. Belle's (1988a) review of the few studies that directly address social support among adolescents led her to conclude that girls seek more help and support from peers than do boys, and the support they utilize tends to be more emotion-focused in nature than the support boys gain. Berndt (1988) and Furman and Buhrmester (1985) include companionship, instrumental aid, esteem support, and affection among the types of support deemed relevant to adolescents. The picture that emerges from the reports of young adolescents reveals that each provision can be gained from more than one category of network members, and that there is specialization in the support extended by mothers, fathers, grandparents, teachers, best friends, and siblings (Furman & Buhrmester, 1985). In this sample of middle class 11–13 year olds, ratings of companionship were higher for friends than for any other category of associates, girls reporting once again that they experienced greater intimacy, affection, and enhancement of worth with their best friend than did boys. For the entire sample, mothers and fathers received the highest ratings of affection, reliable alliance (dependability), esteem enhancement, and practical help.

The majority of the interview measures of adolescents' perceived and enacted support bear a striking resemblance to questionnaires developed for adults (Cohen, Mermelstein, Kamarck, & Hoberman, 1985; Procidano & Heller, 1983; Sarason, Levine, Basham & Sarason, 1983), and therefore should be used with great caution. The psychometric properties of recently developed tools for assessing adolescents' social support are described by Wolchik, Beals, and Sandler (1988). To date, however, none has been based on observations of supportive transactions or on studies of the ways in which youth themselves perceive the support they give to and receive from their associates. As discussed later, this leaves a large gap in our appreciation of the meaning, forms, and functions of social support from the perspective of adolescents.

The extent to which the preceding findings concerning the structure, intimacy, and supportive character of adolescents' relationships apply to youth in contrasting cultural, racial, and socioeconomic groups, as well as to those in nontraditional family contexts, is as yet unknown. Coates' (1987) study of middle class Black adolescents reveals that males tended to see network members more frequently than did females, but there were no sex differences in network size, proximity of members, or duration of relationships. A greater proportion of females than males reported participating in special "chumships" of less than five members, interacting with these peers in private settings more frequently than did males. Girls expressed a preference for female, kin sources of support, while boys favored peers and nonfamily adult sources. But middle class Black youth may have more in common with their White counterparts than they do with their Black peers who live in poverty. Socioeconomic standing is, after all, a powerful determinant of exposure to adversity, opportunities for participation in voluntary organizations and extracurricular activities, and such ecological features as housing and neighborhood quality. As my own study of senior high school boys revealed, it is also a significant determinant of the support provided to youth by the institutions of the community.

With the aim of studying preferred sources of aid and support among White, senior boys, I (Gottlieb, 1975) conducted a series of intensive interviews with boys who were nominated by their peers as central members of four different social subgroups or cliques. My questions probed their preferences for informal sources of help and delved into the nature of the support they actually received from these sources. Briefly, I found striking variations in these respects. For example, members of the group I called the Elites—boys described by their classmates as highly competitive and successful in both academic and athletic domains— prefer the help of adults who are experts and who recognize and reinforce these boys' high social status in the school. The coach epitomizes the authoritative advice and special attention prized by the Elites. In the words of one of the Elites:

> My coach has done everything for me—got a job for me, given me advice during football and stuff like that; helped me extra. You can always count on him to give you some pretty good advice. He knows me too. He's seen me in action.

In contrast, the Outsiders were boys from working class families who were virtually anonymous to their peers. They did not participate in either school or community-based social activities largely because they had already left home and were holding down full-time jobs. They rarely sought the help of teachers and counsellors, instead favoring the support of peers whose life experiences were as different from age-graded norms as their own.

The contrasting preferences for sources and types of support expressed by boys occupying different social niches in the senior class are likely to reflect their family socialization and their cognitive and emotional maturity. However, my interviews in the high school made it abundantly evident that the boys' preferences are also in large measure reflections of the degree to which their subcultural values and norms coincide with those of the adults who are potential donors of support. *Culture not only mediates the stressors to which people are exposed, but also the availability and acceptability of resources in the environment.* The resources in the social environment of the high school—the teachers, coaches, guidance staff, and secretaries—are clearly less responsive and acceptable to some students than to others. Due to differences in their cultural proximity and distance from different students, these adults either invite or discourage youth from seeking their support. Recognizing how impersonal life can be for many students in middle schools, the Carnegie Council's Task Force on the Education of Young Adolescents suggests that "every student needs at least one thoughtful adult who has the time and takes the trouble to talk with the student about academic matters, personal problems, and the importance of performing well" (p. 37).

Although it is imperative to make reforms in the schools and other institutions in which adolescents participate in order to make them equal opportunity systems with respect to the provision of support, it is also necessary to formulate policies and programs that respond to the supportive needs of adolescents whose family and work responsibilities place them on the social sidelines. For example, in the absence of affordable daycare, a large proportion of young adolescents living in single-parent and dual-wage earner families are required to assume responsibility for supervising their younger siblings after school. Opportunities for participation in extracurricular activities, for engaging in community service, or even for casual socializing are thus curtailed. Even when adolescents are not made responsible for supervising younger siblings, they may be part of a growing number of "latchkey children" who are compelled by parents to return home immediately after school and to refrain from inviting friends over. Similarly, due to the absence or prohibitive cost of daycare facilities, large numbers of teenaged parents drop out of school, thus effectively losing the primary basis of their contact with peers.

The support teenagers gain from their participation in the labor force is deficient as well. In their compelling analysis of teenagers' employment in the United States, Greenberger and Steinberg (1986) maintain that the jobs held by almost two-thirds of high school seniors neither equip them with the skills and attitudes necessary for the adult world of work, nor provide them with meaningful feedback about their performance. The majority of the jobs are in fast food outlets, where communication with peer co-workers, much less supervision from adults, is highly constrained. In their survey, adolescent employees gave a resounding negative response to questions about whether they would seek help or advice from adults at work.

In sum, the preceding studies provide valuable information about the widening social context in which adolescents are embedded, emphasizing the developmental bases for the structural differentiation and increased intimacy occurring during this period. To date, investigations of social support have been largely confined to studies of young adolescents, and the concepts and measures adopted have been largely imported from the adult literature on the subject. Virtually no studies have focused on youth in the middle years of adolescence, and little is presently known about the ways in which demographic and ecological differences among adolescents affect the structure and quality of their social ties. Moreover, studies of the structural and relational bases of adolescents' social ties have yet to be joined with studies of their psychological functions both in the presence and absence of stressful events and transitions. By integrating these two topics, we can gauge how adolescents' commerce with their social networks adds to or detracts from their stress resistance, and how it generally affects their feelings about themselves.

Supportive Functions and Processes

Although the research on the stress-related functions of social support among adults can offer instruction to those investigating the subject among adolescents, the translation must be approached with two main considerations in mind. First, researchers must take into account the critical development and ecological differences affecting all aspects of the stress process in childhood as contrasted with adult life. Second, they must take stock of the forms and meaning of social support among adolescents, recognizing that gender, age, socioeconomic, cultural, and ecological differences within this age group have profound effects on the ways support is construed and evaluated. Moreover, these demographic characteristics are bound to shape the types of support that are extended as much as they shape the reactions of the youthful recipients. Both of these considerations are now discussed in greater depth.

Aneshensel and Gore (1990) have identified three broad features of the developmental phase of adolescence that affect psychosocial functioning in the context of stress. First, they observe that differences in the social roles occupied by adolescents and adults expose them to different life stressors. This is substantiated by a number of studies reporting on the types of normative and nonnormative stressful life events typically experienced by younger (Coddington, 1972; Swearington & Cohen, 1985) and older (Johnson & Mcutcheon, 1980; Yeaworth, York, Hussey, Ingle, & Goodwin, 1980) adolescents. Second, they note that adults and youth are likely to differ in the coping resources they can marshall to regulate their emotional states and act on the stressors they encounter. Moreover, differences in the cognitive, social, and emotional development of younger and older adolescents are bound to affect what they deem stressful and how they respond to perceived threats.

Third, Aneshensel and Gore (1990) observe that evidence in the field of developmental psychopathology does not warrant the wholesale application of adult models of disorder to children and adolescents. For example, the nature and timing of pubertal changes may have direct effects on mood and psychological functioning (Rutter, 1980) or they may create behavioral changes such as aggression among boys that affect their peer relations and in turn their access to support. Pubertal changes also directly influence the responses of others, affecting the extent of involvement in dating and sexual activity, and admittance to adult-only settings. Thus, pubertal changes and their interaction with ongoing stressful events may set into motion unique processes that impact on the risk status of youth, both enhancing and detracting from their psychosocial development (Petersen, 1988).

Developmental considerations apply with as much force to the study of social support among adolescents as they do to the study of the broader stress processes outlined above. First and foremost, it is necessary to acknowledge the fundamental contribution that companionship and participation in a peer group make to the self-worth and general well-being of adolescents. Accordingly, *a developmentally valid appreciation of social support at this age level must place strong emphasis on the inclusion, acceptance, and approbation of the peer group.* As noted earlier, it meets needs for a sense of belonging and group identity, offsets feelings of loneliness, and brings stability and continuity to daily life. The status of adolescents immediately improves if they are seen in the company of at least one peer, while social isolation is stigmatizing.

The social network's influence on self-perceptions ranks among its chief supportive functions. There is abundant evidence that social inclusion and peer approbation have profound effects on both adolescents' global sense of self-worth and domain specific self-esteem (Blyth & Traeger, 1989). In this regard, Harter's (1987) work has been particularly instructive. Her studies reveal that the more significant others are perceived to have regard for the self, the higher one's self-regard. Moreover, Harter's (1985) data debunk the myth that parental attitudes wane in their influence on self-esteem as the referent power of the peer group increases in early adolescence. In her study of the relationships among self-worth and different sources of social support, she finds that, among young adolescents, the general support of *both* parents and peers has a greater impact on self-worth than does the support received from the closest friend. More generally, in documenting how the supportive quality of the messages of parents and peers impacts on self-esteem, Harter (1987) has effectively shifted the controversy about the relations between these two constructs to a more productive level. It shifts attention from questions about the causal relations between self-esteem and social support to the study of the psychological processes involved in the individual's interpretation of network members' messages, and their relevance to self-esteem. Harter's (1987) work also calls attention to the inferences made about self-worth on the basis of social comparisons with peers.

Since the network is the crucible in which self-regard is formed, it follows that it should play a significant part in maintaining self-esteem when it is threatened by major life events and developmental transitions. The process whereby it shores up self-esteem and coping in these stressful contexts, however, has yet to be fully understood, although some leads are provided by studies of parental separation (Hetherington, 1989; Wallerstein & Kelly, 1980; Wolchik, Sandler, & Braver, 1984), and the transition to junior high school (Berndt, 1988; Berndt, Hawkins, & Hoyle, 1986; Felner, Ginter, & Primavera, 1982).

For example, in the stressful context of parental separation, Hetherington (1989) reports that girls were heavily overrepresented among children who fell into the highly adaptive cluster of "caring-competent" youth, constituting almost 80% of this more resilient group. Although the majority of them enjoyed a close relationship with mothers who had not remarried, it is intriguing that they were also actively involved in *providing* care and succor to a family member. Hetherington (1989) notes that "This early required helpfulness was the most powerful factor in predicting later membership in the caring-competent cluster" (p. 12). In short, by providing continuing support to others, the donor is afforded protection against maladaptive outcomes of stress. One might speculate that by being useful to others, these girls were able to anchor themselves in one close relationship at a time when parental relationships were in flux. It is also conceivable that a preoccupation with the care of others diverted their attention from their own injuries while also providing an opportunity to exercise control. That is, since the events unfolding in the wake of their parents' separation were largely outside the girls' control, their care and service represented means of exerting some positive effect on others and thereby stabilizing feelings of self-efficacy. These and other processes underlying the adaptive advantage that social support confers on certain youth in stressful situations require careful study. As Rutter (1987) has sagely pointed out, whatever protection is afforded by social support does not lie in the variable itself, but in the process.

Similarly, Brown, Harris, and BiFulco's (1986) research on the genesis of depression in adult women reveals that the most critical link in the complex etiological process they postulate is poor caretaking, or more exactly, a lack of affectionate care in childhood. Specifically, they found that 35% of women exposed to a caregiver who exercised little control and discipline or who showed indifference toward them when they were children were depressed as adults. In contrast, a depressive episode occurred among only 11% of those who were not exposed to such deficiencies in caregiving. Other studies examining the relationship between early parental loss or deficient support and subsequent vulnerability to psychiatric disorders (e.g., Birtchnell, 1980; Sandler, Gersten, Reynolds, Kallgren, & Ramirez, 1988) also suggest that the quality of the compensatory support and care children receive from surrogate caregivers has an appreciable impact on their present and future risk status.

More generally, future research on the stress and support process among adolescents would benefit from prospective studies of the interactions occurring between caregiver and child, with particular attention to the supportive meaning that the child attaches to these interactions. Methods must be developed to discern what people do or say to communicate various types of support to adolescents and how supportive meaning is derived from particular patterns of interaction. The observed interactions and the perceptions of support can then be related to one another and prospectively, to adaptation and mental health status. Moreover, these data can inform the design of interventions aimed to marshall support, especially in programs that involve the introduction of a new supportive relationship and specialization of the support rendered by existing ties.

A second important topic for prospective research concerns the potential impact of support experiences in childhood and adolescence on adult support. Two retrospective studies present data suggesting that the quality of early life attachments prefigures the quality of later life support (Flaherty & Richman, 1986; Parker & Barnett, 1988), and the extent of security and commitment found in adult love relationships (Hazan & Shaver, 1987). Moreover, experiences involving peer rejection, betrayals of trust in confiding communications, and displays of disloyalty may exert as strong an effect on the quality of relationships in adulthood as can experiences in trusting, durable, and mutually respectful relationships. At present, little is known about whether and how parental separation impacts on adolescents' attitudes toward marriage, childbearing, and methods of resolving conflict and communicating support in close relationships. What adolescents learn about the appropriateness and consequences of disclosing personal and work problems from observing their parents has not yet been investigated. Nor have any studies been conducted of the ways adolescents' attitudes toward help-seeking from different sources is shaped by the precepts and practices of their parents. The immediate and future effects of parents' messages about the right and the wrong ways for girls and boys to cope, and particularly about the occasions calling for self-reliance versus interdependence, deserve greater study because they bear upon adolescents' capacity to fully enjoy the benefits of relationships with others.

Reciprocally, as potential providers of support, what lessons do adolescents learn from their networks about being useful to others? Do they have opportunities to observe adults volunteering for community service, rendering informal care to elderly relatives, donating time and money to charitable organizations, or simply taking the time to listen? And the fact is that adolescents are often in a position to respond to the everyday needs of their peers and to demonstrate their alliance with and caring about others. This is perhaps most dramatically illustrated in the literature on youth suicide, which reveals that 25% of preadolescents have considered suicide at least once (Bolger, Downey, Walker, & Steininger, 1989), the proportion mushrooming to between 65 and 70% of high school students (Harkavy Friedman, Asnis, & Boeck, 1987). Suicidal ideation is typically expressed in the company of one or more peers, making those peers critical potential sources of support and referral. More prosaic instances when peer helping can prevent or compensate for psychological injury to the self include failed examinations, family disputes, and humiliating interpersonal events. Little is presently known about the contingencies determining whether adolescents react with support or indifference on these occasions, and about the forms taken by supportive responses. In general, however, we do know that, prior to their teens, adolescents are not likely to verbalize explicit messages of esteem and praise or comment on an associate's handling of a stressful emotional experience. Unlike most adults, they are rarely likely to encourage peers to identify and then vent feelings of sadness or disappointment or to encourage a more hopeful outlook on the future. Moreover, it is only in their late teen years that youth are targeted as consumers of information about human services, making younger groups unlikely agents of referrals to agencies, mental health counsellors, and other professional practitioners.

Furthermore, the acute, sometimes painful self-consciousness of adolescents, combined with their paramount need to be accepted and included by peers, can make them reluctant or unwilling to disclose events that might make them appear deviant, foolhardy, or more generally outside the mainstream. They are therefore less likely than adults to solicit support directly, by disclosing problems that they believe will damage their reputation or standing with peers. Moreover, because it is harder for them to activate support by disclosing their difficulties and emotions, their help-seeking behaviors are likely to be more indirect or disguised, and therefore less effective in mobilizing support early in the coping process. It is more likely to materialize later, when network members observe signs and signals of distress. In sum, the extent and timing of the support adolescents gain depend on the interactions between their skill in soliciting it, the nature of the problem requiring support, and the overt expression of distress.

Adolescents' concern about the embarrassment or stigma resulting from certain problems may account for the difficulty parents, teachers, and helping professionals encounter in their efforts to involve the younger age group in remedial education, personal and family counselling, and other human service programs. Their threshold for defining stigma is low and they are vigilant about their own and others' deviations from normalcy. Universal rather than targeted interventions are therefore more likely to attract and retain adolescents, as are those which advertise their purposes in educational rather than compensatory terms. Parents and siblings are often the objects of teenagers' heightened sensitivity to unconventional behavior or dress; prior to any ego-relevant public appearances with family members, teenagers admonish their parents not to do, say, or wear anything that might be a source of embarrassment. It follows that a tendency should develop to conceal or deny adversities that risk damage to one's reputation, and to inhibit disclosure of feelings of incompetence or dysphoria.

Mobilizing Support for Adolescents

Programs aimed to marshall, augment, or improve the informal support adolescents receive and provide have taken many forms, differing in their structure and content as a function of the developmental level and psychosocial needs of the beneficiaries and the ecological niches they inhabit. Programs also differ with respect to the settings in which they take place, the vast majority occurring in the school and the home. They typically concentrate on either altering structural features of these social environments or optimizing the supportive dimension of relationships. With very few exceptions, these programs focus on the delivery of extra support to youth at risk, either to stabilize them at times when they experience upheavals in their social field or to steer them onto an adaptive path when there are early signs of a downward trajectory. Initiatives bent on equipping adolescents with the skills to provide support to others or that provide opportunities for them to consider moral issues affecting their sense of responsibililty for the welfare of others are rare, largely restricted to college age groups.

Elsewhere (Gottlieb, 1988), I have presented a typology of support interventions that classifies them in terms of their focus on the individual, dyadic, group, social system, or community levels. I defined support interventions as "efforts to optimize the psychosocial resources which individuals proffer and/or receive in the context of relations with their primary social field" (p. 521). My review of the literature on support programs for adolescents suggests that the majority fall at the dyadic and group levels, and within these levels, emphasize strategies of grafting new ties onto their lives rather than specializing the support extended by existing ties in their networks.

One-to-One Support

At the dyadic level, the most widely known example is the Big Brothers/ Sisters organization, a prototype of many other intergenerational support programs designed to improve the life chances of a variety of at-risk youth. The nomenclature applied to the adult providers of support varies, examples being foster grandparents, mentors, coaches, home visitors, and preceptors, as do the frequency, duration, and intensity of the supportive contacts between the two parties. Some programs set limits on the nature, settings, and occasions when the two parties interact, embedding contacts in a more formalized task structure such as supervising academic and employment activities or in the case of teenage parents, improving parenting skills. Since the adults employed in these programs typically bring specialized support to bear on the demands faced by the youth to whom they are assigned, they are usually trained or selected on the basis of the experiential knowledge they have gained in circumstances similar to those presently faced by the youth.

In contrast, programs such as Big Brothers/Sisters offer diffuse support, rarely prescribing its content, the frequency and focus of interaction, or the settings in which contacts take place. These programs typically aim to compensate for a more general deficiency in adult attachments, and therefore concentrate on developing the kinds of support that are gained from such a close relationship. The relationship is the end in itself rather than a means of enlarging particular kinds of coping assistance. Based on his observations of programs in which elderly mentors are paired with teenage mothers, youth who have had conflicts with the law, and students at risk of dropping out of school, Freedman (1988) distinguishes between primary and secondary bonds that adolescents form with their mentors. The former are characterized by unconditional commitment, great intimacy, easy access, and involvement in all spheres of the youth's life. At their best, these primary mentoring relationships take on the qualities of kinship ties, reflecting attachment, closeness, trust, importance, and enjoyment.

To date, there has been no systematic research about how to match adults to adolescents in ways that optimize the likelihood of a relationship developing as a basis for the expression of support. Virtually nothing is known about the personal and interactional variables contributing to the parties' initial receptivity to one another, and to their desire to stay in or withdraw from the relationship. Beyond the stage of relationship initiation, information is needed about the interpersonal processes that predict which matches last and which dissolve. Moreover, as Pearlin (1989) notes, both parties' perspectives must be taken into account because "The forms of support, its reciprocity, the connections between seeking support and getting it, its stability, and even whether or not it is welcomed depend not on the recipient alone, but on the donor–recipient relationship" (p. 248). In Freedman's (1988) qualitative analysis of the factors fostering successful intergenerational pairings, he describes the "receptive youth" as relatively isolated, lonely, and emotionally intact, and the elderly mentors as also lonely, but eager to make an investment in the mentoring relationship as a way of leading more socially fulfilling lives. Apparently, the loneliness and marginal status they share with youth endow them with empathy that overcomes cultural and age differences. In addition, the elders' attractiveness to the youth stemmed from special aspects of their role. They were not perceived as authority figures, and as nonprofessionals and volunteers, they were viewed as freely choosing the relationship.

Although these observations are based on Freedman's (1988) interviews with the participants in only five intergenerational support programs serving youth in particular stressful situations, they underscore some of the desirable social psychological features of helping relationships identified by Fisher, Goff, Nadler, and Chinsky (1988). Specifically, support providers whose aid is seen to be voluntarily tendered rather than constrained by role obligations are liked more, and their support is more highly valued and accepted. Related to this point, when nonprofessional helping relationships are structured in a way that permits bidirectional expressions of support, they are more attractive. The youth Freedman interviewed frequently commented on the ways their relationships with their mentors drew out their own instincts and abilities to be helpful. In addition, the mentoring relationships did not trigger the kinds of threatening social comparisons that might have been produced had the mentors been peers who were handling their difficulties more adeptly or who had not experienced the same difficulties at all. This latter point, concerning the advisability of developing peer helping relationships for adolescents is stressful circumstances, merits separate consideration because a number of programs have attempted to optimize support by temporarily embedding adolescents in a set of new peer ties or by introducing them to a peer helper.

The most popular dyadic peer helping strategy has been to train adolescents as peer counselors (Buck, 1977; McManus, 1982). Many secondary schools and colleges have recruited and trained students to engage in personal and academic counseling with their peers, assigning senior students to new entrants as a way of smoothing the latter's adjustment to a novel environment. Although peer counseling has also been widely implemented in substance abuse and teen parenting programs (e.g., Halpern & Covey, 1983), the reports issuing from these programs rarely shed light on the impediments to recruitment and retention of the participants. An exception is Coupey, Doctors, and

Boeck's (1987) account of the difficulties encountered in creating a peer helping program for a minority inner-city group of chronically ill teenagers. Their efforts to recruit both counselors and counselees with chronic health conditions met with several kinds of resistance.

First and perhaps most important, they had considerable difficulty recruiting counselors with chronic illnesses because the youth they contacted through physicians and hospital clinics did not see themselves as ill and did not feel that their chronic condition should form the basis for establishing a counseling relationship with peers. They may have felt stigmatized by a recruitment strategy that focused mainly on their illness. This source of resistance was later overcome by offering training to both ill and healthy teenagers. The latter were recruited by asking the ill teenagers to bring friends along, and their presence seemed to improve program retention. Second, because the evaluation design called for random assignment of the youth who were trained to be peer counselors into an experimental and a control group, the staff could not promise all of them that they would be counselors. However, it became apparent that the youth's enthusiasm was based on their desire to put their training to use as helpers rather than to contribute to the baseline control data. Third, the teenagers' busy schedules interfered with their training, only a small proportion of them completing enough sessions to be considered adequately trained. Moreover, poor attendance was also deemed to reflect the fact that the youth associated the hospital with sickness and unpleasant experiences. Finally, they found that some of the youth trainees, mainly boys and teenagers with poorer verbal skills, were not comfortable with the counseling role. Consequently, other kinds of helping activities that depended less heavily on verbal ability were made available, including tutoring activities and jobs in the nursing home and infant nursery.

The preceding observations suggest that peer counseling programs are more likely to be successful in attracting and retaining adolescents if they provide opportunities for the expression of mutual rather than unidirectional aid, and if they recruit participants on the basis of their abilities rather than their handicaps or deficiencies. Universal rather than targeted strategies are likely to be more productive. Both the training and the counseling should be introduced as jobs, and retention is likely to improve if friends are included and wages are paid. Moreover, if the benefits of peer helping accrue as much if not more to the helper as to the helpee, then a variety of helping activities need to be available to suit the preferences and the talents of the trainees. Peer counseling is therefore only one of a number of helping and human service activities that deserve more systematic study, particularly with respect to the developmental gains produced by opportunities to be useful to others.

Group Support

Support groups have proved to be a ubiquitous strategy of marshalling help for older adolescent substance abusers, victims of domestic sexual abuse, and those involved in raising children at an early age. Typically, the groups are convened and led by professionals who combine skills in facilitating the process of mutual aid with expert knowledge about the stressors members face and productive ways of coping with them. Support groups average 8–10 youth, who meet for a fixed number of weekly or biweekly sessions. The most detailed information about their process, structure, and outcomes has come from reports of groups created for adolescents whose parents have separated or divorced (Kalter, Schaefer, Lesowitz, Alpern, & Pickar, 1988; Pedro-Carroll, Cowen, Hightower, & Guare, 1986). In general, the findings reveal that the groups speed the process of adjustment by normalizing the youth's feelings and family status, by counteracting their tendency toward self-recriminations with respect to the causes of parental separation, and by enhancing their ability to cope with troublesome family interactions and new emotional experiences.

Unfortunately, these studies have not been explicitly designed to illuminate the support process. They offer much less guidance about the processes that animate the development of relationships and mutual aid among the participants than they do about the content of the sessions. Aside from advising that the members should be roughly matched in age, they do not inform decisions about ways of composing the group that stimulate mutual identification, disclosure, and helping. Should boys and girls participate in the same or in separate groups? Should youth who are living in single-parent households be combined with those who are living with a remarried parent? Could the social comparison process work against the development of supportive ties in a group composed of youth who occupy very different social positions in the peer culture of the school? Little is known about the characteristics of those who drop out of these groups or about those who benefit most and least from participating.

It would also be informative to discern whether the salutary effects reported for support groups are directly attributable to the group's process or whether they result from the interaction between the skills gained in the group and the stressful external demands placed on the youth. Moreover, the interplay between the support group and the larger ecology may be reflected at the network level, impacting on relationships in the participants' natural social orbit. Are the ties germinated in the support group transplanted in the social network or kept segregated from it? Is there any risk that new relationships formed in the support group will displace formerly valued peer ties, or can they be smoothly integrated in the social fabric? Should the support group be planned as a temporary support system functioning in parallel with the natural network or as a specialized milieu from which new relationships can be recruited as sources of continuing support? These questions can be answered by systematically varying the structure of support groups and the degree of connection they have to the participants' lives at home and at school.

Some programs for adolescents have offered a sequence of dyadic and group strategies of marshalling support. For example, the Preventive Intervention Research Center at Albert Einstein College of Medicine has been particularly creative in its approaches to the enhancement of support for children with chronic illnesses and their families (Stein, 1988). They have introduced lay case coordinators, deployed nurse practitioners who offer homecare support, and, as described above, assigned older adolescents who are coping well with their condition to newly diagnosed younger adolescents. Sandler and his colleagues (Sandler et al., 1988) have been equally creative and thoughtful in designing support interventions for bereaved adolescents. In the planning process he asked the intended beneficiaries to comment on the potential helpfulness and appeal of several alternative formats for a bereavement program, including written and filmed material on bereavement, discussions about how to handle grief, support groups, professional counselors, and home visitors. Acting on their preferences, he developed a Family Bereavement Program in which peer and intergenerational group support was followed by the introduction of a lay helper. Specifically, Sandler began by convening a three session family grief workshop in which the parents and children participated in joint and separate activities designed to help them learn about grief and share the feelings and changes precipitated by their own bereavement. This was followed by the assignment of a Family Advisor, a support provider who has had a personal grief experience and has been trained to work with bereaved families. Chiefly, the advisors attempt to meet the surviving parents' needs for specialized, supplemental support and guidance so that the parents, in turn, can better meet their adolescents' supportive needs.

Enlarging Support in the Family and School

Sandler's approach forces recognition of the fact that when adolescents lack family support, it is likely that the support available to their parents is deficient as well, suggesting the need for interventions that are responsive to the needs of both generations. The absence of support is a risk factor, hampering family adjustment, as much as it is a protective factor that facilitates it. Children and adolescents are at risk of deficient parental support for many different reasons. First, their parents may not be well enough themselves to meet their children's needs for care and support, as in the case of parents who suffer from major mental illnesses or alcoholism. Second, parents may be preoccupied with their own personal problems, making them less available to their children or causing them to behave inappropriately with their children. For example, separation and divorce can entail not only the loss of one parent's support, but can result in parents making supportive demands of adolescents that are impossible for them to meet on the basis of their developmental maturation. Other stressful family contexts that call for equal measures of support to parents and children include the death of a parent or sibling through illness or suicide, chronic unemployment or repeated episodes of job loss, and the diagnosis of a serious or chronic illness occurring to the parent or child. Each of these life events and chronic hardships imposes special needs and demands for support on parents and children alike, and so collectively they form an agenda for planning initiatives that augment *family* support.

The family, however, is only one of the primary socializing contexts in which adolescents are embedded. As noted earlier, the school and the workplace are two additional settings in which support can be improved. Among the recommendations offered in the Carnegie Foundation's study of middle schools, the most prominent involve initiatives that counteract the impersonality of the social environment, according a high priority to meeting young adolescents' needs for intimacy. They include the creation of "houses" or "schools-within-schools," smaller learning environments that afford greater stability and familiarity among students and between them and teachers. A second recommendation that goes even further toward dispelling the anonymity of the middle school is for teachers to collaborate with one another in teams, thereby gaining the support of their own peers. Each team of at least 5 teachers would become a part of a larger "community of learning," composed of teachers and students who would remain intact for the duration of the middle school period. Third, recognizing the huge caseloads carried by guidance counselors, the Carnegie report calls for the assignment of an adult advisor to each student, a teacher or other staff member who would use his/her knowledge of adolescent development and principles of guidance to marshal school and community resources on behalf of the student. In this way, the credo that "Every student should be well known by at least one adult" could be realized.

It is noteworthy that certain aspects of the Carnegie Report's vision of how to transform the social environment of the middle school have already been implemented and evaluated by Felner, Ginter, and Primavera (1982). In an effort to smooth students' transition to junior high school, they added certain guidance and administrative duties to the homeroom teacher's role, including responsibility for maintaining contact with the students' families. In addition, at the structural level, they stabilized relations among the students by allowing the same set of students to attend all four core academic subjects together. Students who were not assigned to the demonstration followed the usual system of rotating between classes composed of different students. The empirical data on the effects of these efforts to generate greater peer and adult support revealed that, relative to a matched control group of students in another urban school, students in the intervention had significantly better academic and attendance records, developed more positive self-concepts, and viewed the school's social climate more favorably. On the latter score, they perceived its expectations and structure more clearly, and assigned higher ratings to the level of teacher support.

Schools can also host more broadly interpreted support interventions. As Rutter (1987) points out, they can enlarge opportunities for success in extracurricular activities, afford students equal access to positions of responsibility in school clubs, and involve them in tutoring other students. Such experiences cultivate leadership skills and engender feelings of self-worth arising from the positive appraisals of others. Finally, Aronson and his colleagues (Aronson, Blaney, Stephan, Sikes, & Snapp, 1978) have shown that the everyday learning process that occurs in the classroom can be shaped to foster cooperative rather than competitive interaction. He has found that his method of classroom instruction, known as the "jigsaw classroom," in which students teach each other portions of each lesson to be learned, facilitates empathy and friendliness.

Conclusion

In every day life and during times of adversity, people's supportive needs are met through the intimacy afforded by close relationships, the affirmation and stability derived from the feedback and social comparisons offered by the larger social world, and the sense of identity and belonging gained from the personal community they inhabit. Adolescence is a developmental period when the capacity increases to form both casual and intimate ties and to weave them into a network that can ease the passage through this time of life. Whether this capacity is fully developed is determined by both the personal resources that youth bring to their commerce with others, and the resources extended by the primary agents and institutions of socialization. They are in critical positions to offer guidance by precept and example, and to make provisions to abet the full expression of adolescents' ability to give aid and comfort to others and, reciprocally, to gain support from others.

Numerous challenges attend efforts to marshall support on behalf of adolescents. In order to embed them in supportive relationships we will need to develop a contextual understanding of support as it is experienced by adolescents. In fact, each program will have to gain a special understanding of the meaning of support to its intended beneficiaries and of the unique developmental and ecological factors that shape both opportunities for and perceptions of supportive relationships. Equally important, each program will have to discern the kinds of support that are required by adolescents facing different stressful circumstances and then determine, from a relationship perspective, who is best suited to render these provisions. Moreover, the work of planning supportive environments for youth involves creating opportunities for all youth, not just the privileged and successful, to render service and support to others. By thoughtfully planning alternative avenues for youth to display and develop their helping and caregiving skills, we can promote their personal and social development and help prepare them for meaningful and satisfying relationships in adulthood.

Four centuries ago, one of the keenest social observers of the day, William Shakespeare, had this to say about the adolescent years:

> I would there were no age between ten and three and twenty, or that youth would sleep out the rest; for there is nothing in the between but getting wenches with child, wronging the ancientry, stealing, (and) fighting.

Although there is no denying the timelessness of his words, it is important to remember that his dark view of adolescent turmoil reflects the dismal health, economic, and social conditions characterizing the lives of urban youth in sixteenth-century England. Today, a commitment to enhancing the life prospects of adolescents should preclude the existence of an underclass of young people cut off from the mainstream. Any comprehensive strategy aimed to realize that commitment must begin with initiatives that bring social support to bear on the settings and networks that adolescents inhabit.

References

Aneshensel, C., & Gore, S. (1990). Development, stress and role-restructuring: Social transitions of adolescence: In J. Eckenrode (Ed.), *The social context of coping.* New York: Plenum.

Aronson, E., Blaney, N., Stephan, C., Sikes, J., & Snapp, M. (1978). *The jigsaw classroom*. Beverly Hills, CA: Sage.

Asher, S. R., Markell, R. A., & Hymel, S. (1981). Identifying children at risk in peer relations: A critique of the rate-of-interaction approach to assessment. In J. D. Wine & M. D. Smye (Eds.), *Social competence* (pp. 125–157). New York: Guilford Press.

Beardslee, W. R., & Podorefsky, D. (1988). Resilient adolescents whose parents have serious affective and other psychiatric disorders: Importance of self-understanding and relationships. *American Journal of Psychiatry, 145,* 63–69.

Belle, D. (1988a). Gender differences in children's social networks and supports. In D. Belle (Ed.), *Children's social networks and social supports* (pp. 173–188). New York: John Wiley.

Belle, D. (Ed.) (1988b). *Children's social networks and social supports*. New York: John Wiley.

Berndt, T. J. (1982). The features and effects of friendship in early adolescence. *Child Development, 53,* 1447–1460.

Berndt, T. J. (1988). Obtaining support from friends during childhood and adolescence. In D. Belle (Ed.), *Children's social networks and social supports* (pp. 308–331). New York: John Wiley.

Berndt, T. J., Hawkins, J. A., & Hoyle, S. G. (1986). Changes in friendship during a school year: Effects on children's and adolescents' impressions of friendship and sharing with friends. *Child Development, 57,* 1284–1297.

Birtchnell, J. (1980). Women whose mothers died in childhood: An outcome study. *Psychological Medicine, 10,* 699–713.

Blyth, D. A., & Traeger, C. (1988). Adolescent self-esteem and perceived relationships with parents and peers. In S. Salzinger, J. Antrobus, & M. Hammer (Eds.), *Social networks of children, adolescents, and college students*. Hillsdale, NJ: Erlbaum.

Bolger, N., Downey, G., Walker, E., & Steininger, P. (1989). The onset of suicidal ideation in childhood and adolescence. *Journal of Youth and Adolescence, 18,* 175–189.

Brown, G. W., Harris, T. O., & BiFulco, A. (1986). Long-term effects of early loss of parent. In M. Rutter, C. E. Izard, & P. B. Read (Eds.), *Depression in young people: Developmental and clinical perspectives* (pp. 251–297). New York: Guilford Press.

Buck, M. R. (1977). Peer counseling in an urban high school setting. *Journal of School Psychology, 15,* 362–366.

Buhrmester, D., & Furman, W. (1987). The development of companionship and intimacy. *Child Development, 58,* 1101–1113.

Carnegie Council on Adolescent Development (1989). *Turning points: Preparing America's youth for the 21st century*. New York: Carnegie Corporation of New York.

Coates, D. L. (1987). Gender differences in the structure and support characteristics of Black adolescents' social networks. *Sex Roles, 17,* 667–687.

Coddington, R. D. (1972). The significance of life events as etiologic factors in the diseases of children: II. A study of a normal population. *Journal of Psychosomatic Research, 16,* 205–213.

Cohen, S., Mermelstein, R., Kamarck, T., & Hoberman, H. M. (1985). Measuring the functional components of social support. In I. G. Sarason & B. R. Sarason (Eds.), *Social support: Theory, research, and applications* (pp. 73–94). Dordrecht, The Netherlands: Martinus Nijhoff.

Coie, J. D., & Dodge, K. A. (1983). Continuity of children's social status: A five year longitudinal study. *Merrill-Palmer Quarterly, 29*, 261–282.

Coie, J. D., Dodge, K. A., & Cappotelli, H. (1982). Dimensions and types of social status: A cross-age perspective. *Developmental Psychology, 18*, 557–570.

Coupey, S. M., Doctors, S., & Boeck, M. (1987). *Preventive intervention research with adolescents: A study of a peer counseling program for teenagers with chronic health impairment.* Paper presented at the annual meeting of the Society for Research in Child Development, Baltimore, MD.

Felner, R. D., Ginter, M., & Primavera, J. (1982). Primary prevention during school transitions: Social support and environmental structure. *American Journal of Community Psychology, 10*, 277–290.

Fisher, J. D., Goff, B. A., Nadler, A., & Chinsky, J. M. (1988). Social psychological influences on help seeking and support from peers. In B. H. Gottlieb (Ed.), *Marshaling social support: Formats, processes, and effects* (pp. 267–304). Newbury Park, CA: Sage.

Flaherty, J. A., & Richman, J. A. (1986). Effects of childhood relationships on the adult's capacity to form social supports. *American Journal of Psychiatry, 143*(7), 851–855.

Freedman, M. (1988). *Partners in growth: Elder mentors and at-risk youth.* Philadelphia, PA: Public/Private Ventures.

Furman, W., & Buhrmester, D. (1985). Children's perceptions of the personal relationships in their networks. *Developmental Psychology, 21*, 1016–1024.

Garmezy, N. (1983). Stressors of childhood. In N. Garmezy & M. Rutter (Eds.), *Stress, coping, and development in children* (pp. 43–84). New York: McGraw-Hill.

Gottlieb, B. H. (1975). The contribution of natural support systems to primary prevention among four social subgroups of adolescent males. *Adolescence, 10*, 207–220.

Gottlieb, B. H. (1988). Support interventions: A typology and agenda for research. In S. Duck (Ed.), *Handbook of personal relationships* (pp. 519–541). Chichester, UK: Sage.

Greenberger, E., & Steinberg, L. (1986). *When teenagers work: The psychological and social costs of adolescent employment.* New York: Basic Books.

Halpern, R., & Covey, L. (1983). Community support for adolescent parents and their children: The parent-to-parent program in Vermont. *Journal of Primary Prevention, 3*, 160–173.

Harkavy Friedman, J. M., Asnis, G. M., & Boeck, M. (1987). *Suicidal behavior in adolescents: A high school sample with replication.* Paper presented at the annual convention of the American Psychological Association.

Harter, S. (1987). The determinants and mediational role of global self-worth in children. In N. Eisenberg (Ed.), *Contemporary topics in developmental psychology* (pp. 219–241). New York: John Wiley.

Hartup, W. W. (1983). Peer relations. In P. H. Mussen (Ed.), *Handbook of child psychology* (Vol. IV, pp. 103–196). New York: John Wiley.

Hays, R. B., & Oxley, D. (1986). Social network development and functioning during a life transition. *Journal of Personality and Social Psychology, 50,* 305–313.

Hazan, C., & Shaver, P. (1987). Romantic love conceptualized as an attachment process. *Journal of Personality and Social Psychology, 52,* 511–524.

Hetherington, M. (1989). Coping with family transitions: Winners, losers, and survivors. *Child Development, 60,* 1–14.

Hofferth, S. (1985). Updating children's life course. *Journal of Marriages & the Family, 47,* 93–115.

Holinger, P. C. (1978). Adolescent suicide: An epidemiological study of recent trends. *American Journal of Psychology, 135,* 754–756.

Hunter, F. T., & Youniss, J. (1982). Changes in functions of three relations during adolescence. *Developmental Psychology, 18,* 806–811.

Johnson, J. H., & McCutcheon, M. (1980). Assessing life stress in older children and adolescents: Preliminary findings with the Life Events Checklist: In I. G. Sarason & C. D. Spielberger (Eds.), *Stress and anxiety* (Vol. 7, pp. 111–125). Washington, DC: Hemisphere.

Kalter, N., Schaefer, M., Lesowitz, M., Alpern, D., & Pickar, J. (1988). School-based support groups for children of divorce. In B. H. Gottlieb (Ed.), *Marshaling social support: Formats, processes, and effects* (pp. 165–186). Newbury Park, CA: Sage.

McManus, J. L. (1982). Comprehensive psychological services at the secondary level utilizing student paraprofessionals. *Journal of School Psychology, 20,* 280–298.

Norton, A., & Glick, P. (1986). One parent families: A social and economic profile. *Family Relations, 35,* 9–17.

Parker, G., & Barnett, B. (1988). Perceptions of parenting in childhood and social support in adulthood. *American Journal of Psychiatry, 145*(4), 479–482.

Pearlin, L. (1989). The sociological study of stress. *Journal of Health & Social Behavior, 30,* 241–256.

Pedro-Carroll, J., Cowen, E., Hightower, A. D., & Guare, J. C. (1986). Preventive intervention with latency-aged children of divorce: A replication study. *American Journal of Community Psychology, 14,* 277–290.

Petersen, A. C. (1988). Adolescent development. *Annual Review of Psychology, 39,* 583–607.

Procidano, M. E., & Heller, K. (1983). Measures of perceived social support from friends and from family: Three validation studies. *American Journal of Community Psychology, 11,* 1–24.

Rutter, M. (1980). *Changing youth in a changing society: Patterns of adolescent development and disorder.* Cambridge, MA: Harvard University Press.

Rutter, M. (1983). Stress, coping, and development: Some issues and some questions. In N. Garmezy & M. Rutter (Eds.), *Stress, coping, and development in childhood* (pp. 1–42). New York: McGraw-Hill.

Rutter, M. (1987). Psychosocial resilience and protective mechanisms. *American Journal of Orthopsychiatry, 57,* 316–331.

Salzinger, S., Antrobus, J., & Hammer, M. (1988). *Social networks of children, adolescents, and college students.* Hillsdale, NJ: Erlbaum.

Sandler, I., Gersten, J. C., Reynolds, K., Kallgren, C. A., & Ramirez, R. (1988). Using theory and data to plan support interventions: Design of a program for bereaved children. In B. H. Gottlieb (Ed.), *Marshaling social support: Formats, processes, and effects* (pp. 53–84). Newbury Park, CA: Sage.

Sarason, I. G., Levine, H. M., Basham, R. B., & Sarason, B. R. (1983). Assessing social support: The Social Support Questionnaire. *Journal of Personality and Social Psychology, 44,* 127–130.

Selman, R. (1980). *The growth of interpersonal understanding.* New York: Academic Press.

Stein, R. E. K. (1988). *Renewal application for preventive intervention research center for child health.* Department of Pediatrics, Albert Einstein College of Medicine, Bronx, N.Y.

Sullivan, H. S. (1953). *The interpersonal theory of psychiatry.* New York: Norton.

Suls, J., & Sanders, G. (1982). Self-evaluation via social comparison: A developmental analysis. In L. Wheeler (Ed.), *Review of personality and social psychology* (Vol. 3, pp. 91–113). Beverly Hills, CA: Sage.

Swearington, E. M., & Cohen, L. H. (1985). Measurement of adolescents' life events: The Junior High Life Experiences Survey. *American Journal of Community Psychology, 13,* 69–85.

U.S. Bureau of the Census (1982). *Statistical abstract of the U.S.: 1982–1983* (103rd ed.). Washington, D.C.

Waller, A. E., Baker, S. P., & Szocka, A. (1989). Childhood injury deaths: National analysis and geographic variations. *American Journal of Public Health, 79*(3), 310–315.

Wallerstein, J., & Kelly, J. (1980). *Surviving the breakup.* New York: Basic Books.

Wolchik, S. A., Beals, J., & Sandler, I. N. (1988). Mapping children's support networks: Conceptual and methodological issues. In D. Belle (Ed.), *Children's social networks and social supports* (pp. 191–220). New York: John Wiley.

Wolchik, S., Sandler, I., & Braver, S. (1984). *The social support networks of children of divorce.* Paper presented at the American Psychological Association meeting, Toronto.

Yeaworth, R. C., York, J., Hussey, M. A., Ingle, M. E., & Goodwin, T. (1980). The development of an adolescent life change scale. *Adolescence, 15,* 93–97.

Youniss, J. (1980). *Parents and peers in social development: A Sullivan-Piaget perspective.* Chicago: University of Chicago Press.

Biographical Sketches of the Contributors

Hortensia de los Amaro is an Associate Professor of Social and Behavioral Sciences at the School of Public Health, and the Department of Pediatrics at Boston University School of Medicine.

During the last decade, Amaro's research has brought attention to the prevalence and impact of substance abuse among women, adolescents and Hispanic and Black populations in the United States. Her investigations on HIV infection among high risk pregnant women, and on HIV-related knowledge and its affect on attitudes and risk behaviors among Hispanics have provided innovative models for community-based prevention research.

With support from the William T. Grant Foundation's Faculty Scholars Program, she is working on the development of a community-based drug prevention program targeted for inner city adolescent girls.

Robert H. Aseltine, Jr. is a doctoral candidate in Sociology at the University of Michigan, Ann Arbor, and a research associate with the Center for Survey Research, University of Massachusetts, at Boston. He is currently completing his doctoral dissertation on family disruption and adolescent functioning.

Linda Asmussen is a Visiting Research Associate in Human Development and Family Studies, at the Center for the Study of Reading at the University of Illinois. She is interested in adolescent and family relationships. Her current research examines interaction in families with a child at risk for academic failure.

Judith L. Braeges recently received her Ph.D. from the Graduate School of Education and Human Development at the University of Rochester. Her research focuses on communicative competence in normal and atypical children and adolescents.

Jeanne Brooks-Gunn is Senior Research Scientist and Director of the Adolescent Study Program in the Policy Research Division at the Educational Testing Service and is an Adjunct Associate Professor of Pediatrics at the University of Pennsylvania. A developmental psychologist, she studies families and children, with a special emphasis on the biological and social factors that render children and youth at risk for school, relational, and emotional problems. Her recent books include *Adolescent Mothers in Later Life, The Encyclopedia of Adolescence*, and *The Development of Depression during Adolescence*

Zeng-yin Chen is a doctoral candidate in the Department of Sociology at Stanford University. She is interested in cross-cultural perspectives of social psychology.

Mary Ellen Colten, a psychologist, is Director of the Center for Survey Research at the University of Massachusetts at Boston. Her research has been focused on sex roles, mental health and substance abuse. Together with Susan Gore, she is engaged in a longitudinal study funded by the National Institute of Mental Health to investigate the stress and mental health of high school aged adolescents, focussing on both protective and harmful features of social relationships.

Bruce E. Compas is Associate Professor of Psychology at the University of Vermont. His research interests focus on stress and coping processes in children, adolescents, and families, and preventive interventions to enhance coping skills in these groups. His current research includes a longitudinal study of families coping with the extreme stress of cancer in a mother or father.

Sanford M. (Sandy) Dornbusch has been a Professor at Stanford since 1959. Educated at Syracuse and the University of Chicago, he previously taught at Harvard and the University of Washington. He is currently Reed-Hodgson Professor of Human Biology and Professor of Sociology and Education. He is also Director of the Stanford Center for the Study of Families, Children and Youth. He has received the Walter J. Gores Award for Excellence in Teaching at Stanford.

He was recently elected President of the Society for Research on Adolescence, the first non-psychologist to receive that honor.

Dornbusch is the author of numerous articles and the author or editor of six books. The most recent volume is *Feminism, Children, and the New Families*, which appeared in 1988.

Maurice J. Elias is Associate Professor of Psychology and Coordinator of the Internship Program in Applied and Community Psychology at Rutgers University. He is the co-chair of the William T. Grant Foundation-supported Consortium on the School-Based Promotion of Social Competence. For his action research project, the Improving Social Awareness-Social Problem Solving Project, he has received the Lela Rowland Prevention Award from the National Mental Health Association and the National Psychological Consultants to Management Award from Division 13 of the American Psychological Association. His book, *Social Decision Making Skills: A Curriculum Guide for the Elementary Grades*, (1989) received validation as a national model of educational excellence by the Program Effectiveness Panel of the U.S. Department of Education's National Diffusion Network.

Susan Gore is Associate Professor of Sociology at the University of Massachusetts at Boston. She has written on stress, support systems and mental health and is especially concerned with processes that promote resilience in the face of stress. Together with Mary Ellen Colten, she is recipient of a grant from the National Institute of Mental Health to investigate the stress and mental health of high school aged adolescents focusing on both protective and harmful features of social relationships. She is co-author of the volume *Stress between Work and Family* (1990).

Dr. Gore is also co-organizer of a consortium on stress research supported by the William T. Grant Foundation.

Benjamin H. Gottlieb is Professor of Psychology at the University of Guelph and Chair of the Child, Youth and Family Policy Research Center of Ontario (Canada). He is presently conducting research with populations at early and late stages of the life cycle, examining the process and outcomes of a variety of mentoring programs for at-risk youth, and the impact of respite programs for family caregivers of persons with Alzheimer's Disease. His edited books include *Social Networks and Social Support* and *Marshaling Social Support*, and he is the author of *Social Support Strategies: Guidelines for Mental Health Practice*.

Melodie Wenz-Gross is a Research Associate at the Center for the Study of Social Acceptance, University of Massachusetts/Boston. She is interested in the contribution of social support to the child's development and ability to deal with stress. She was recently awarded an Initial Career Award by the Office of Special Education and Rehabilitative Services to conduct a longitudinal study of the role of social support in mentally retarded children's adjustment to school transitions.

Robert E. Kennedy is Research Associate at The Pennsylvania State University. His research interests include the development of depression and delinquency during adolescence and gender differences in these problems. Recent publications include "Effects of Depression and Anxiety on a Learning Task" (*Behavior Therapy*, 1988) and "Delinquency" (in *Encyclopedia of Adolescence*, in press).

Cheryl Koopman is Assistant Professor of Clinical Psychology at Columbia University. She is Research Director for the Adolescent AIDS Awareness Project of the HIV Center for Clinical and Behavioral Studies. Her research examines the relationship of goals, perceived risks, and beliefs to decision-making and behavior in high risk situations.

Reed Larson is an Associate Professor of Human Development and Family Studies and Kinesiology at the University of Illinois, Urbana/Champaign. He is author with Mihaly Csikszentmihalyi of *Being Adolescent*, a book that describes the daily emotional lives of high-school-aged adolescents. His chapter in this volume is from the first phase of a longitudinal study on the relationship between daily experience and the development of psychological health and disturbance in adolescence.

Randy Mont-Reynaud is a Research Associate at the Stanford Center for the Study of Families, Children and Youth. She is interested in cross-cultural perspectives on adolescent development and minority adolescent issues, particularly education, identity and development of the self.

Anne C. Petersen is Professor of Health and Human Development and Women's Studies, and Dean, College of Health and Human Development at The Pennsylvania State University. Her books include *Promoting Adolescent Health: A Dialog on Research and Practice* (1982), *Girls at Puberty: Biological and Psychosocial Perspectives* (1983), *Adolescence and Youth: Psychological Development in a Changing World* (3rd Ed., 1984), *Brain Maturation and Cognitive Development: Comparative and Cross-Cultural Perspectives* (1991).

Angela Restrepo has a Master's degree in Human Development from the University of Rochester. She is currently working as a clinician with disturbed children at a community mental health agency.

Philip L. Ritter is a Research Associate in the Stanford Center for the Study of Families, Children and Youth and Lecturer in the Department of Anthropology. He is currently studying family and peer influences on adolescent achievement, particularly among minority youth. He has also done research on the relations between demographic change and family and social organization.

Mary Jane Rotheram-Borus is Associate Professor of Clinical Psychology of the College of Physicians and Surgeons at Columbia University. Her research focuses on preventive interventions with high risk adolescents. She has developed and evaluated the effectiveness of social competency training for reducing suicide and HIV risk behaviors among minority youth, and investigated the development of ethnic identity in adolescents.

Margaret Rosario is a postdoctoral fellow at Columbia University's HIV Center for Clinical and Behavioral Studies. Her research with nonadult high risk populations includes the effects of stress and social supports on adaptation.

Gary N. Siperstein is Professor of Psychology at the University of Massachusetts/Boston, founder and Director of the Center for the Study of Social Acceptance. The Center is a research and development institute, concerned with the participation of individuals with disabilities within the mainstream of our society. He has written numerous articles on the critical aspects of children's social relationships. Dr. Siperstein is also a consulting psychologist at the Developmental Evaluation Clinic, Children's Hospital in Boston. He is Associate Editor and Consulting Editor to national scientific journals, and is recently a recipient of a merit award from the National Institute of Child Health and Human Development.

Judith G. Smetana is Professor of Education, Psychology, and Pediatrics at the University of Rochester. Her research interests focus on social-cognitive development, including children's conceptions of moral and social rules, relations between judgments and actions, the developmental origins of morality, and the contextual basis of social judgments. Her current research is on adolescents' and parents' conceptions of rules, conflicts, and authority relations.

Laurence Steinberg is Professor of Psychology at Temple University. His research examines familial influences on adolescent development and adjustment. Dr. Steinberg is the author of numerous scholarly articles on adolescent development.

Patricia A. Sullivan is a graduate assistant in Human Development and Family Studies at the Pennsylvania State University. As part of a longitudinal study concerning the development of mental health across adolescence, her current research focuses on gender differences in stress and coping.

Barry M. Wagner is Assistant Professor of Psychology at the Catholic University of America. His primary interests center on the family context of child and adolescent stress, competence, and coping. He is also currently engaged in research on the etiology and prevention of adolescent suicidal behavior.

Cathy Spatz Widom is Professor of Criminal Justice and Psychology at Indiana University, Bloomington. She is a graduate of Cornell University and holds M.A. and Ph.D. degrees in psychology from Brandeis University. She edited *Sex Roles and Psychopathology* (1984) and has carried out research and has written on a variety of topics, including child abuse and neglect, juvenile delinquents, incarcerated and noninstituionalized psychopaths, female criminality, prostitution, and victimization in the United States and abroad. A former faculty member in the Department of Psychology and Social Relations at Harvard University and a former Chair of the Department of Criminal Justice at Indiana University, she serves on the editorial boards of psychology and criminology journals. Her current work focuses on violent criminal behavior as one consequence of early childhood victimization.

Jenny Yau is Assistant Professor of Educational Foundations at Buffalo State College. Her research focuses on adolescent-parent conflict in Chinese-American families.

Barry Zuckerman, M.D. is Professor of Pediatrics and Public Health at the Boston University School of Medicine and Director of the Division of Developmental and Behavioral Pediatrics at Boston City Hospital. He is a member of the National Commission on Children, Chairman of the Section of Developmental and Behavioral Pediatrics of the American Academy of Pediatrics and a member of many state and national organizations. He has conducted research and written articles on the impact of biological and environmental factors on the health and development of young children, especially those living in poverty.

Author Index

Aboagye, K., 225
Abramowitz, R. H., 100
Achenbach, T. M., 157, 170
Adelson, J., 10, 44
Adrian, C., 75
Alapack, R. J., 37
Albee, G. W., 262
Alers, J. O., 181
Alessi, N. E., 158
Alfaro, J., 202, 203
Allen, V. L., 135
Alpern, D., 298
Alpert, J. J., 225
Amaro, H., 7, 11, 155, 223, 224, 225, 228
American Humane Association, 203
Ames, M. A., 216
Aneshensel, C., 3, 16, 289–290
Anglin, D., 230, 233
Anthony, E. J., 2
Antrobus, J., 283
Arey, S. A., 113
Aronson, E., 301
Asher, S. R., 283
Asmussen, L., 8, 11, 17, 18, 91
Asnis, G. M., 293
Atkinson, T., 247
Attie, I., 135, 136, 143

Bachman, J. G., 1, 223–224, 226
Bader, B., 262
Bak, J. J., 239, 242, 243, 245–246

Baker, S. P., 282
Baltes, P. B., 131
Band, E. B., 245
Barnes, H., 43
Barnett, B., 292
Barrera, M. Jr., 10, 187
Basham, R. B., 286
Bauchner, H., 225
Baydar, N., 136–137
Bayley, H., 239
Beals, J., 286
Beard, J., 96
Beardslee, W. R., 223, 282
Beck, A. T., 158
Beck, N. C., 166
Belle, D., 9, 127, 286
Bemis, K., 166
Bentler, M. D., 158
Bentler, P. M., 1, 99, 164, 190
Bergman, A. B., 112
Bergman, L. R., 160
Berndt, T. J., 68, 74, 285, 286, 291
BiFulco, A., 291
Biglan, A., 185
Birtchnell, J., 292
Bjork, J. P., 23, 75
Black, A., 45
Blaney, N., 301
Block, J., 159, 166
Block, J. H., 159
Bloom, B., 262
Blos, P., 133, 143

Blumstein, A., 204
Blyth, D. A., 5, 9, 101, 135, 137, 166, 257, 284, 290
Bock, R. D., 181
Boeck, M., 293, 296–297
Boike, M., 112, 244
Bolger, N., 293
Bolton, F. G., 202
Boskind-Lodahl, M., 166
Bowerman, C. E., 28
Bowlby, J., 249
Boyce, T. W., 112
Boyd, J. H., 113
Bradley, J., 182
Braeges, J. L., 11, 17, 44
Branden, L. R., 262
Braver, S., 291
Broadhead, W. E., 134
Bronfenbrenner, U., 87–88
Brooks-Gunn, J., 2, 11, 22, 52, 91–92, 131, 132, 133, 134, 135, 136, 137, 138, 139, 140, 141, 142, 143, 151, 167
Brophy, J. E., 241
Brown, G. W., 291
Browne, A., 212
Brownell, A., 245
Brownley, B., 243
Buchanan, C. M., 140
Buck, M. R., 296
Bucy, J., 182
Budoff, M., 238
Buescher, T. M., 104
Buhrmester, D., 246, 285, 286
Burge, D., 75
Burgeson, R., 5, 61
Burke, R. J., 69
Buros, O. K., 113
Burrow, C., 136
Burt, C. E., 23, 75
Bush, D. M., 9, 10, 126, 166
Bushwall, S. J., 56

Cabral, H., 225, 228, 230
Camara, K. A., 56–57, 58
Camarena, P. M., 99
Canter, R. J., 166

Cantwell, D. P., 158
Caplan, M., 263
Cappotelli, H., 283
Carlsmith, J. M., 56
Carlson, G. A., 158
Carlton-Ford, S., 5, 143
Carpenter, R. A., 224
Carrieri, V. L., 226
Casper, R., 22
Cassell, J. C., 112
Caton, D., 182, 183, 184–185, 196
Cauce, A. M., 10, 242
Chadwick, O. F., 138
Champion, L., 96, 99
Chase, J. A., 230
Chelimsky, E., 182, 183
Chen, Z., 11, 88
Children's Defense Fund, 182, 183
Chinsky, J. M., 296
Cicchetti, D., 248, 249–250
Clabby, J. F., 264, 265, 269, 270, 273, 274
Cleary, P. D., 116–118, 126, 159
Cleland, C. C., 243
Coates, D. L., 286
Cochran, U. L., 243
Coddington, R. D., 289
Cohen, E., 183
Cohen, J., 204
Cohen, L. H., 23, 75, 76, 190, 289
Cohen, S., 134, 286
Coie, J. D., 283
Coleman, J., 97
Collier, A. M., 112
Collins, W. A., 37
Colten, M. E., 9, 166
Commins, W. W., 264
Committee on Adolescence, 228
Compas, B. E., 5, 8, 10, 11, 16–17, 18, 23, 67, 69, 70, 76, 77, 78, 79, 93, 98, 104, 134, 160, 164, 244, 245, 250
Condon, S. M., 51, 52
Condran, G. A., 103
Conger, J., 94
Connell, J. P., 80
Cooper, C. R., 51, 69, 141

Cornelius, S., 51
Costos, D., 69
Council on Scientific Affairs, 183
Coupey, S. M., 296–297
Covey, L., 296
Cowan, P. A., 27
Cowen, E. L., 112, 244, 264, 298
Craighead, W. E., 166
Cramer, P., 99
Crnic, K. A., 240
Crockett, L. J., 95, 99, 100, 137
Cross, C., 113
Crouter, A. C., 100
Csikszentmihalyi, M., 2, 22, 140, 141
Cullinan, D., 239
Cummings, S. T., 239

David, T., 182
Davidson, P., 45, 46, 47
Davies, M., 158, 159, 166, 171
Davis, G. E., 70
D'Arcy, C., 69, 73, 99
Deci, E. L., 80
Deisher, R. W., 196
Derogatis, L. R., 70, 162
DeRougemount, D., 37
Deykin, E. Y., 10, 18, 160
D'Augelli, A. R., 185
DHHS (Department of Health and
    Human Service, U.S.), 1, 181
Doctors, S., 296–297
Dodge, K. A., 283
Dohrenwend, B. P., 112, 113, 126,
    127, 262
Dohrenwend, B. S., 112, 113, 126,
    127, 262
Donovan, J. E., 230
Dooling, E., 225
Dornbusch, S. M., 2, 11, 56, 58, 59,
    88, 89, 90–91, 151
Douvan, E., 10, 44, 127, 162, 167, 168
Downey, G., 293
DuPont, R. L., 228
Dweck, C. S., 80

Earls, F., 160
Eastman, G., 51

Ebata, A. T., 94, 95, 97, 98, 101, 102,
    168
Eccles, J. S., 105, 140, 141
Eckenrode, J., 11
Edelbrock, C. S., 157, 170
Ehrhardt, A. A., 187
Eichorn, D. E., 137
Einbender, A. J., 203
Eisenberg, J. G., 112
Elder, G. H., 133
Elias, M. J., 10, 11, 257, 258, 259,
    262, 263, 264, 268, 269, 270,
    273, 274
Elkind, D., 34
Elliot, D. S., 224
Elliott, E. S., 80
Emde, R. N., 95
Emery, R., 7
Epstein, M. H., 239
Epstein, S., 23
Erikson, M. T., 240
Exner, T. M., 187

Fagan, J., 203
Fagan, T., 183
Farberow, N. L., 192
Farrington, D. P., 204
Feld, S., 43
Felner, R. D., 2, 10, 112, 160, 242,
    291, 300–301
Fergusson, D. J., 75, 76
Finkelhor, D., 212
Fischer, C. T., 37
Fisher, J. D., 296
Fishman, D., 264
Flaherty, J. A., 292
Flanagan, C., 58, 59
Fletcher, B., 244
Folkman, S., 21, 80, 81, 93, 99, 242,
    244, 247
Follansbee, D. J., 52, 69
Fondacaro, K. M., 245
Ford-Somma, L., 203
Forman, S. G., 264
Forsythe, C. J., 70, 164
Fox, R., 135
Frank, D. A., 225, 228

Frederick, C. J., 105
Freedman, M., 296
Freud, A., 22, 43
Fried, L. E., 225
Friedrich, W. H., 203
Friedrich, W. L., 240
Friedrich, W. N., 240
Furman, W., 246, 256, 285, 286
Furstenberg, F. F., Jr., 133, 181, 225

Gara, M., 268, 274
Garbarino, J., 202
Gardner, W. I., 239
Gargiulo, J., 135
Garmezy, N., 2, 88, 93–94, 160, 240, 244, 282
Gayle, H. D., 181
Geller, M., 203
Gersten, J. C., 112, 126, 292
Gfroerer, B. A., 230, 233
Gibbs, J., 126
Gilligan, C., 70, 72
Ginter, M., 10, 291, 300–301
Girgus, J. S., 133
Gittleman, R., 101–102
Giunta, C. T., 77
Gjerde, P. F., 60, 159, 166
Glick, P., 282
Glueck, E., 202
Glueck, S., 202
Goding, M. J., 241
Goff, B. A., 296
Gold, J. J., 139
Goldman, H., 262
Goldston, S., 262
Goodwin, T., 289
Gordon, D., 75
Gore, S., 9, 16, 289–290
Gottlieb, B. H., 9, 10, 11, 155, 257, 258, 259, 281, 287, 294
Gove, W. R., 159, 166
Graber, J. A., 99, 101
Graham, P., 138, 244
Graham, S., 37
Gray, E., 201, 202, 209, 274
Green, A. H., 217
Greenberg, M. T., 240

Greenberger, E., 288
Greene, A. L., 24, 25
Greenwald, H., 212
Gretton, M. E., 75
Grief, E. B., 132
Grimson, R. C., 226
Gross, R. T., 56
Grotevant, H. D., 51, 70–71, 141
Gruen, R. S., 187
Grumbach, M. M., 139
Guare, J. C., 298
Gutierres, S. E., 202, 203

Haboush, K., 274
Haggerty, R. J., 98
Hall, G. S., 131, 133
Halpern, R., 296
Ham, M., 22, 23
Hamburg, B. A., 2, 196, 131
Hamilton, L. H., 136
Hammen, C., 75, 76
Hammer, M., 283
Hampton, R. L., 202
Hansen, K., 203
Hanson, E. A., 141
Harding, R., 185
Harkavy Friedman, J. M., 293
Harmon, R. J., 95
Harre, R., 21
Harris, P. L., 24, 27
Harris, P. W., 112
Harris, T. O., 291
Harter, S., 284, 290–291
Hartstone, E., 203
Hartup, W. W., 141, 245, 284
Hastort, H. A., 56
Hauser, S. T., 2, 44, 52, 55, 60, 61, 69
Hawkins, J. A., 291
Hays, R. B., 284
Hazan, C., 292
Heller, K., 286
Helwig, C. C., 46
Herb, T. R., 159, 166
Hermann, R. C., 182, 183
Hersch, P., 193
Hetherington, E. M., 56–57, 58, 59, 60, 61, 291

Hetrick, E. S., 192
Hightower, A. D., 298
Hill, J. P., 43, 44, 51, 53, 99, 126, 135,
    141, 143, 166
Hindelang, M. J., 204
Hingson, R., 225, 225, 228
Hiroto, D., 75
Hirsch, B. J., 10
Hirschfeld, R. M. A., 113
Hirschi, T., 204
Hoberman, H. M., 286
Hofferth, S., 282
Hoffman, L., 43
Hoffman, M., 32
Holahan, C. J., 75–76
Holinger, P. C., 282
Holmbeck, G. N., 53
Holmes, T. H., 111, 247
Holzer, C. B., III, 113
Hornbeck, D. W., 105
Horne, M., 241
Horowitz, A. V., 159, 166
Horwood, L. J., 75
Howell, D. C., 76, 77, 78
Hoyle, S. G., 291
Hser, Y., 230, 233
Huba, G. J., 1, 99, 164, 190
Huberman, M., 264
Hughes, M., 113
Hundleby, J. D., 224
Hunter, F. T., 284
Hunter, J., 191
Husaini, B., 126
Hussey, M. A., 289
Hymel, S., 283

Ingle, M. E., 289
Inhelder, B., 24, 31, 43
Inoff-Germain, G., 140
Iosimovich, J., 139
Irwin, C. D., 263

Jaccard, J., 246
Jackson, A. W., 105
Jacob, T., 51, 55

Jacobson, A. M., 52, 69
Jaenicke, C., 75
James, J., 212
Jenkins, R. L., 203
Jensen, E. W., 112
Jessor, R., 152, 155, 185, 224, 230,
    231, 233
Jessor, S. L., 155, 185, 224
Jewell, L., 22
Johnson, J., 112, 127
Johnson, J. H., 67, 164, 186, 226, 289
Johnston, L. D., 1, 223–224, 226
Joreskog, K. G., 76

Kagan, J., 37, 126
Kallgren, C. A., 292
Kalter, N., 298
Kamarck, T., 286
Kandel, D. B., 158, 159, 166, 171,
    224, 225, 228, 230, 231, 233,
    233
Kanner, A. D., 21
Kanter, J. F., 181
Kaplan, B. H., 226
Kashani, J. H., 158, 166
Kayne, H., 225, 225, 228
Keating, D. P., 133
Keirn, W. C., 240
Kellog, P., 185
Kelly, J., 112, 291
Kelly, J. B., 57, 58, 61
Kelly, J. G., 162, 265
Kennedy, J., 184
Kennedy, R. E., 11, 88, 101, 104, 137,
    250
Kessler, R. C., 70, 72, 99, 126, 127,
    128, 134, 158, 159
Kessler, R. C., 224
Ketterer, R., 262
Killen, M., 46
Kilner, L. A., 2, 44
Kinch, J. W., 28
King, L., 126
Klerman, G. L., 1, 10, 18, 158, 159,
    160
Knop, J., 205
Koopman, C., 11, 182, 184

Kovacs, M., 158
Kratcoski, P. C., 202, 203
Kruks, G. N., 192
Kulka, R. A., 127

Lampman-Petraitis, C., 22, 25
Landesman, S., 246
Langner, T. S., 112
Larson, A., 43
Larson, R., 2, 8, 11, 17, 18, 22, 23,
    24, 25, 28, 30, 91, 140, 141
Launier, R., 134
Laursen, B., 37
Lawrence, R. A., 225
Lazarus, R. S., 21, 80, 81, 93, 99, 104,
    134, 242, 244, 247
Ledoux, N., 76
Leiderman, H., 56
Leland, J., 166
Lesowitz, M., 298
Lessor, R., 157
Levenson, S., 225
Levin, H. M., 106
Levine, H. M., 286
Lewin, K., 87–88
Lewinsohn, P. M., 166
Lewis, C. E., 113
Lewis, D. O., 202, 203
Lewis, M., 25
Lewis, M. A., 113
Lieberman, M., 43
Lieberman, M. A., 98
Liem, J. H., 126, 247
Liem, R., 126, 247
Lindbergh, C., 58
Lindsey, A. M., 226
Lipsitz, J., 95
Locksley, A., 162, 167, 168
London, P., 263
Lorion, R., 264
Lotyczewski, B. S., 112, 244
Low, H., 140
Luftig, R. L., 243
Lutz, C., 21
Lye, D. N., 103
Lynch, J. H., 51, 53
Lynch, M. E., 99, 126, 135, 166

Maccoby, E. E., 51, 248
Macdonald, D., 228
MacKenzie, R., 183
Magnusson, D., 135, 137, 160
Mahler, M., 37
Malcarne, V. L., 245
Mandler, G., 21
Mannis, J., 43
Manoff, S. B., 181
Margulies, R. Z., 158
Markell, R. A., 283
Marsh, J. C., 166
Martin, A. D., 185, 192
Matson, J. J., 239
Mattson, A., 140
Maughan, B., 96, 99
Mays, M. A., 181
McAdoo, H., 126, 127
McCord, J., 202, 203
McCubbin, H., 43
McCutcheon, M., 289
McCutcheon, S., 112, 164, 186
McDill, E. L., 106
McGlothlin, W., 230, 233
McKinney, K. L., 135
McLeod, J. D., 70, 72, 126, 159
McManus, J. L., 296
Mead, M., 38
Meadows, L., 58
Mechanic, D., 116–118
Mednick, S. A., 205
Menaghan, E. G., 98
Mercer, G. W., 224
Mermelstein, R., 286
Merrit, T. A., 225
Metz, J. R., 244, 245
Meyer-Bahlburg, H. F. L., 187
Meyers, C. E., 240
Michaelson, L., 25
Midgley, C., 105
Mikesell, J., 104–105
Miles, M., 264
Miller, F. T., 226
Miller, H. G., 184
Miller, W. H., 240
Mink, I. T., 240
Mirowsky, J., II, 113

Mitchell, J., 228
Monahan, J., 262
Montemayor, R., 44, 69, 141, 143
Mont-Reynaud, R., 11
Moore, E. G. L., 181
Moos, R. H., 76
Morelock, S., 225, 228
Morgan, S. B., 248
Morgan, S. P., 103
Morse, B. J., 224
Moses, L. E., 184
Mullan, J. T., 98
Munoz, R. F., 265
Murphy, G.E., 1
Muxen, M., 43
Myers, H. F., 126

Nadler, A., 296
Naeye, R. I., 225
Nannis, E. D., 27
National Network of Runaway and
       Homeless Youths, 183
Neff, J., 126, 127
Neighbors, H. W., 127, 128
Neigher, W., 264
Nesselroade, J. R., 131
Newberger, C. M., 202
Newberger, E. H., 202
Newcomb, M. D., 99, 113, 158, 164,
       190
Newman, D., 142
Nihira, K., 240
Nisbett, R., 81
Noam, G. G., 52, 69
Nolen-Hoeksema, S., 99, 105, 133
Norbeck, J. S., 226
Norton, A., 282
Novick, L. F., 184
Nucci, L. P., 45–46, 47

O'Grady, D., 244, 245
Offer, D., 43, 69, 74
O'Malley, P. M., 1, 223–224, 226
Olson, D., 43
Olthof, T., 24
Olweus, D., 140
Oppenheimer, E., 225

Orvaschel, H., 166
Oxley, D., 284

Padilla, E. R., 112
Pagelow, M. D., 216
Paikoff, R. L, 133, 138–139, 142, 143
Palleja, J., 196
Parker, G., 292
Parker, S., 225, 228
Paroski, P. A., 185
Paton, S., 225
Pearlin, L. I., 43, 98, 127, 295
Pedro-Carroll, J., 298
Pennbridge, J., 183
Petersen, A. C., 2, 4, 10, 11, 22, 88,
       89–90, 91, 93, 94, 95, 96, 97,
       98, 99, 100, 101, 102, 103, 104,
       134, 137, 138, 151, 166,
       167–168, 170, 250, 290
Phares, V., 76–77, 78
Phelps, E., 133
Piaget, J., 24, 31, 43, 237
Pickar, J., 298
Pines, A., 212
Plantz, M. C., 202
Podorefsky, D., 282
Politser, P., 264
Powers, S. I., 2, 44, 52, 55, 59–60, 61,
       69
Price, R. H., 99, 134, 262, 264, 276
Price, V., 184
Primavera, J., 10, 242, 291, 300–301
Procidano, M. E., 286
Pryor Brown, L., 112–113
Puig-Antich, J., 158–159

Quarforth, G. R., 217

Rabkin, J., 111, 112
Radloff, L. S., 162, 226
Rahe, R. H., 111, 247
Raimey, C. T., 112
Rajanpark, D. C., 52
Ramirez, R., 292
Ramos-McKay, J., 264
Reef, M. J., 61
Reich, J. A., 202, 203

Reich, R. B., 106
Reid, M., 246
Reiter, E. O., 131, 137, 138
Remafedi, G., 96, 185, 186, 191, 192
Restrepo, A., 11, 17, 52
Reynolds, K., 292
Ricci, C. S., 247
Richards, M. H., 22, 23, 28, 30, 94
Richman, J. A., 292
Rie, H., 239
Ritter, P. L., 11, 56, 88
Robbins, D. R., 158
Robertson, M. J., 182, 183, 184, 185, 196
Roesler, T., 196
Rogers, M. F., 181
Rohsenow, D. J., 112
Rook, K. S., 9
Rorty, A. O., 21, 29
Rosario, M., 11
Roseman, I. J., 21, 29
Rosemier, R. A., 239
Rosenbaum, M., 230, 233
Ross, C. E., 113
Ross, L., 81
Ross, R. A., 224
Rosso, J. T., 136
Rothbaum, P. A., 274
Rotheram-Borus, M. J., 7, 11, 154–155, 182, 184
Rothman, J., 182
Rubenstein, J. L., 158
Ruble, D., 132, 142
Ruggiero, M., 112
Rutter, M., 2, 5, 69, 88, 93, 98, 138, 158, 160, 166–167, 217, 240, 243–244, 282, 290, 291, 301
Ryan, R. M., 51, 53, 80

Safer, D. J., 105
Salzinger, S., 283
Samelson, M., 135
Sameroff, A. J., 238
Sandberg, S., 160
Sanders, G., 284
Sandler, I. N., 286, 291, 292, 299
Santrock, J. W., 58, 59

Sarason, B. R., 286
Sarason, I. G., 226, 286
Sarason, S. B., 264, 269
Sarigiani, P. A., 99, 100, 101, 102, 137
Schaefer, M., 298
Schalling, D., 140
Scherer, K. R., 21
Schilling, R. F., 196
Schinke, S. P., 196
Schneider, M., 185
Schneider, S. G., 192
Schneider-Rosen, K., 248, 249–250
Schoenbach, V. J., 226
Schulsinger, F., 205
Schuyler, T., 265, 274
Schwartz, J. M., 52
Scott, C. K., 243
Seifer, R., 238
Seligman, M. E. P., 133
Selman, R. L., 68, 284
Selye, H., 111, 247
Shaffer, D., 182, 183, 184–185, 196
Shane, P. G., 183
Shannon, F. T., 75
Shanok, S., 202
Shantz, C. U., 43, 46
Shaver, P., 292
Shumaker, S. A., 245
Shure, M. B., 244, 265
Siddique, C. M., 69, 73, 99
Siegel, J. M., 113, 226
Signorielli, N., 94
Sikes, J., 301
Silbert, M., 212
Silverberg, S. B., 28, 54, 59, 69, 74
Simcha-Fagan, O. S., 112
Simmons, R. G., 5, 9, 10, 29, 61, 98, 101, 126, 135, 136, 137, 166, 257
Single, E., 224
Siperstein, G. N., 11, 155, 238, 239, 241, 242, 243, 245–246
Sirey, J. A., 52
Sivo, P., 263
Sizonenko, P. C., 139
Slaby, R. G., 217
Slavin, L. A., 23, 69

Small, S. A., 51, 59
Smetana, J. G., 8, 11, 17–18, 44–45,
    46, 47, 67–68, 141, 142, 143
Smith, A. H., 112
Smith, C., 274
Smith, R. S., 2, 88, 167
Smith, S., 264
Snapp, M., 301
Snowden, L. R., 265
Solarz, A. L., 183
Soloman, R. C., 21
Sorbom, D., 76
Sorenson, J. R., 228
Speisman, J. C., 69
Spiga, R., 2, 97
Spivack, G., 244, 265
Stein, R. E. K., 299
Steinberg, L., 11, 27, 28, 54, 59, 69,
    74, 88, 288
Steinberg, L. D., 141, 143
Steininger, P., 293
Stephan, C., 301
Sterling, S., 112, 244
Stolberg, A. L., 112
Stolz, S. B., 264
Strattin, H., 135
Streuning, E., 111, 112
Stricof, R., 184
Strommen, E. F., 191
Suffi-Krenke, I., 104
Sullivan, H. S., 285
Sullivan, P., 11, 88, 250
Sullivan, T., 185
Suls, J., 244, 284
Susman, E. J., 96, 139, 140
Swearington, E. M., 190, 289
Szocka, A., 282

Talbert, L. M., 141
Tanner, J. M., 100
Taylor, B., 22, 138
Terwogt, M. M., 24
Thoits, P. A., 93, 112
Thomas, M. E., 113
Thomson, B., 75
Timperi, R., 225, 228
Tizard, J., 243–244

Traeger, C., 284, 290
Treder, R., 246
Troidan, R. R., 185
Turiel, E., 44–45, 46
Turner, C. F., 184
Turner, J. L., 239, 251

USDHHS (U.S. Department of
    Health and Human Service), 1,
    181
Ubriaco, M., 268, 274
Udry, J. R., 141
Ulman, K. J., 132

Vannatta, K., 23, 69
Vaux, A., 76, 112
Veroff, J., 43, 127
Vicary, J., 100
Vinci, R., 225

Wagner, B. M., 5, 8, 11, 16–17, 18,
    23, 69, 70, 134, 250
Wagner, E. H., 226
Walker, A. E., 282
Walker, E., 293
Wallerstein, J. S., 56–57, 58, 61, 112,
    240, 291
Warheit, G. J., 113
Warren, M. P., 22, 135, 135, 136, 137,
    139, 140, 141, 142
Washak, R., 58
Wayment, H. A., 239, 243, 245, 246
Webster, T. G., 245
Weiner, B., 37
Weiner, I. B., 158
Weir, T., 69
Weis, J. G., 204
Weisfuse, I., 184
Weiss, B., 69
Weiss, R. S., 56, 58, 60
Weissberg, R., 112, 244, 263, 264,
    265, 276
Weissman, M. M., 1, 113, 158, 159
Weiss-Perry, B., 52
Weisz, J. R., 245
Wells, B., 160
Wells, V. E., 10, 18

Wenz-Gross, M., 11, 155, 246
Werner, E. E., 2, 88, 167
Wertlieb, D., 7–8
Weston, D., 45
Wethington, E., 126
Wetzel, R. D., 1
White, H. R., 159, 166
White, K. M., 69
Widom, C. S., 11, 153–154, 201, 202,
      203, 205, 213, 216
Williams,, R. A., 76–77
William T. Grant Commission on
      Work, Family, and
      Citizenship, 263, 264
William T. Grant Foundation, 181
Wills, T. A., 134, 230, 231, 233
Wilson, J., 100
Wilson, M., 43
Winegard, J. A., 1

Witmore, K., 244
Wolchik, S. A., 286, 291
Wortman, C. B., 99, 134

Yates, G., 183, 184
Yau, J., 11, 17, 44
Yeaworth, R. C., 289
Yin, R., 264
York, J., 289
Youniss, J., 2, 68, 284
Yule, W., 138, 244

Zahaykevich, M., 52, 142, 143
Zayas, L. H., 196
Zelnick, M., 181
Zetlin, A. G., 239, 243, 245, 246, 251
Zins, J. E., 264
Zuckerman, B., 11, 155, 223, 224,
      225, 228, 230, 233

Subject Index

Accountability, 275
Action-research
  dialectic in, 270–271
  graduate training for, 275–276
  perspective of, 263–265
  principles of, 272–275
  structure of, 269–270
Adolescence (*See also* Change in
    adolescence)
  adolescent-parent conflict in,
    prevalence of, 17
  adult concerns during, 237–238
  biological growth in, 100
  cognition in, 100
  depression in, 92, 101–102
  developmental transitions in, 96
  early, 96–99
  interpersonal processes in, 67–68
  intrapersonal processes in, 67–68
  late, 99–100
  life stresses during, 4–5
  literature on, 22
  of mentally retarded child, 250–252
  and relationships, 68–69
  self-concept in, 100
  self-consciousness during, 29
  stressful life events in, 93
  stress in, 95
  transition to, 43–44
Adolescent development (*See also*
    Developmental transitions)
  characterization of, 103–104

of mentally retarded children and
    adults
  adolescence, 250–252
  background, 247–249
  early childhood, 249
  middle childhood, 249–250
  and stress, 4–5
Adolescent love, 37–38
Adolescent mothers (*See* Adolescent
    pregnancy)
Adolescent-parent conflict
  conceptual framework of, 44–46
  conclusions about, 61
  in divorced, single-parent families
  and family social interaction,
    59–61
  hypothesis of, 56–57
  methods of study of, 57
  and ratings of conflict, 57–58
  and reasoning about conflict,
    58–59
  and types of conflict, 58
  empirical investigation of
  design and methods of, 47–48
  and family social interactions,
    51–56
  interview findings of, 48–51
  methodological implications of,
    46–47
  on mental health, 7
  prevalence of, in adolescence, 17
  and pubertal changes, 91

Adolescent Perceived Events Scale
(APES), 70, 71, 79
Adolescent pregnancy
problem of, 223
and profile of drug users during,
229–230
and runaways, 183
and social context of drug users
during, 230–233
substance use during, 225–228
Adolescent stress (*See also* Stress)
concept of, 1
and developmental
psychopathology, 93–94
gender differences in, 89–92
increase in, 1
and person-situation interaction,
87–88
research on, 2–8, 95, 112–113
Adolescent Study Program, 139
Affect, 162
Affective constraining, 52
Affective enabling, 52
Affiliation, 30–31
Aggression, 140–141
AIDS, 194, 237 (*See also* HIV)
Albert Einstein College of Medicine,
299
Alcohol offenses, 207
Anxiety, 162
APES (Adolescent Perceived Events
Scale), 70, 71, 79
Arizona Social Support Interview
Schedule, 187
Arousal states, 24–25
Arrest records, 204–205, 207
At-risk populations, 3, 152–153, 238
(*See also* specific types of)

"Beeper study", 18–19
Behavior of others, 31–32
Big Brothers/Big Sisters, 295
Biological changes, 142
Biological growth, 100
Boys (*See* Gender differences)

Carnegie Council on Adolescent
Development, 282
Carnegie Foundation's study of
middle schools, 300–301
CECS (Constraining and Enabling
Coding System), 52
Center for Epidemiologic
Studies-Depression scale
(CES-D), 161, 162
Change in adolescence (*See also*
Stressful life events)
and coping style, 99
coping with, 104–106
effects of, on developmental
patterns, 102–103
extensiveness of, 93
negative trends, 101–102
positive trends, 100–101
sequential, 97
simultaneous, 97
social support for, 94, 99
Child and adolescent mental health,
2–3, 7, 16
Child Behavior Checklist, 70
Child development research, 4
Childhood victimization
and criminal behavior, 203–204
and delinquency
juvenile sex offenders, 212
prostitution, 212
race in, 209
research on, 201–203
as risk factor, 208–209
sex in, 209
types of deliquent behavior,
209–212
violent juvenile offenders, 213
and ethnic backgrounds, 214–215
study of
design, 204–208
discussion, 214–218
findings, 208–214
Circumstances of others, 32
Cognition, 37, 100, 142–143
Cognitive constraining, 52
Cognitive enabling, 52
Cognitive evaluation theory, 80

Communication, 53
Conflict (*See also* Adolescent-parent conflict)
  and biological changes, 142
  and cognition, 142–143
  counterargument, 49–50
  frequency of, 55–56
  justification, 47–48, 49
  mother-daughter, 143
  in parental relationships, 141–142
  personal reasoning about, 53–54, 58–59
  and psychodynamic processes, 143
  and self-definitional changes, 142
  severity of, 54–55
  types of, 48–49, 58
Constraining, 52
Constraining and Enabling Coding System (CECS), 52
Convention, 45, 46
Conventional counterargument, 50–51
Coping
  with change in adolescence, 104–106
  and developmental stress, 9–12
  and interventions, 257
  of mentally retarded children and adolescents, 244–247
Coping style, 99 (*See also* Coping)
Cornell Medical Index, 113
Counterargument, 47–48, 50–51
Criminal behavior, 203–204 (*See also* Delinquency)
Cultural groups, 21
"Culture of schools", 269–270
Curriculum, 269–270
"Cycle of violence" hypothesis, 213

Dehydroepiandrosterone (DHEA), 140
Dehydroepiandrosterone sulfate (DHEAS), 140, 141
Delinquency
  and childhood victimization, study of
    juvenile sex offenders, 212

  prostitution, 212
  race in, 209
  research on, 201–203
  as risk factor, 208–209
  sex in, 209
  types of delinquent behavior, 209–212
  violent juvenile offenders, 213
  definition of, 207
  as measure of mental health problems, 162, 163
Depression
  in adolescence, 92, 101–102
  and coping style, 99
  and externalizing problems, 158–159
  in female adolescence, 139–140
  gender differences in, 102, 159
  and hormones, 138, 139
  increases in rate of, 1
  masked, 158
  measure of, 162
  and negative emotions, 36
  and other behavioral problems, 170–171
  and stress, 16
Desensitization, 217
Developmental stress, 8–12
Developmental stressors, 8
Developmental transitions (*See also* Adolescent development)
  in adolescence, 96
  adolescence to adulthood, 99–100
  childhood to adolescence, 96–99
  definition of, 95–96
  examples of, 95
  and research on adolescent stress, 5–7
  stress of, 43–44
DHEA (dehydroepiandrosterone), 140
DHEAS (dehydroepiandrosterone sulfate), 140, 141
Disagreement, 51–52 (*See also* Conflict)
Disorder (*See* Distress and disorder)
Distress and disorder

conclusion of study of, 176
and externalizing versus
    internalizing problems,
    157–158
methods of study of, 160–164
research on, 159–160
results of study of
    distribution of problems, 164–168
    dominance of problems, 171–173
    multiple problems to stressors,
        relationship of, 173–176
    relationship among problems,
        170–171
Divorce, 56–57, 237
Divorced, single-parent families
    adolescent-parent conflict in
    and family social interactions,
        59–61
    hypothesis of, 56–57
    methods of study of, 57
    and ratings of conflict, 57–58
    and reasoning about conflict,
        58–59
    and types of conflict, 58
    justification in, 59
Domains of problems, 162–164,
    171–173
Drinking, 162, 163 (*See also* Substance
    use)
Drug use, 162, 163. (*See also*
    Substance use)
DSM-III, 154, 183

Eating disorder, 162
EMIT (Enzyme Mediated
    Immunoassay Technique), 226
Emotional state, 24–25
Emotional tone, 101
Emotions, 21, 22, 38 (*See also*
    Negative emotions)
Enabling, 52
Enzyme Mediated Immunoassay
    Technique (EMIT), 226
Ethnic backgrounds
    and childhood victimization,
        214–215
    and runaways, 183

and stressful life events
    discussion of study of, 125–128
    findings of study of, 116–125
    research on, 112–113
    sample and measures of study
        of, 113–116
Events to self, 164
Experience Sampling Method, 18, 22
Externalizing problems
    and depression, 158–159
    distinction between, and
        internalizing, 157–158, 161
    examples of, 16–162
    and mentally retarded children and
        adolescents, 244–247
External social support, 10

Family (*See also* Adolescent-parent
    conflict)
    and coping with adolescence, 106
    disagreement in, 51–52
    nature of, 15
    and negative emotions, 26
    of runaways, 183
    social interactions
        CECS, 52
        and disagreement, 51–52
        in divorced, single-parent
            families, 59–61
        and frequency of conflict, 55–56
        and personal reasoning, 53–54
        and rating of conflict, 52–53
        and severity of conflict, 54–55
    and social support, 299–301
    social system of, 45
    stress, 239–240
Family Bereavement Program, 299
Family events, 164
Family Social Interaction Task, 47, 52
Feedback, 269
Feelings of others, 33–34
Feelings towards others, 31
Female adolescence
    aggression in, 140–141
    characterization of, 131–133
    depression in, 139–140
    emotions in, 38

Female adolescence (cont.)
  and hormones, 132
  mood lability in, 140
  and parental relationships, 141–143
  research on, 131–133
  storminess in, 133, 138–141
  and stressful life events, 134–138
Follicle-stimulating hormone (FSH),
    139, 140
Formative evaluation, 269
Friend events, 164
Friends, 26 (*See also* Peer support)
FSH (follicle-stimulating hormone),
    139, 140

Gays
  data on, 185
  and risk taking behaviors, 185–186
  and school problems, 185
  social support for, 193–195
  stressful life events of
    assessment of study of, 186–187
    differences of stresses
      experienced in study of,
      190–191
    positive events in study of,
      192–193
    social support in study of,
      193–195
    subjects of study of, 186
    types of stresses experienced in
      study of, 187–190
  stress of, 191–192
Gender differences
  in adolescent stress, 89–92
  in depression, 102, 159
  in domains of problems, 171–173
  in negative emotions, 38
  in pubertal change, 102–103
  in runaways, 183
  in stressful life events, 119–122
General adaptation syndrome, 111
Girls (*See* Female adolescence;
    Gender differences)
Goals, 80
Grades, bad, 162, 164
Grant Foundation report (1988), 105

Group support, 298–299
Growing Up Forgotten (Lipsitz), 95

HIV, 154, 184
Homeless youths, 182
Hormones
  and aggression, 140–141
  and depression, 138, 139
  and emotions, 22
  and female adolescence, 132
Hostility, 162

Identity formation, 67
Ifaluk, 21
Illicit drugs (*See* Substance use)
Impact evaluation, 269
Improving Social Awareness-Social
    Problem Solving Project (*See*
    ISA-SPS Project)
Internalizing problems
  distinction between, and
    externalizing, 157–158, 161
  examples of, 161
  and mentally retarded children and
    adolescents, 244–247
Internal social support, 10
Interpersonal processes
  in adolescence, 67–68
  and life event stressors, 16
  model of, 79–83
  and psychosocial stress, 67–68
Interpersonal stress, 68–74
Interventions
  and coping, 257, 257
  interest in, 261
  ISA-SPS Curricular, 270
  from multilevel, action-research
    perspective, 263–265
  from prevention/social competence
    promotion perspective,
    262–263
  research on, 261
  school-based
    dialectic of action-research,
      management of, 270–271
    ecology of action-research,
      267–269

graduate training for
action-research, 275–276
perspective of action-research,
269–270
principles of action-research,
272–275
research on, 257–258
stressful transition to middle
school, 265–267
social support
enlargement of, 299–301
function of, 289–294
group, 298–299
mobilization of, 294
one-to-one, 295–297
peer, 284–289
processes of, 289–294
relevance of, 281–283
research on, 258–259
and social circles, 284–289
Intrapersonal processes
in adolescence, 67–68
model of, 79–83
and psychosocial stress, 67–68
ISA-SPS (Improving Social
Awareness-Social Problem
Solving) Project
beginning of, 265
curricular intervention, 270
as example of school-based
intervention, 261
purpose of, 257–258
results of, 273
working relationships in, 271, 273

Justification, 40, 47–49, 59
Juvenile deliquency (*See* Delinquency)
Juvenile sex offenders, 212
Juvenile violence, 213

Kovacs Child Depression Inventory,
36

Leisure pursuits, 26
LH (luteinizing hormone), 139
Life events, 16 (*See also* Stressful life
events)

Life stress, 4–5, 262
Life transitions, 4 (*See also*
Developmental transitions)
Likert response scale, 187
Love, 37–38
Luteinizing hormone (LH), 139

Masked depression, 158
Mastery and Coping scale, 104
Matched cohorts design, 204
Media, 26
Mediating processes, 8
Mentally retarded children and
adolescents
coping of, 244–247
development of
adolescence, 250–252
background, 247–249
early childhood, 249
middle childhood, 249–250
and externalizing problems,
244–247
and internalizing problems,
244–247
research on, 237–239
social support for, 245–247
stressors of, 239–244
Minority youths
gays, 185–186
runaways, 181–185
MMPI profiles, 239–240
Moderator variables, 8
Modification, 269
Mood lability, 140
Morality, 45, 46
Moral justification, 48
Mother-daughter conflict, 143
Multiple regressions, 122–125
Multiple stress arenas, 5–8

National Cohort Study of High
School Seniors, 223–224, 226
National Institute of Mental Health,
262
National Study on Child Neglect and
Abuse Reporting (AHA), 215

National Study on the Incidence and Severity of Child Abuse and Neglect (NCCAN), 215
Negative emotions
and cognition, 37
and depression, 36
domains that elicit, 25–29
and family, 26
gender differences in, 38
increase in, 22–23
and love, 37–38
occurrence of, 21–22
perceived causes of, 29–34
pool of, 24–25
and psychological problems, 22
and "what matters", 23–24
Neglect, 205, 213 (*See also* Childhood victimization)
Nondevelopmental stressors, 8

Observational techniques, 18
One-to-one support, 295–297
Order offenses, 207

Parental relationships, 141–143 (*See also* Adolescent-parent conflict)
Peer stress, 242–244
Peer support, 15, 258, 284–289
Personal autonomy, 67
Personal choice justification, 48
Personal issues, 45–46
Personal stress, 74–79
Person-situation interaction, 87–88
Physical abuse, 205 (*See also* Childhood victimization)
Populations at risk, 3, 152–153, 238 (*See also* specific types of)
Positive states, 34–36
Preadolescence, 38
Pregnancy (*See* Adolescent pregnancy)
Preventive Intervention Research Center, 299
Problem behavior, 101
Progesterone, 141
Property crimes, 207
Prostitutes, 212

Protective factors, 5, 8, 9, 88
Prudential justification, 48
Psychoactive substance use (*See* Substance use)
Psychodynamic processes, 143
Psychological justification, 48
Psychopathology, 93–94, 262
Psychosocial stress
interpersonal domains of, 67–68
intrapersonal domains of, 67–68
model of, 79–83
Psychosomatic symptoms, 162, 163
Pubertal changes, 91, 102–103
Pubertal events, 135–136
Puberty, 94

Rejection, 30
Relationship events, 164
Relationships, 68–69, 91–92 (*See also* Adolescent-parent conflict; Peer support; Social support)
Resilience, 2, 4, 88
Risk, 2, 4, 88
Risk-taking behaviors, 88, 152, 162, 164, 185–186
Rites of passage, 94
Role problems, 162
Romance, 37
Runaway children, 182
Runaways
categories of, 182
ethnic backgrounds of, 183
factors associated with, 183–185
families of, 183
gender differences in, 183
increase in number of, 181–182
and pregnancy, teenage, 183
social support for, 193–195
and stressful life events
assessment of study of, 186–187
differences of stresses experienced in study of, 190–191
positive events in study of, 192–193
social support in study of, 193–195

subjects of study of, 186
types of stresses experiences in study of, 187–190
and substance abuse, 183

Samoan girls, 38
School, 26, 299–301 (*See also* Interventions, school-based)
School achievement, 98, 101
School behavior problems, 162, 163, 185
School performance problems, 162, 164
School stress, 241–242
School system, 105–106
School transition, 102
SCL-90R (Symptom Checklist 90 Revised), 70, 73, 162
Self, 25–26, 29, 164
Self-concept, 100
Self-consciousness, 29
Self-definitional changes, 142
Self-esteem, 98
Self-Image Questionnaire for Young Adolescents (SIQYA), 104
Self-reported drug use, 228–229
Self-system theory, 80
Sequential change, 97
SES (socioeconomic status), 53, 72, 74
Sex offenses, 207
Sexual abuse, 205 (*See also* Childhood victimization)
Sexual Risk Behavior Assessment Schedule—Youth Baseline Interview, 187
Sexual risk taking, 162, 164, 184
Simultaneous change, 97
Simultaneous developmental changes, 5
Singular developmental events, 5
SIQYA (Self-Image Questionnaire for Young Adolescents), 104
Social circles, 284–289
Social convention, 45, 46
Social-conventional justification, 48
Social emotions, 24

Social events, 135–136
Social rejection, 30
Social Services for Children Bureau, 182
Social support
  for change in adolescence, 94
  for coping with change, 99, 105–106
  and developmental stress, 9–12
  external, 10
  and family, 299–301
  for gays, 193–195
  internal, 10
  and interventions
    enlargement of, 299–301
    function of, 289–294
    group, 298–299
    mobilization of, 294
    one-to-one, 295–297
    peer, 284–289
    processes of, 289–294
    relevance of, 281–283
    research on, 258–259
    and social circles, 284–289
  for mentally retarded children and adolescents, 245–247
  for runaways, 193–195
  and school, 299–301
Socioeconomic status (SES), 53, 72, 74
Status offenses, 207
Storminess, 133, 138–141
Street kids, 182
Stress (*See also* Adolescent stress)
  in adolescence, 95
  and adolescent development, 4–5
  and culture, 113
  and depression, 16
  developmental, 8–12
  of developmental transitions, 43–44
  ethnic-specific sources of, 112–113
  family, 239–240
  of gays, 191–192
  and health, 111–112
  interpersonal, 68–74
  and life events, 111
  peer, 242–244

Stress (cont.)
  psychosocial, 67–68, 79–83
  research on, 112, 201
  school, 241–242
Stress-buffering factors, 8
Stressful life events (*See also* Change
      in adolescence)
  in adolescence, 93
  cumulative effects of, 136
  and ethnic backgrounds
    discussion of study of, 125–128
    findings of study of, 116–125
    research on, 112–113
    sample and measures of study
        of, 113–116
  and female adolescence, 134–138
  frequency of occurrence of, 116–119
  gender differences in, 119–122
  and interaction of pubertal and
      social events, 135–136
  novelty of, 136–138
  occurrence of, 134
  problem of, 98
  relativity of, 136–138
  research on, 134–135
  of runaways and gays
    assessment of study of, 186–187
    differences of stresses
        experienced in study of,
        190–191
    positive events in study of,
        192–193
    social support in study of,
        193–195
    subjects of study of, 186
    types of stresses experienced in
        study of, 187–190
  scale of, 113–114
  type of, 136–138
Stressors
  developmental, 8
  life event, 16
  of mentally retarded children and
      adolescents, 239–244

and multiple problems,
    relationship of, 173–176
nondevelopmental, 8
Stress-related interventions (*See*
    Interventions)
Substance use
  during adolescent pregnancy,
      225–228
  as measure of mental health
      problems, 162, 163
  research on, 223–225
  and runaways, 183
  and self-reported drug use,
      228–229
Suicidal thoughts, 162–163
Suicide, 1
Summative evaluation, 269
Symptom Checklist 90 Revised
    (SCL-90R), 70, 73, 162
System kids, 182

"Terrible twos", 37
Throw-away children, 182
Turning Points, 282
Type A personality, 88

UMDNJ-CMHC (University of
    Medicine and Dentistry of
    New Jersey-Community
    Mental Health Center), 265,
    269, 271–273
"Uplifts", 34–36

Victimized children, 182 (*See also*
    Childhood victimization)
Violence, 207, 213
Violent crimes, 207
Violent juvenile offenders, 213

"What matters", 21, 23–24

Youth Self-Report (YSR), 70, 73